Under the Cap *
A Nurse's Memoir

Peggy Newton, RN retired

*It's not what's on your head but what's in it.

Special thanks to:

Carolyn Johnston for her sincere and insightful critique, encouragement, and guidance.

Cheryl West for her writer's and editor's eye.

January 2019

© 2019 Peggy Newton, St. Petersburg, Florida
ISBN: 978-0-578-424-29-3

All patient names herein are pseudonyms.

Page iv: Florence Nightingale photo 1858 by Goodman Public Domain.

Cover, Book Design & Layout: Kristie Kempker, Visually Speaking!

For more information or permission contact: arkangel16@verizon.net.

Dedicated to the memory of
Sister Mary Beatrice, O.S.F.

Who said in her thick Boston accent:

I'm going to tell you, so you'll know, Mahgret.

You've got to do good and be brave.

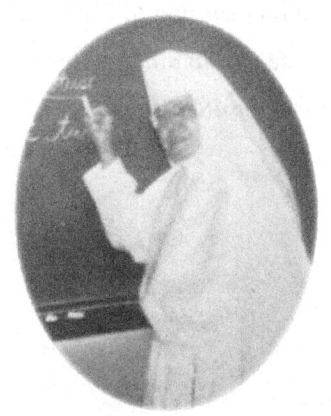

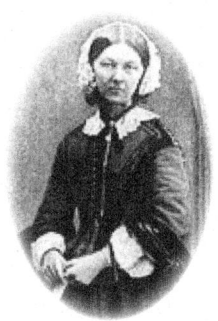

The Nightingale Pledge

I solemnly pledge myself before God and in the presence of this assembly, to pass my life in purity and to practice my profession faithfully. I will abstain from whatever is deleterious and mischievous and will not take or knowingly administer any harmful drug. I will do all in my power to maintain and elevate the standard of my profession and will hold in confidence all personal matters committed to my keeping and all family affairs coming to my knowledge in the practice of my calling. With loyalty will I endeavor to aid the physician, in his work, and devote myself to the welfare of those committed to my care.

Lystra Gretter 1893

The unique function of the nurse is to assist the individual,
sick or well, in the performance of those activities contributing to health or its
recovery (or to a peaceful death) that he would
perform unaided, had he the necessary strength, will or
knowledge—and to do this in such a way as to help him
gain independence as rapidly as possible.

Virginia Henderson, *The Nature of Nursing*, 1966

. . . here on earth God's work must truly be our own.

Last words of John F Kennedy's Innaugural Address
January 20, 1961

Ode to Patient Care

(Adapted from Corinthians 1:13)

If we speak with the tongues of specialists and consultants, and have not love, we will have nothing more than the noise of our own voices and the clanging of pet ideas.

If we develop new methods, write new curriculums, and learn new techniques, and if we understand all about the five stages of dying so that we are not surprised when a patient is angry or depressed; and yet we have not love, we are useless.

If we give up our old anxieties about talking with patients concerning their true feelings, but we have not love, we gain nothing.

Love never ends. As for tumor conferences, they will pass away; as for workshops, they will cease; as for in-service training, it will change. For our methods are always imperfect and our plans often don't work out.

When I first became a helper, I thought like an idealist and talked like an expert. As I began to mature, I realized that I, too, was afraid, and that the patient often taught me.

For now, we see only reflections of sickness and death, but someday we will see them face to face. And the time will come when we will know for sure what it is like, and we will be sorry we ever judged.

So, methods, techniques, case conferences, care plans, seminars, small group experiences, counseling—there is all of this and much more we would suggest for gaining insight and increasing effectiveness; But greater than all of these is love.

The Rev. Dan H. McEver, Director Chaplaincy Services
Wellborn Baptist Hospital, Evansville, Indiana

Table of Contents

Illustrations

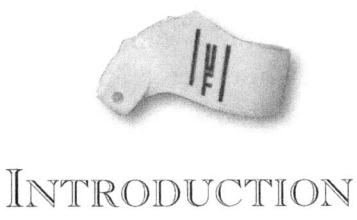

Introduction

My practice of nursing will seem quaint to nurses of the future. Mary Roberts Rinehart's description of early twentieth century nursing seemed equally quaint to me when, as a child, I read her nurse-centered mysteries.

When I chose my profession, nursing and education were practically the only professions open to women. *Now* a woman can be what she chooses . . . provided she can afford the education.

Then nursing was almost exclusively female. The Women's Movement happened. *Now* men take their place beside us, changing the communicative patterns between health professionals which held us captive for so many years.

Then doctors were scientists, healers, blusterers and often poor communicators. Nurses were the empathizers, the nurturers, the glue holding diverse elements of care together. We communicated—patient needs and conditions to other professionals; healthcare education to patients and families. If the patient received the wrong diet or the wrong respiratory treatment, the nurse took the heat—even when the responsibility lay with other departments. *Now* it is mishmash with some in each discipline being excellent communicators—but specialists unable to appreciate the patient in his entirety. *Now* the concept of a family/friend advocate sitting by a hospitalized patient to protect him from staff mismanagement is not unusual. Hospitals employ patient ombudsmen and risk managers. There are law suits . . .

Then a hospitalized patient's job was to fit into the pre-existing rigid hospital structure in return for receiving care. Like it or not, needing it or not, he was bathed daily. *Now* the patient could be discharged after several days' hospital stay without a bath!

Cultural revolutions concerning beginning and end-of-life care surfaced in the nineteen sixties, seventies and eighties with the family-centered maternity and hospice movements. Revolutionists were initially outspokenly hostile to anything smacking of conventional care. They epitomized consumer mistrust— sometimes rightfully so. *Now* hospice and family-centered maternity concepts are well integrated into hospital care and have extended to extrinsic community centers.

Then hospital stays were counted in weeks, sometimes months. *Now* Diagnosis Related Group categories (DRG's) determine payment and abbreviate hospital stays. Care is extended via home health care or skilled nursing facilities. *Then* International Categories of Disease (ICD) codes were used to track public health issues. *Now* much-expanded ICD codes form the basis for reimbursement. *Cost Effectiveness* and *Outcomes* are all-important buzz words. They did not used to be. *Then* it was more the *process* than the result.

One constant from *then* to *now*—economics determine the type, availability and quality of health care. Educators might believe they shape the profession, but economics remain a more likely determinant.

Lay opinions about nurses range between motherly, all-knowing and compassionate angels of mercy to cold, insensitive women. I am neither. As an adolescent, I believed that nurses walked on water. My perceptions have changed. I've formed my own ideals but never fully reached them. Even in my most nurturing and heartfelt moments with patients, even while educating students and practicing nurses, I have been fraught with self-doubt. I have never felt that I knew exactly the right thing to do in a given situation. What I did was the best I was able to do in the moment. I didn't hold back from stepping into the water for fear of drowning. Though I have never been completely satisfied with my nursing, I have used dissatisfaction with myself to teach others and to dream of systems which could impact an even broader group of patients.[1] I have hoped to help others avoid my mistakes.

Bottom line: nursing has been a consuming profession for me. I have been awake and alert at the wheel throughout and have given each of the many roles it offered my best shot. To some, nursing is merely a job or a way up and out of a bad debt, a bad marriage or a bad life. There are folks like this in all professions.

Despite factors which conspire to prevent it, many nurses persevere to make a significant difference.

Nurses are ordinary people with ordinary sensibilities and humanity. We share the natural aversions and prejudices that anyone has. We override them in the interest of helping. Nurse and patient. The patient is pivotal. The patient has need. It might be a need for self-maintenance; it might be a need for treatment. It might be a need for education. It might be a need for recognition of achievement, of dignity, of individuality, of humanity.

Then and *now*: to be a nurse, it takes an open mind and an open heart.

Endnote

1. The term *patient* has been in and out of favor in nursing for years. *Client* is politically correct and is very appropriate in non-traditional settings. But I will use *patient* throughout. The word *client* implies a transaction like buying a used car. The *patient*—nurse relationship is much more personal and visceral. At its best, the nurse and *patient* relate to each other authentically.

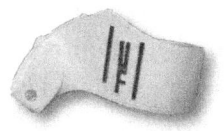

CHAPTER ONE
The Dream: 1951-1964

Childhood

A woman in white with white-seamed stockings, and a navy-blue cape lined in red walked by us one evening while my grandfather and I watched a Pittsburgh parade featuring presidential candidate Dwight D. Eisenhower. Bup Bup explained that she was a nurse at a nearby hospital.

From that moment, I wanted to be a nurse—a very solid fashion-based decision! I was five. Not long after the parade, Bup Bup suffered a heart attack. Armed with my toy nurse kit, toy stethoscope and thermometer, my mother drove me to Bup Bup's where I could "be his nurse, take care of him and make him well." Scared and super-serious, I protested hysterically. I had no earthly idea what to do and was afraid of the responsibility.

I had a dream that I was a fairy living underground with other fairies, rescuing wounded soldiers and taking care of them. It was an impressive dream that I believed and secretly remembered. It was word from on High that my destiny was to be a nurse. In my teens, during the Cuban missile crisis, I considered the dream an omen that I would care underground for survivors of a nuclear Armageddon. Perhaps it was overly dramatic, but that seed grew secretly within me—something between me and God.

Grade School

It is impossible to quantify the huge influence of twelve years of Catholic parochial education. My home life with an agnostic mother and a barely practicing

Catholic father provided little in the way of religious education. My mother had promised at marriage to raise children (just one—me) Catholic. At home, we practiced the letter but not the spirit of Church law. School was different. Every class began and ended with a prayer led by beautiful, self-denying women, married to God, insisting that we girls strive to be Mary-like. Like Jesus' mother, we were to be compliant, submissive, modest and nurturing. Others' needs took priority over our own. Imagine future husbands, children. We were to practice the corporal works of mercy—visit the sick; bury the dead; comfort the sorrowful. "Whatever you did for one of the least of these brothers of mine, you did it for me." (Matthew 25:40) Remember Jesus' example of washing the feet of the apostles? No task was beneath us. If it were difficult or painful, "Offer it up for the poor souls in purgatory." No humility could be too much. We were encouraged to be modest and self-effacing. I was stunned in high school when Sister Beatrice cautioned us against *false* modesty. "Don't hide your light under a bushel. If you have a talent, let it shine." The same nun in her quavering Boston accent also admonished us to "Do good and be brave." Her simple advice would become a subtitle to my nursing career.

For twelve years, those elements were inextricably woven into the fabric of my personality. They were the basis upon which the most minor day-to-day decisions were made. Don't get me wrong, I was no saint. I just accepted that a giving, compliant and modest person was the person I should strive to be. Don't think that I didn't inherit my mother's fire; didn't inwardly struggle or resent-authority. An invisible presence, these spiritual strands were tied to my nursing aspirations. Nursing became *doing the right thing*. I *should* care about everybody before myself.

My family, aware of my interest in nursing, kept me supplied with books about a child's patron saint of nursing, Cherry Ames. Written in the 1940s, Cherry Ames was a series of stories like the Hardy Boys mysteries which took young and beautiful Cherry Ames through several years of nursing school and into several careers—the one most remembered, *Cherry Ames, Flight Nurse*. Once I *was* a nurse, the series would seem overly dramatic and simplistic. But in elementary and junior high school, I was enthralled. Joining the armed service as a nurse might be just what that dream had been about!

High School

St. Paul's Catholic all-girls high school solidified my beliefs and expanded my opportunities through Future Nurses Club. From sophomore year on, not only did I belong with a passion, but I volunteered after school at St. Anthony's Hospital two days a week. I walked fifteen blocks from school to the hospital. In a basement employee-lounge adjacent to the morgue, I donned a green stripe pinafore (sewn by yours truly) over a white blouse and sprinted up to the DON (Director of Nurses) office to be given my floor assignment. Once there, I gathered and filled water pitchers with ice water and returned them to owners— no hand washing in between was mentioned. When trays arrived, we fed the patients—without ever having been told how!!! Some of the patients were old and probably demented—strapped down with leather wrist restraints. Others had cataract surgery and were to remain flat with sandbags on either side of their head—a practice now passé. If some of these folks didn't develop aspiration pneumonia, it would really surprise me. But then I was blissfully ignorant. And, I suspect, the nursing staff might have been too. At that time, folks remained in the hospital for weeks. I remember observing a Foley (urine) cath-

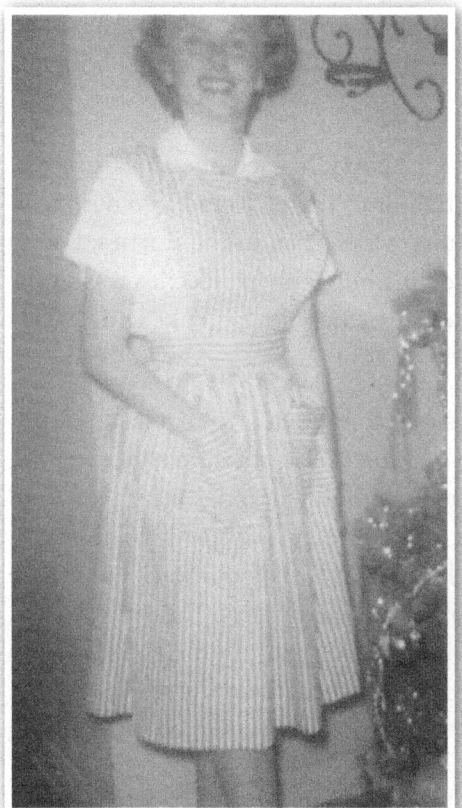

Figure 1 *High School Sophomore wearing the handmade green striped pinafore. My father managed to chop my head in this picture.*

eter tube caked with gunk and wondering why the patient's condition deteriorated. Once, one of my fellow candy stripers was caught filling a urinal with ice water. Coming from a girl's school, how would she know? The containers then were both metal—the urinal lidless. As president of the club in my senior year, I was sure to provide orientation which included the differences between the two.

One evening, I leaned my elbows on an over-bed table before realizing that the urinal on it had spilled its contents, covering the table with warm fluid. Though my favorite floor was 3 North, I was also sent to the Villa (the original hospital built in the 1920s) and the Mayflower (an old hotel converted to patient rooms and a convent). The facilities in the older sections were less than pleasant, and odors abounded. Only what I called the *Rich Floor*, a small unit on the fifth floor, was air conditioned. Elsewhere, sweat, stool, urine mixed with food odors wafted everywhere. On the Villa, a nurse gestured to one room indicating that those patients had cancer. From that room emanated a strong camphor-like odor which I equated with the *odor of cancer*. Only later did I realize that cancer is odorless unless it becomes necrotic (dead) or infected. The odor emanating from that room was a deodorizer probably placed to over-lay the odor of stool.

Other observations left impressions. There was the obviously (not then) demented old white woman named Susie who was lifted from a malodorous bedside commode to her chair for me to feed. Feeding her amidst the odor, it struck me in my innocence that she was monkey-like (about that cognitive level). She was there for life gratis the Sisters of Allegheny who owned the hospital. On the third floor, there was an infant with hydrocephaly whose father had threatened to shoot him. Billie. This child lived to be more than two with an unbelievably huge head, skin stretched thin with prominent veins. The nuns, believing in the sanctity of human life, underwrote his care. At St. Anthony's, I witnessed the beliefs which I had been taught translated into action.

In my teens, I used the St. Pete Beach public library, housed one block south of Corey Avenue in a small concrete-block building. There I found a gold mine in a 1930s era nursing school text book. I discovered that, in the thirties, taking blood pressure was a skill reserved for doctors but applying leaches was in the nurse's purview. Photos were with the text. Leaches? Bugs? Yuk! Did I really want to do this? . . . resolve . . . If that's what it took . . .

My father was unimpressed by my nursing aspirations. My maternal grandmother referred to him and his family as "refined." He couldn't conceptualize his daughter sloshing bedpans and doing very unrefined things which he could only imagine. Had I professed the desire to become a prostitute, it would probably have evoked the same response. Volunteering two days a week over three school years eventually convinced him of my determination. The girl who had vomited when asked to clean up her Collie's poop had become the teen who minded it no less but was grimly determined to become a nurse. Tales from the hospital held my father in thrall of the nitty gritty to which I was being exposed.

In my junior year, without telling me, he typed inquiries to colleges of nursing throughout the country. I might be going into nursing but, by God, I would have a college degree! I only discovered his endeavors when the replies arrived.

At the time, there were three avenues to nursing. The traditional three-year nurses' "training" program had originated early in the profession when hospitals needed inexpensive labor and nursing was learned more through apprenticeship than education. Acquiring the skills through repetition meant exceeding by far the repetition required to become proficient. This was the type of school attended by Cherry Ames, my idol. It was attractive. A child, I did not appreciate its economic basis. Traditionally, hospital schools were a low cost means for a girl with few funds to "make something of herself." I also didn't see, although later I experienced it in action, that the diploma school forged a propensity for blind adherence to institutional policy rather than for patient-centered problem-solving. Think Nurse Ratchet; Hot Lips Houlihan. Because they did not understand the *whys*, they adhered to the rigid *hows*. When I was in high school, hospital nurses were primarily from diploma schools. Not all

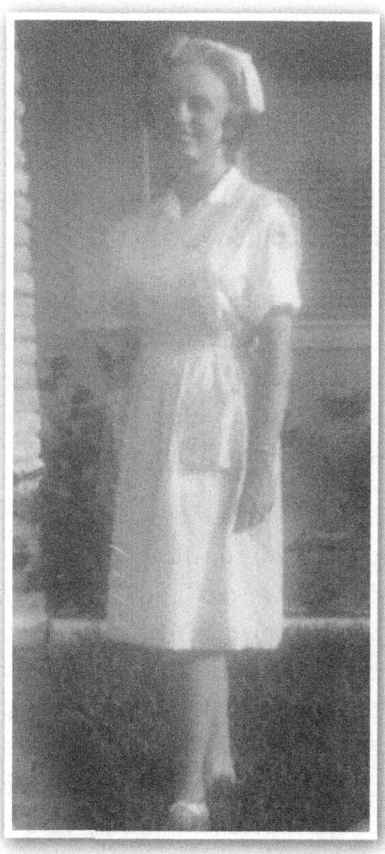

Figure 2 *Sixteen and proudly wearing a cap and blue-striped Red Cross pinafore while summer volunteering at Mound Park Hospital.*

diploma school grads became the narrow-minded Nurse Ratchet. But if they did not, it was more a tribute to their personal humanity, intellect and use of common sense than it was to their education. Likewise, not everyone who graduates from college lives up to their fortunate potential. *You can't make a silk purse out of a sow's ear.*

The two-year nursing program emerged from the hospital-based institution and was developed in the junior college system. St. Petersburg Junior College (SPJC) was nearby and would have been perfectly acceptable to me. I *did* wonder, since the SPJC program had emerged from the original Mound Park Hospital (diploma) School of Nursing, how a program could shrink yet offer the same quality of education. The caps of this fledgling program looked like a French fry container! And the student uniforms were not half as nice as they had been in Mound Park School of Nursing. See, I really hadn't grown up yet. But my father had set different goals for me.

The college four-year program had been around since the 1920s but represent-ed a very small proportion of graduate nurses. My father sent for information from the three Florida universities offering nursing programs at that time. He also queried the University of Pittsburgh from which he and my mother were alums, and the University of Hawaii. There could have been others. It was ex-pensive to attend any of them—more so Pitt. The University of Hawaii would have been the least expensive but getting there was another story. My folks were not wealthy. My dad's job was a secure one for the government. He was a Social Security Field Rep. My mother was an eighth-grade teacher at St. John's parochial school which paid less than public school. It was a tribute to them that they would contemplate sending me to college rather than the less expen-sive diploma or two-year programs. That my father took the time to request catalogs after his conversion to my great desire, I will never forget.

That summer, we vacationed driving around the state, stopping at FSU, UF and U Miami. I liked FSU caps the best. They looked like "real" nurses. I don't even remember how we chose UF. Maybe because it was only a three-hour drive away. Maybe because the curriculum appealed. Maybe I liked the campus. Though teens appear mature, in fact, their cerebral cortex is still developing. I know mine was.

A bit of luck came my way. Since Florida was so desperate for nurses and teachers, the state offered scholarships to people who passed a test and prom-ised to practice in the state of Florida for the number of years they attended school. No problem. To make a long story short, I *did* qualify for the scholar-ship which paid approximately half of my total college expenses.

While I awaited the test results, one of my classmates, Sheryl, remarked, "Peg-gy, you are so smart you should be a doctor (not a nurse)." Out of my mouth flew the words, "I don't want to be a doctor. I want to be a nurse." The response was automatic. That night, I considered why. Doctor or nurse. One was no better than the other—just different—no more than the husband is better than the wife. Comforting, soothing, caring—I had been acculturated to consider these as more feminine attributes. If performed well, nursing would require great intelligence. I wanted to be a great nurse. Years later, I would view the doctor/nurse relationship on a continuum. At its best, it was a Yin/Yang, a Fred and Ginger where Ginger did the same but in high heels and backwards. A partnership. At its worst, it could be bully/victim. Usually it was somewhere in between. But, in high school, I believed that nursing was as worthy as doctor-ing and my resolve to be a great nurse remained undiminished.

I approached college with a mixture of excitement and apprehension, looking to the future with bright and hopeful eyes, blissfully unaware of factors
already shaping an ever-emerging person. There was a strong Catholic ethic,
summarized succinctly by Sister Beatrice's admonition: *Do good and be brave.*
There was the legacy of parents who valued education and constantly challenged themselves to learn more. There was the secret dream through which I
felt God's finger pointing the way. And there was the gnawing fear that I would
not be good enough.

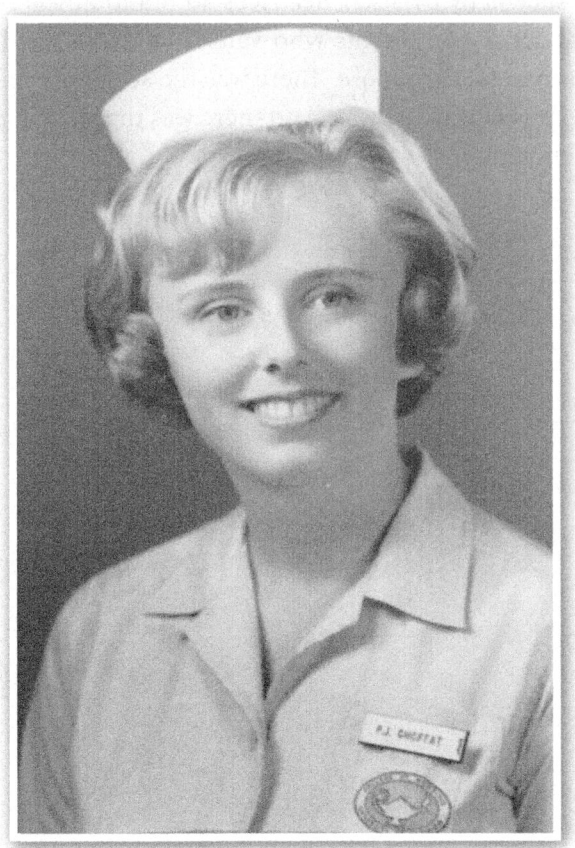

Figure 3 *College Sophomore and a cap at last!*

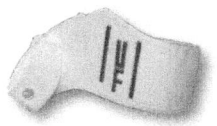

CHAPTER TWO
Can the Dream Become Reality?
1964-1967

College

The University of Florida was at once an awesome and a scary place. I was on my own. And, though I had tested in the ninety-ninth percentile of graduating high school seniors, I was in the sixty-fifth percentile of entering freshmen according to the freshman assessment exams. Adding insult to injury, I discovered that, of the hundred and fifty applicants to the College of Nursing, only sixty would be accepted for sophomore year. Well into my thirties and forties I had nightmares about not being accepted or failing the program.

The introductory nursing classes were not clinical but laid the groundwork for the heavily weighted psychosocial approach that was de rigueur at the college at that time. We were required to write what seemed to be endless reaction papers to various topics, plumbing our values and emotional depths. Worse—revealing them to our instructor. A history of nursing course was taught by the founding Dean, Dorothy Smith. Her presentations contained irony and dissonance of which I was only vaguely aware. We were not to be like the diploma school nurses who learned via endless repetition of skills. We were to be *educated* <u>not</u> *trained*. Ironically, at that time, most of our instructors were diploma school grads who had "tacked on" their degrees. Often, they taught as they had been taught. We were to become change agents, but Dean Smith never elucidated HOW. We could idealistically identify needs after educated assessment only to be puzzled about how to effect change from within the system.

After two trimesters of predominantly non-nursing related classes, My English professor recommended that I become a writer. My dorm advisor thought I should pursue the arts. ***But I wanted to be a nurse!*** Somehow, in-spite-of a lowly 2.7 average (I discovered social life, too!), I was admitted to the College of Nursing for my sophomore year—and, at last, a cap! The sophomore cap had only the UF insignia on the right side. Each of the next two years a bar would be added.

Freshman year had proved a seminal point in my personal development. Though I was known by my dorm-mates, the university was huge. I felt anonymous. There were more than twenty thousand UF students from all over the world studying a multitude of different majors. I was just one of them. How different from my homogenous high school class of sixty! There I had been president of Para Meds (*Future Nurses* had become *Para Meds*), editor of the yearbook, salutatorian, a member of National Honor Society, Quill and Scroll, Mathettes and GAA. Here I was just another body walking to class. I loved it. Thus, began my lifelong quest to travel below the radar, reveling in invisiblity.

Summer Break

That summer at home while suffering withdrawal pains from a passionate romantic entanglement with my Frostproof UF boyfriend, I applied for a summer job at St. Anthony's as a Nursing Assistant. At the time, anyone off the street could be an NA without educational preparation. There was no certification. Mrs. Veasy, the ADON, took one day to teach another teenager and me all that we needed to know about being an NA. She took us to empty beds on the third floor of the Villa (circa 1928). There we learned to boil water for the baths. Hot water didn't reach the top two floors. She taught us how to make a bed with either squared or mitered corners. At that time, tight sheets were a must. There was no such thing as a fitted sheet. She taught us to move people in the bed using a draw sheet. And she taught us how to give backrubs. We were not allowed to do vital signs. We could empty bedpans and measure urine though. And best of all, we wore white dresses and white stockings with seams. No pants. No cap.

At the time, the hospital was still unair-conditioned and it was hot, humid Florida summer. Though I worked the evening shift (traditionally not bath time), most of my patients required a complete bed change and cleanup considering the sweat and other excretions and secretions. My home unit was Third North (there was no west building) though at times I "floated" to other floors. Each evening, we received our floor assignment from the DON office after signing in with a time card in the basement. Often, I was asked to return to the basement with a stretcher to pick up clean linen. The linen room was unlocked by the evening ADON herself, Miss Mott. Linen would "disappear" unless closely monitored. Linen was hoarded on the units—one of the ubiquitous subplots which affect patient care everywhere to this day.

I was in heaven and gloried in the job. I worked eagerly and hard. With the squared body type of Julia Childs wearing immaculate, starchy white, the Charge Nurse on Third North was Mrs. Goodwin. For most of the shift, she sat at the desk. There were no unit secretaries. Mrs. Goodwin made rounds once a shift. For this nursing assistant, rounds were like standing at inspection for latrine duty in the film *No Time for Sergeants*. Mrs. Goodwin admonished me if the patient's room was anything but spotless and the bed wheels were not pointed in the right direction. I never figured the latter out. I was known as Miss Choffat—not always correctly pronounced.

The Med Nurse was another RN, Mrs. Henninger, with an interestingly pointed cap like a witch. (Each school or college of nursing was known by its unique cap. Only later did "universal" caps become popular before caps disappeared altogether.) Mrs. Henninger was the good witch—soft spoken and kind. An RN, Miss Emmert, or an LPN, Mrs. Mudway, were designated as Treatment Nurse. Aware that I was in nursing school, sometimes they allowed me to watch a "procedure."

My experiences furnished constant surprise. There was an Italian woman who had been in an auto accident, her jaw was wired shut, forcing her to speak a bit like the Godfather through clenched teeth. We kept trying to get her to walk into the hall. When finally, she did, the woman let out a screech after glancing down the hall to a statue of the Blessed Mother with St. Anne. Apparently, she recognized it as having been on her husband's unit when he died. Until then, it had not dawned on her that she was on the same unit. It took time to cajole her out of her room again.

A gentleman put his light on in his semi-private room and asked me for the emesis basin. I left it with him, running to take the Italian woman off the bedpan. When I returned, his body was contorted, his face frozen. He was unresponsive. I rushed to tell Mrs. Goodwin who called a primitive code. CPR was not yet in widespread use. Up from the ER bounded Dr. Sotolongo, a Cuban expatriate, oxygen tank & mask in hand. (Oxygen was not yet piped in through the walls.) He swiftly pronounced the gentleman dead. At the beginning of the shift, Mrs. Goodwin had given me one-on-one report, directing me to watch for anything unusual from this patient. She never told me what was wrong with any of my patients, including him, and never told me what "unusual" might be. The episode taught me the value of including the entire team in shift-to-shift report, making certain that everyone knew the patient's diagnosis and what to observe and report.

I held my composure—even helped wrap the man's still-warm body for the morgue. I believed that stiff-upper-lip behavior was what nurses did. It contrasted with my overly feelings-saturated beginning at UF. This was how actual working nurses operated, I thought. No one in this workplace would have dreamt of a touchy/feely approach. Years later, concerned about the impact of similar situations on young nurses, I offered classes about care of the dying. In class, a wise LPN, Susie Swain, remarked, "We nurses eat our young." When unexpected or grotesquely negative events occurred in my later practice, I felt a strong responsibility to help staff or students vent and debrief.

One of my duties was to boil the night's used rectal tubes in a narrow, lidded rectangular pan over a two-burner hot plate. Often, the tubes were still mucky from the lubricant. I wondered how boiling them for ten minutes would help dislodge the excrement—albeit microscopic—which must have been lodged inside the tubes.

I remember a very nice, buoyant guy, probably in his fifties, admitted with an ulcer. A long-timer, he was known to have his wife bring treats for the staff. One night, he vomited bright red blood. He survived that night but did not survive a subsequent episode on the day shift.

A woman was admitted after a severe stroke. She was totally unconscious and remained so for almost a month. We were fastidious about turning her every two hours to prevent bedsores. I don't remember but I assume she had a feeding tube—usually nasal then. One day, she began purposeful movement; soon she was speaking and was eventually discharged—without a pressure ulcer.

From both—the man with an ulcer and the woman with a stroke—I learned that things will not always go as expected. We probably need a little more hope when there seems to be none and should consider that, even in the most hopeful case, things can go wrong.

College Sophomore Year

Having survived the summer with some concrete experience under my belt, I felt much more self-assured returning to UF to begin the clinical part of nursing. I now wore a washed-out pale blue A-line shirtwaist dress with the College of Nursing insignia over my left breast pocket and a starched white cap with the "UF" pin on my head. The shoes were mandated white Florsheim laced flats. We wore beige stockings. My name tag announced: P.J. Choffat, garnering lots of teasing about the PJ. Of course, the required non-nursing courses continued. I endured them—excepting Humanities which I loved.

Both sophomore trimesters concerned basic nursing skills—bed-making, vital signs, medicine administration, catheterization. Former diploma school grads Dorothy Luther and Carol Hayes taught these fine arts as *they* had been taught. Passing scrutiny meant making the perfect bed with perfect corners, tight enough to bounce a coin on it. I spent many hours in the learning lab at night perfecting my skills, dragging non-nursing dorm mates down the hill to practice making an occupied bed.

We learned the steps of perfection needed to properly cleanse a thermometer—literally up one side and down another with the appropriate friction. The thermometers were in Centigrade, so we learned the different norms. Heart rate was always by palpable pulse—not apical. (Pulses are palpated in carotid, brachial, radial, ante-cubital, and pedal sites. The apical pulse of the heart is heard with a stethoscope.) We left apical pulse and lung sounds for the doctors.

Blood pressures were taught first globally (why we take them and what they mean). More time was devoted to how to take them. We practiced with another student. Then it was off to the units to take BP's under supervision. With my instructor watching, I pumped the patient up with the sphygmomanometer but, though my practice had been previously successful, now the valve stuck! Panic! *If I didn't get that cuff off soon*, I thought, *the woman's arm would turn blue and fall off!* So, I did what I had been taught—pull the tubing apart to release the air. I thought that I had handled the crisis very well, not ruffling the patient—until I was pulled away by my instructor. She was convinced that my extreme action signaled a nervous breakdown on the spot. No, I assured her—just couldn't get the valve to work. Privately I mulled that maybe my English professor and dorm adviser had been right—I should consider writing or art. They came so naturally. This nursing had to be practiced and practiced—and still I was all thumbs!

Anatomy Lab

Interestingly, the College of Nursing required sophomore students to take an anatomy & physiology course—not an official course in the catalog—counting toward our nursing grade. For two trimesters, groups of eight or nine nursing students walked up to the med students' area of the health center on the second floor for an hour each week. There, a senior med student dissected and demonstrated anatomical sites on a corpse, a cadaver—the same one for two trimesters!

My group met at night. I walked down the hill to the med center in the dark to the dimly lit second floor hall where other nursing students congregated outside a series of dissection rooms. A glass display case with jars of preserved fetuses representing each month of a term pregnancy adorned the alcove where we waited. There was also a jar containing a term baby with anencephaly, a birth defect in which there is a brainstem, no cerebral cortex and no skull. To a somewhat sheltered nineteen-year-old, the wait alone was like a ghoulish horror movie.

Once summoned, we walked through a dark room of tables covered with shrouded dark figures wreaking of formalin. In daylight hours, current med students dissected their own corpses there. Our lighted room beyond it had one figure only on the table with a substance the consistency of a convenience store Icee® clinging to it, stinking of formalin.

Apparently, this gentleman, probably in his thirties when he died, had been a chain-gang prisoner when there was an altercation. He was struck in his sternum which cracked and punctured his aorta. It bled out quickly into his pleural space and collapsed his lung. He died either from blood loss or asphyxiation. The body was over ten years dead. The first night, probably in a state of shock, we listened to the med student expound upon the skin. We would eventually dissect all layers of skin, subcutaneous tissue, muscle, bones, and organs. (Later we used the donated lower extremity and semi-pelvis of a seventy year old woman to dissect her atrophied female anatomy.) I couldn't restrain my morbid curiosity asking, "Is he black because he is dead or because he is Negro?" (Negro was a polite term then.) He was black because of his race although being dead didn't help. After a month, we gave our first injection to this gentleman in the ventral gluteal site, identifying anatomic landmarks for correct placement. It was like trying to throw a dart through tanned leather!

That leads to skills lab and my first injection. I learned that there were three types: intra-dermal, subcutaneous and intramuscular. I spent hours agonizing over memorizing the needle lumen and length, site, and proper angle for each. Thinking about it made me ill. I had not been able to bring myself to puncture a high school classmate's finger for blood typing in biology. How could I do this?

I was literally sick for that day's clinical experience and spent my day vomiting in the dorm bathroom.

Fate eventually caught up with me and I was nabbed to give an injection when we were on the unit taking vital signs or making beds. I don't remember what the medication was or how I drew it up. It was intramuscular. We used the dorsal gluteal site (upper outer buttock quadrant). Fortunately for me, the patient was an unconscious, obese black woman. She was on her side facing away from me. I outlined the site for the instructor using anatomic landmarks, then held my breath and slammed—expecting that tanned leather resistance that I had felt on the cadaver. But it sunk into marshmallow instead! Whew! The instructor talked me through the rest, but it was done! I had given my first shot—woops!—wrong terminology—injection. It helped that the patient had been black because it did not look like the skin I was used to seeing. I would not begrudge a black student saying the same about me if she had given me her first injection. Whatever gets you through . . .

That was my modus operandi—a gritty determination to get through. I was not insensitive. In fact, I was extremely sensitive. Not in the sense of one who can react to even a cross-eyed look or a correction. I would never have been assertive. My premise was that if something didn't work, it was my fault and I had to correct my behavior or response. Frightening or disgusting or shocking as something could be in nursing, I was poised not to react but to function and get through it as best I could.

Dog Lab

Determination was sorely tried when time came to "practice" surgical technique by assisting with doggie surgery. You read correctly—D-O-G. At the time, UF did *not* have a College of Veterinary Medicine. But deep in the bowels of the medical center, there was an "operating room" with multiple trough-like tables where dogs and possibly other animals had surgery. Operations were performed for research by fourth year medical students or residents. Our "surgeon" later became a prominent plastic surgeon. But then he was involved with studies to measure the effects of certain drugs on gastric secretions.

The purpose of our assisting was to implement what we had learned about sterile technique and to familiarize ourselves with the names of surgical instruments and operating room procedures. It was token. We would never, as part of our UF education, scrub-in for human surgery—that was for *technical* nurses.

(*Technical* was a term being used for two-year nurses—ironic since they had no more practice at technical skills than we.) But at least we could say we had scrubbed in.

My problem was not the educational objectives. My problem was that we would be operating on living, breathing, precious dogs—dogs who had done nothing to cause this to happen and who would not understand it at all. I was very close to freaking out. But grim determination prevailed. We were told to be sure to have breakfast beforehand. I did.

After scrubbing my hands and arms raw, I broke through several gloves, plunging into them as they were held open for me. I finally succeeded after causing gaping holes in several of them. There were multiple tables in process. The dogs had been tethered on their backs and were being administered ether through a cone. At least one student fainted. I was the scrub nurse tasked with passing instruments correctly—don't stab the surgeon or force him to look up; slap the instruments in the surgeon's palm. Unfortunately, his Spanish accent combined with the mask over his face prompted my repeated requests for clarification. I required constant reminders to keep everything, including suture threads above the level of the sterile field (surface)to avoid contamination.

The other nursing student, my partner, was his assistant, holding retractors, dabbing at blood, etc. Once "in" the surgeon pulled up the dog's uterus which looked like a large intestine. It had bumps in it. She was pregnant. Ohhhh. I almost cried beneath my mask. She would lose her puppies! He assured me that she would not. Then he went about the business of inserting a metal device into her stomach and through her abdominal wall so that samples could be taken of gastric secretions through a metal nipple-like device. Then he closed. Now I knew what animal experimentation entailed—something I could have done without. Yes, I returned a few days later and, yes, he was correct, the dog did not lose her pups.

Not long after dog surgery, we were exposed to human surgery. My assignment was a sixty-something male having a prostatectomy. I remember a spacious, well-lit amphitheater, spotless, predominant colors pastel green and white; multiple masked and gloved people. There was an anesthetist, surgeon, surgical assistant, scrub nurse and circulating nurse. There could have been more (beside the patient) but it is a blur. Again, instructed to eat breakfast beforehand, I did. My chief concern was to avoid contaminating the sterile field. I was not "scrubbed in" but wore a paper shower cap over my hair, scrub suit, mask and booties. It felt unreal, but I was far more comfortable here than in doggy surgery. *Here*, the man had a prostate problem, he had *decided* what to do about it—*and he wasn't pregnant!!!* My patient was the grandfather of one of my nursing classmates. Following up with him the next day on the unit, I read his chart. He had developed congestive heart failure (CHF). I was aghast! Was he dying? It sure sounded like it to me but I was very careful not to say much to my classmate—doctor's prerogative. I remember little else about my first surgical patient except being astonished when, more than a year later, I encountered him tooling around the Jennings Dorm parking area with his wife, looking for his granddaughter and a place to park. I discovered that CHF can be controllable, and that people who have it can live a normal life.

In February of my sophomore year, I was called to the dorm phone very early one morning. It was my mother. My father had a heart attack and died at home while preparing for work. His heart problems dated to before my birth. Still, it was a shock. After returning to school from his funeral, I grieved alone. I had a single room. My dorm/floor mates, though kind, were engaged in their own studies—not nursing.

My mother and I discovered that, with government compensation for dependent children (me), my mother's part time new job as a substitute teacher, and my scholarship, I could continue my studies. Serendipitously, the College of Nursing made it easier. UF anticipated change from the trimester to quarter system. Because of its effects on curriculum, we who should (hopefully) graduate in June of '68 would graduate in August of '67. That meant being at the college for two summers in addition to the regular school year and increasing slightly the number of credit hours each term. I was game. From my perspective, the sooner a nurse, the better. One of my friends was graduating from SPJC in nursing when I was only finishing my skills lab. I envied her. I would just turn twenty-one at graduation and I would no longer be considered a dependent child by the Social Security Administration. So, I would earn an RN (initially Graduate Nurse, GN), salary by the age of twenty-one—a whopping four hundred dollars a month. I would be a nurse. I would be self-supporting.

A Summer of Maternity

To this point, visions of Cherry Ames still danced in my head. So did that very early fairy dream. I would care for soldiers with medical or surgical problems. Now, in wicked-hot summer, I was to take maternal infant nursing. What did I know about babies? Absolutely nothing. I was an only child. Our freshman class had toured the J. Hillis Miller Health Center's Shands Teaching Hospital (Shands) and had peeked into the newborn nursery. I was so naïve that I thought those thick cords with a clamp on them just above the top of the diaper were penises. *Oh, that must be a boy!* I thought. Beginning maternity nursing, my greatest fear was that I would be lost.

I was lucky on two counts—Betty Mitchell and Miss Betty Hilliard. Betty Mitchell was a very plain, quiet classmate who studied very hard and became aggravated when she didn't score well on tests. I did not study as hard as she did and often achieved the better score. Still I had no doubt that she was the brighter of the two of us. One thing we had in common—we were both as chicken as they come! Both in Miss Hilliard's section, we stuck together for moral support. Where I was, Betty would not be far behind and vice versa. The beauty of that moment in time was that litigiousness had not yet reared its bloody head. We were welcome to go down to the Health Center and participate in patient care or read charts as much as we were able, being sure to communicate well with the nursing staff on the unit. That was in addition to our scheduled clinical time. Betty and I spent hours in the newborn nursery. If one of us was not visible Bessie, the rotund lead nursery aid, would ask, "Where's your partner?" We spent hours in labor and delivery (L&D) coaching patients, cleaning them after delivery, taking their vitals, etc. In short, we were fearful but committed to learning. We survived by mutual support.

Fortune smiled upon us in our instructor, Miss Betty Hilliard, a masters–prepared nurse midwife via Massachusetts General, the Navy and Yale. She was probably in her forties, mature and single. Miss Hilliard was low key. In lecture, she gestured with her two fingers (forefinger and adjacent) bolstering my fancy that they were permanently fused from performing so many vaginal exams. She was slow, thoughtful and understanding when she probably felt like laughing outright at our naïve questions. In short, she was just what we needed. Her manner with patients turned my life around to a completely new course. You would never know that she was childless. Instead, to the vulnerable new mother and father, she was a warm, reassuring presence. She took time with them. She was very skilled at newborn care. No one would question her credibility. She inspired confidence by being slow and steady. I am willing to bet that most of her patients thought she was a mother of eight . . . well, maybe not that many. Inspiration! If she could be so wonderful and skilled a nurse, then I could be, too. I would learn to nurse in the way that Miss Hilliard nursed. What's more, if I did, I could truly make a difference, impacting the lives of young families.

Maternal infant content was a revelation. At first, I focused on what I later realized was obstetrics not maternal infant nursing. I memorized all the pelvic diameters in *Zabriskie's Obstetrics*[1], only flummoxed to discover that we would never be tested on them! Later I was told that obstetrics is the art of getting the head through the pelvic diameters safely. Maternal infant nursing represented so much more.

Reva Rubin[2] wrote an article claiming that new mothers experienced various stages of bonding with their babies. This was an era when most mothers were not awake at the time of birth—gratis nitrous oxide. To them, it was as though the baby had just appeared and their abdomen had deflated. Rubin posited that there were two stages: 1) *Taking in*; 2) *Taking hold*. Betty and I conducted a small study for which we took babies from the newborn nursery to their mothers over a several-day period. We extended the baby to each mother, allowing her to choose where to place it. Sure enough, the moms first kept the infants at arm's length. Only on subsequent days were the babies embraced. Before embracing, we observed an instinctive compulsion to undress the baby and examine it from head to toe. Only after the *taking in* period were the mothers able to *take hold* and perform some basic newborn care. Betty and I utilized our best Miss Hilliard approaches while interacting with the new moms.

That simple concept applied to us, too. As students we were in the process of taking in before we could take hold. In later parts of my nursing career, I expanded the theory to patients and families dealing with serious illness or death.

The UF College of Medicine had been the recipient of multiple government grants. It was the era of the Johnson Presidency. We had Maternal Infant Care Project (MIC) funds and a full-time nurse for the project geared toward cutting peri-natal mortality and morbidity. The program followed mothers at risk—usually poverty stricken, often very young, often unmarried.

Shockingly the United States ranked tenth or greater in world-wide maternal/infant mortality and morbidity statistics. *How could we as a country endure such high morbidity/mortality statistics, have sick hungry children who were born to other sick hungry children and expect them to grow up to become productive members of society?* It seemed clear that the poverty cycle could be broken if nipped in the bud, starting with mothers and babies. The MIC project provided these women with formula and instructions. Their nurse, along with the OB Residents, counseled them about birth control methods. Often the same women returned again and again pregnant, sicker with hypertension, diabetes, toxemia or other complications of pregnancy. The complications and their residuals became a permanent problem after delivery. In the case of repetitive, health-damaging pregnancies even after counseling, a choice for family planning could be a post-partum hysterectomy or tubal ligation—both permanent. Enter the civil rights movement and Black Panthers. One Sunday an activist held a rally in Gainesville at which he accused the Health Center doctors of committing genocide. I wondered what that activist thought of the ten-year-old girl who had given birth.

Our Maternal Infant faculty invited an eccentric anthropologist to lecture about the *mother-daughter axis* in the African American community. Her name was Carol Taylor, undoubtedly a PhD, fiftyish, with short, limp, white hair. She wore rubber flip flops and a polyester muumuu scarred with cigarette burns. Lecturing while holding a burning cigarette in each hand—way before the Clean Air Act—she was hard-put to use chalk for the blackboard! I had trouble suppressing my giggles throughout the hour. Betty, too. But Taylor's description of the mother-daughter axis was riveting. Since slavery, poor black men had been transient. They had sex and moved on. The woman was left to care for and support her baby. Since there was no father in *her* house, her own mother *really* cared for the baby while the baby's mother worked to support them. But the grandmother could have health problems of her own relating to *her* previous pregnancies. In the cycle of poverty, there was nothing much to do—except sex and childrearing. Poor black women would say *I needed a knee baby* to justify their pregnancy. Once the children outgrew toddler stage, moms needed more knee-high babies. Everyone needs to love and be loved. My care study, Dorene, further opened my eyes to that different world.

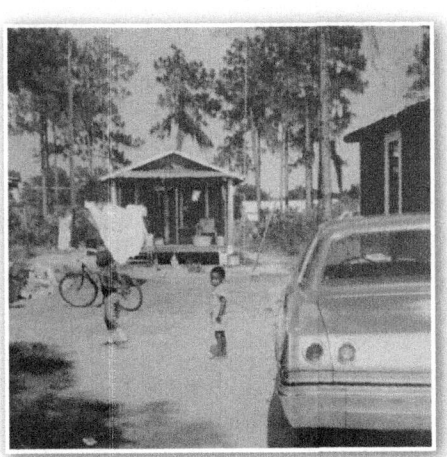

Figure 4 *Care Study Dorene's children and home.*

The sociologic/anthropologic approach to nursing was a revelation. I began to understand a culture living right here in America, previously foreign to me. The doors to empathy were opened with the recognition that it is important to view the patient contextually. She was not just the primigravida (first pregnancy) in room 302 but someone with a culture, a family, expectations, beliefs and fears. If I did not prioritize understanding *her* as well as her diagnosis, then any health education I could offer would fall on deaf ears. Oh, yes. In addition

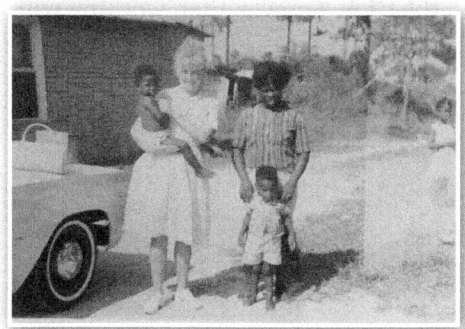

to being care providers, we were also educators according to this fascinating course. Teaching was absolutely nothing that I had ever wanted—or else I would have applied for a state teachers' scholarship, right? Yet, I watched Miss Hilliard, seamlessly integrating education into care. I found it—delicious!

Figure 5 *Care Study Dorene and children.*

There are other vivid memories—like meconium. Meconium is the first stool passed by the newborn. It reflects his in-utero ingestion plus his GI system's contribution. Bottom line, Uncle Remus wasn't the only one who knew a Tar Baby. Meconium is black and thick and sticky just like tar. I swore that Bessie in the nursery saved those tar babies just for us. We were charged with taking the babies out to their moms for feeding. We changed their diapers, wrapped them tightly like a papoose and took them out expeditiously. But what do you do when you are holding little ankles up with one hand as you expose the buttocks only to see black tar exuding like an unending tube of black toothpaste? No sooner did I wipe it away and apply a new diaper (cloth) but more oozed out as though on cue. It was unending. Eventually I learned, when it began, to put that baby down and work on another until baby #1 was finished. It saved diapers and saved time. But in the beginning, I hovered over the crib, eternally wiping, changing, wiping, changing . . .

Nursery technique was sacrosanct. Before entering the newborn nursery, we were required to scrub to our elbows. But once there, we were cautioned to avoid passing infection from one child to another. Each was already colonized with his and his mother's bacterial flora. If we were not careful, we could start an epidemic. Miss Hilliard had a wonderful way of explaining it. Each baby in his bassinet is covered with invisible jelly. Strawberry jelly on this one, grape jelly on that one, peach preserves on that

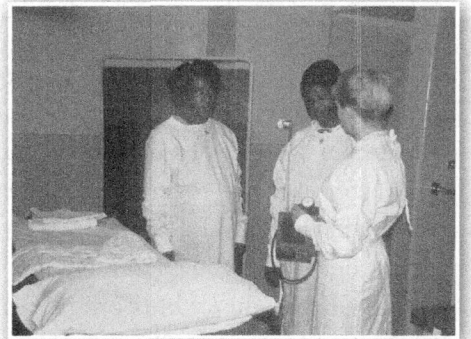

Figure 6 *Touring expectant mothers in L&D.*

one. The name of the game: don't get the jelly mixed up. She helped us visualize and form an aseptic conscience. It did the trick. Forever after, working with one baby, I sensed his jelly on my hands compelling me to wash them before moving on to the next.

The first time I brought a newborn to his mom from the nursery was confusing. The protocol for matching the right baby with the right mom was to match the number on his bracelet with the mom's bracelet. But one look at the mom, without checking the bracelet, told me that this was not the right match. She was a very dark-skinned black woman and the baby was white! I excused myself to the mom retreating quickly to the nursery. Miss Hilliard asked if I had checked the numbers. No, I told her, the mom was black. "Look at this baby's fingers." There was a darker band around each joint. She explained that African American babies can be pale when newborn and darken with time. They can have Mongolian spots on their sacrum—bruised looking pigmentation on their lower back. Sure enough. Miss Hilliard was right. This baby was black and, indeed, the mother I had visited had been the correct one. The numbers matched.

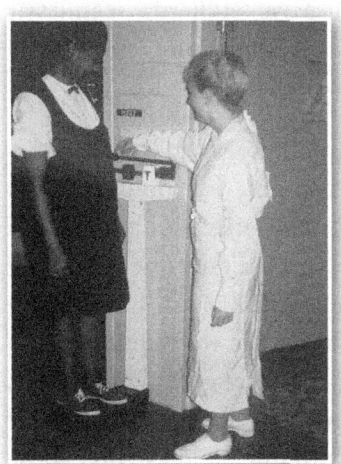

Figure 7 *Admitting to labor.*

My first delivery was mind-boggling. I had not been part of this woman's labor but was placed behind the obstetrician who faced the woman's perineum. The patient's legs were up in stirrups, a huge light shone brightly on her perineum which faced the door and hall. This was a teaching hospital and privacy was apparently not of much concern.

We were in masks and gowns. I was very careful not to contaminate anything—standing in terror of moving. The fully-gowned, masked and head-dressed obstetrician sat on a stool, face not far from her perineum, commanding the patient to push. She reared up her head, arching over her abdomen, holding her breath, face flushed red with each push. With each push, a dusky almost hairless head emerged incrementally. The contrast was great—mother's beet red face—baby's dusky blue one. A person with a head at each end! Bizarre! I was gripped by fear! Dusky meant cyanotic. Cyanotic meant without oxygen. Was this baby dead? Ohhh. I felt tears behind my mask. With the mom's one last ear-splitting grunt, the baby's flaccid body spilled out into the obstetrician's hands with a torrent of fluid. He held the slippery newborn upside down, suctioning its mouth with a bulb syringe. There was a small sound—finally erupting into a full-blown cry. Dusky turned to crimson! Oh, he was not dead. I expelled a breath. Thank heavens. The mom was no longer a two headed monster! I remember little else but the afterbirth (placenta). It was placed in a refrigerator for placentas awaiting further study. Employee's bagged lunches were in there too.

We observed a caesarian section. It was more like an operation than a delivery. The room was bigger. Everyone was gowned and masked with head covering, including Betty and me (Frick 'n Frack). The mother was administered general anesthetic only after her abdomen was painted with betadine and drapes were placed over the area not to be incised. The rationale: once general anesthetic was administered, it travelled right to the baby. There were only a few minutes to get that baby out before his heart and respirations were depressed—potentially fatally. The pediatric team (residents and med students) waited to care for the anticipated infant. They were sequestered in the corner around an incubator, suction and intubation equipment at the ready.

Once anesthesia was administered, the two obstetricians and all present went berserk, frantically incising, stopping bleeders, and struggling madly to get to that uterus, to carve a window and GET THAT BABY OUT!!! Anxiety flashed through the room like an electric current. With frenzied clumsiness, the baby was ripped from the womb. Shakespearian lines repeated over and over in my head, "I was from my mother's womb untimely ripped." I wasn't just observing. I felt it to my toes. There was blood everywhere and mild cramps reminded me that I, too, was bleeding (menstruating). Another Macbeth quote surfaced, "Who would have thought the old man (read: mother) to have SO MUCH blood in him!" Once the placenta was delivered and the major bleeders were staunched, the previously frenzied, frenetic OR took on a lazy southern pace for "closing." The danger was over. The baby was fine.

One Saturday, mid-July, I worked in L&D for several labors, deliveries and recoveries. It was extra time on the unit but, with practice, I was finally getting the hang of it, even feeling part of a team. I was elated. Jennings, my summer dorm, sponsored a dance in the rec room that night. I ascended the hill and joined the party, dancing with many young strangers with abandon for I had been made privy to the secrets of the universe!

By entitling this section A Summer of Maternity, I might have implied that Maternity was my only course. It wasn't. Pediatric Nursing was also on the agenda. Unfortunately, I found it uninspiring—maybe because I was so enthralled with maternity. The instructor for my pediatric section was Polly Barton, a PhD whose style was more appropriate for graduate school where her heart was. She was zaftig and a wee bit stern. Never let it be said that she would bother coming to the unit with us. We were given an assignment and left to the floor nurses to deal with our questions. Since they were busy with their own work, I was loath to interrupt them. Instead, I floundered.

Dr. Barton's primary interest was human growth and development. Her focus was awareness of normal range for a child at each age—newborn to adolescent. She included the Freudian oral, anal, genital phases and Erikson's stages of developmental challenges (i.e.: identity versus role diffusion of adolescence) but also physical and cognitive abilities. This I found helpful. For example: a mother cannot expect her child to be potty-trained at nine months when he lacks the physiologic capability of controlling his bowels. That was interesting. But—diseases of childhood and how they were treated or how to customize procedures to a child—not so much.

Polly Barton had a developmentally delayed adult child of her own. She was interested in mental retardation (now called developmentally disabled, delayed or challenged). One day we were trundled off to the Gainesville campus of Sunland. Sunlands were homes scattered throughout Florida housing the mentally retarded. It was heartbreaking to realize that many of these children's parents, learning that their children were imperfect, had sent them away to Sunland. Some retained interest but possibly could not provide the specialized care. Abortion was illegal and amniotic fluid testing before birth was only in an experimental stage at the university. There was no way of knowing that the baby a mother carried was not normal. Even if she knew, she would not be able to end the pregnancy legally. Some women died trying to do it illegally with unqualified "backstreet" abortionists.

Sunland's campus was composed of a series of cottages. Each cottage, not as small as the word implies, was filled with children of the same age and sex. Bedrooms were at each end and the dayroom/playroom was in the middle. We were toured through several, including one for older adults. I had been raised with an adult mentally retarded uncle, Buddy. My grandmother had been ashamed of him as though his condition were her fault. From my earliest memory, Buddy was always there—a loving and predictable friend. We always communicated even though he was unable to speak a complete sentence and punctuated his thoughts with jumps or claps. Being with "retarded" adults was not at all disturbing to me.

We—yes Betty was there, too—were paraded through a cottage of about twenty pre-kindergarten age boys. The aid in charge stood to the side of the great room, arms folded. There were no toys at all in evidence. A herd of wild children were clothed only in diapers. One of the children had a face wider than my own but a profile no wider than a book's spine. The condition, craniosynostosis, involves a premature knitting of the suture lines in a newborn's head. The brain grows but it is compressed by the skull. When recognized early, it can be surgically corrected.

Walking through, I noticed that Betty stopped to chat with one child. When we were outside, Betty showed me what the child had placed in her hand. She opened it to reveal his BM. This was all that he had to give her. She had said thank you for her "present." It was testimony not only to Betty's empathy and kindness but also to the brutality of the state system of warehousing children.

At Shands, we were required to participate in play therapy with a child before a procedure. My four-year old was to have a cardiac catheterization. The evening before the event, I explained what to expect in child terms. You will take a ride on a stretcher. People will wear masks. They will give you an injection, etc. Then the child was to do some of these things: don a mask, place the doll on the stretcher, give her or me an injection. My arm was black and blue from multiple very vehement injections. Fortunately, it was from the hub of the needle-less syringe. Having been an adult practically since the day I was born, the experience did nothing to endear me to the field of pediatrics. I had no idea in hell how to deal with a bratty, albeit stressed, kid.

I rocked a two-year-old African American girl on my lap administering a tube feeding. The child had crawled under her family's sink and swallowed the lye stored there. It had scarred and constricted her esophagus. She was hospitalized to dilate it. Hospitalized children can experience sensory deprivation. They can also developmentally regress. During the feeding, I was doing my part to cuddle and love her. I felt something warm on my lap (her) but then over my own perineum. She was urinating in two-year-old quantities that her cloth diaper couldn't hold. Her urine ran over my perineum like a river. I took care of her, changed the diaper and got her situated in her crib. But when I left, I was still close enough to my own childhood to fear that someone else—med student or resident—would think I had wet my pants—front and back.

The only other memorable event in Pediatrics was our lecture session, taught by Virginia Strozier, a quietly passive middle-aged southern lady. For some reason, she thought that we should tour the morgue and crematory. On one wall opposite the crematory, there was a large refrigerated closet in which corpses were kept until they were released to the family funeral home. One little girl went unclaimed for years. The diener (morgue assistant) explained that he kept her fondly (like a pet).

Med-Surg Nursing

After a brief end-of-summer respite, Med-Surg rotation began. Medical–Surgical Nursing was the type of nursing which I had always envisioned. Enthralled as I had been with maternity nursing, I was determined to keep an open mind. It didn't take long to close it. At the time, the instructors within the Med-Surg section were consumed with politics. The old guard was represented by Miss Kordana who occasionally lectured. The younger members of the section, also known as "Young Turks," were recently masters-prepared nurses, young and probably inexperienced. One was Linda Aiken who later became nationally prominent. Another was Sue Thomas. My clinical instructor, like Polly Barton, was not much of a presence on the unit. Overweight and mournful, she complained constantly about the state of nursing. I had the impression that she knelt at the foot of Dean Smith and absorbed the Dean's frustrations about nursing without ever putting in the work or effort to earn them. Fortunately, I was placed in a clinical group which included seasoned RN's earning their BSN. They were very good about helping those of us who were inexperienced. One of the RN students was Marian Oppy, my future sister-in-law. The others were Minerva Kozma, a wise, jocular southern lady who didn't mince words; Maude Royals, a very pretty, demure southern young woman; and Joyce Middleton, a mother probably in her mid-thirties.

Med-Surg nursing represents a huge swath of medicine with a plethora of unrelated diseases, different interventions and prohibitions. Understanding and surviving it was one tall order. The only clinical day I remember was being assigned a woman with a new, double-barreled colostomy. My assignment was to give her morning care including bed bath, and bed change. The pièce de resistance was that I was to irrigate her colostomy so that she would have a BM.

In those days, the theory was that irrigating a colostomy every day would establish a bowel pattern to prevent "accidents" during the day. There was a special pouch sleeve with a convex clear plastic dome which fit over the stoma (an abdominal opening lined with pink bowel, sometimes called a rosebud because it looks like one). The plastic dome had a central hole through which the irrigation (enema) was administered. In this lady's case there were two stomas (double-barreled). Hopefully eventually the bowel could be reconnected. One stoma led to the rectum where there was no stool. One stoma led to the upper colon where there was stool. If you are a reader with no nursing experience and feel confused, you understand how I felt.

I read about the colostomy in our text. The equipment was in the room. Without an instructor to explain, I was to figure it out while appearing to know what I was doing. I walked the patient to the bathroom; applied the special dome, directed the chute into the toilet and began to irrigate. Only I irrigated the wrong stoma. Soon, the soapy irrigant poured from her rectum. The patient became very anxious at the unexpected. We both did. I calmed her, repositioned the equipment, placed it in the correct stoma and waited. We waited an eternity. Nothing happened. Was this not the right stoma either? The patient was tired. She had been up too long. I helped her back to bed where I planned to bathe her and change the occupied bed. Only, in my anxiety, I had forgotten to secure the linen. Once she was back in bed but pouch-less, I left to gather linen, planning to place the new pouch after I had bathed her. I returned to find her covered in feces. The irrigation had finally worked! Obviously a more experienced nurse (or instructor) would know: just like not leaving a newborn without a diaper, you don't leave an ostomy without a pouch. Also, a seasoned person would have secured the linen before touching the patient. Lucky for me, almost in tears, the older RN students helped me clean and console the patient.

Psychiatric Nursing

Having survived Med-Surg and decided Maternity Nursing was probably for me, I embarked upon a spring term of Psychiatric Nursing. The experienced RNs were on another track. My friend Betty; tiny Gila Levin, a campus activist's wife; Evelyn Moore, later the first African American graduate of the College of Nursing, and I became a motley crew of car mates on the road to Macclenny, site of a state mental institution.

Our clinical instructor was Joanne Waugh—a young and intense masters-prepared nurse who lived with two other psychiatric instructors—Jo Snyder and Jody Irving. Another mature, less intense instructor was Gretchen Lagodna, whom I dearly wished was mine.

Crazy, nuts, insane. The nineteen fifties and sixties of my youth did little but stigmatize those needing psychiatric care. Institutionalization and drugs to control behavior were big—psychotropic restraints. There was no Baker Act. Institutionalization could be indefinite. As a high school candy striper, I had seen locked psych units at both Mound Park and St. Anthony's. I had also watched a late-night movie starring Olivia De Havilland called *Snake Pit*. The movie stimulated empathy as had *Lust for Life*, the Vincent Van Gogh film starring Kirk Douglas. But that was my sole awareness of psychiatric issues.

Lectures entailed all manner of psychopathology. In the clinical setting—Macclenny—each student was assigned a male and a female patient to follow for the months we were there. David, a fifteen-year-old schizophrenic from north Florida, was my primary patient. He was shorter than I, blonde with an Elvis Presley pompadour, protuberant tongue and shuffling gait. The last two were side-effects of his antipsychotic medication.

My secondary patient, Darla, was a schizophrenic black woman in her late twenties or early thirties from St. Petersburg. A major issue—she thought she was pregnant (pseudocyesis). Her pregnancy test was negative. I must have spent four months asking her in a variety of ways why she needed to be pregnant. Increasingly she assumed the lordotic posture of pregnancy while her abdomen enlarged. Only in the last week of our rotation did I discover that she was, indeed, pregnant despite her psychiatrists' former pronouncements to the contrary. Sometimes I wondered *who* had the psychiatric disorder.

Macclenny afforded a bizarre introduction to a psychiatric institution. On our first day in the parking lot, a teenage male flew out at us, arms elevated in the air, growl-screaming, "Aaaaarrraugh." The term "stark raving mad" crossed my mind. Our instructor reassured us that this was Joe. He initiated each new nursing class that way. It spoke volumes about what he thought of himself, where he was, and the perceptions others held of him.

I spent hours in occupational therapy with David, trying to get him to communicate with me—which he did minimally while lethargically tooling his leatherwork. The occupational therapy room where multiple other patients worked on leather tooling was permeated with the incessant twang of country music. Naturally. Most of these folks, staff included, were rural north Floridians. The music grated on my ears and, to this day, when I hear country music, I remember Macclenny.

Macclenny's campus was locked and secure. There were a series of one story dormitories, outwardly reminiscent of my Florida grade school buildings, scattered throughout the campus. Some were locked. Some were not. Joe, an adolescent like David, had come from one of the unlocked ones. The buildings segregated the males and females—like good Catholic schools—but far from it. We were each given a key to the locked units when we arrived. I kept the key warm in my left breast pocket behind the UF Nursing logo. I touched it often—reassuring myself that I could get out.

Miss Waugh chose a day for our small group of eight to observe ECT/EST (Electroconvulsive Therapy /Electric Shock Therapy). We were taken to a classroom-sized room with an examining table. A pre-medicated but alert patient was already on the table, his limbs restrained. Someone prepared a padded tongue blade. Another person at the head of the table could have been a nurse anesthetist. I don't remember how the shock was delivered but I do remember what followed. The patient's entire body tensed and began to turn blue; jerking convulsions ensued until the patient was calm but unresponsive. Repeated episodically on the same patient over several weeks, ECT's purpose was to alleviate severe depression.

After the event, Miss Waugh brought us to a small room, sat us in a circle and asked each of us, rounding the circle as though for a spelling bee, "How do you feel about that?" Most of us couldn't respond. Silence. Eventually, some of the more talkative students gave Miss Waugh what she sought. I was fairly in shock. It had been barbaric. At that point, I was unable to feel indignation. I could dissociate and intellectualize, "Oh, that is what a grand mal seizure looks like—tonic followed by clonic movements." I could appear the impassive "good nurse." But inwardly, I was repulsed. I learned that after ECT, people can forget or lose track of the basics of their lives. I thought: to forget about what was depressing you is fine—but to lose track of who you are . . . ? And to have someone extrinsically manipulate who you are . . . ?

There were other uncomfortable situations. I was sent into the men's day room on an assignment to interview one man. I kept asking him questions, trying to keep eye contact but my eyes were drawn to his hands in the pocket of his pants where he masturbated. I had no idea what to do about that . . . I just kept on asking my assigned questions.

If we students sat in the glass-enclosed nurses' station working on charts and a psychiatrist entered, we were to rise and give him our seat just as the regular staff did.

A middle aged male patient obsessed about his idea that there should be a rubber bumper around cars so that when they hit a tree, occupants would remain unhurt. His obsession was ripe for Freudian interpretation by our faculty—mother was the rubber bumper, the tree a phallic symbol. I remembered this man years later when automakers did, indeed, begin to place rubber on bumpers (and later air bags in cars). Was it lunacy or invention?

One fateful Monday morning, our small group discussion session met at the health center for "how do you feel about it?" sessions which I abhorred. The "how do you feel about it" had become so mechanical and hackneyed that we parroted it in a sing song voice to one another. This particular morning, Miss Waugh looked directly across the table at me accusing, "Your patient, David, got hold of a female patient in the parking lot and raped her over the weekend. How do you feel about that?" Sixteen-year-old, zombie-fied David and I had barely communicated. He had been in another (drugged) world. I was astonished! The only reply I had for her was a stunned, "I didn't know he had the ego strength to relate to other people." Miss Waugh retorted contemptuously that rape was not a relationship. In my small corner of the world, initiation of any interaction was surprising from David. She went on that because my patient had raped another patient, the adolescent wards would now be locked—a supreme injustice according to Miss Waugh.

I thought I would fail my psych clinical. I could parrot theory well enough. But, obviously, I did not do well in practice. I was still at a point where, if a patient told me she saw the Blessed Mother behind my right shoulder, I would turn and look. But, thankfully and only by the grace of God, I passed with a C. Ironically, psych was my highest score on the State Board of Nursing Exam post-graduation.

In Miss Waugh's defense, perhaps she had been trying to push a naïve, repressed goody-two-shoes into being something more. Still in her twenties, Miss Waugh died a few years later in an automobile accident.

The Last Hurdle—Public Health

It was our last summer. Hopefully we would graduate in August. There would be no formal university cap and gown graduation. Dean Smith, who did not believe in pinning ceremonies or caps, had struck down a pinning ceremony. Her rationale was: "It is what's in your head, not what's on it that is important." There would be no formal closure for us—the ultimate irony for such a psychosocially oriented program!

Most of us were exhausted. It probably showed. I have recounted only a portion of our nursing education. There had been many more non-nursing classes. The end was in sight. For me it was the Promised Land which I had sought most of my life.

All Public Health Nursing classes were held at the Public Health Department in town near Alachua General Hospital. Unlike the hidden-agenda-ridden, Freudian, complicated psych instructors, the public health professors were open, honest, forthright and practical. Hallelujah! But my encounters while making home visits would be as foreign as anything I had experienced so far.

That summer, I developed mononucleosis requiring a week in the infirmary. My friend Betty was zealous in her support, keeping me current with assignments. A relationship with the man who would become my husband was also escalating. We would later become engaged on August 12, 1967. It was the date of my official graduation. But there was no graduation and we were not in Gainesville.

Each section of public health students sat together at long tables in a large office behind the public health building. Each section was responsible for a given number of home visits—most of them in rural Alachua county. Most patients were poor—black or white. Some could not read. Others read at grade school level. This was a point which our instructor, Mrs. Virgie Pafford, addressed. Her approach was similar to my maternity role model, Miss Hilliard's. Virgie's task was to teach graduating senior nursing students, worn bone weary from completing a four-year curriculum in three. She gave each of us in her section coupons to get "made-over" at the Mary Kay cosmetics store on University Avenue.

Until then, our university experience had required scholarly communication, using convoluted sentence structure, million-dollar words and medical lingo. We called ourselves BSNs—Bull Shit Nurses because of all the papers we had written versus hands-on. Now our task was to synthesize and express ourselves in the most common terms. This, Virgie opined, was the mark of a truly educated nurse. Aha! The pieces continued to fall into place. Unless I could "translate" into common English, did I really understand at all?

I remember only glimpses of actual field (community) work. Often it entailed visits to recent discharges from mental facilities—monitoring their ability to safely care for their families. Were their children at risk? At one home, children played barefoot in their front yard of sand and broken glass. I encountered homes with broken screens and flies swarming on baby bottles. Some homes had no indoor plumbing. Occasionally, I had the pleasure of monitoring an MIC Project's newborn baby at home. I weighed him in a diaper tied into a sling and suspended from a fish scale—careful to place an open palm just inches below him. Was he gaining or losing weight?

A mystical element of public health nursing was bag technique. Ever the potential for the nurse to transmit microbes from one home to the other, bag technique was essential. These were mighty dirty homes. The potential was real! We each carried newspapers to place under our bags in the homes. We were also taught how to make disposable bags out of newspaper to hold discarded tissue or dressings. The same pattern, modified, created newspaper slippers for a patient without shoes. Our bags—black leather, a bulkier rectangular version of the small, rounded traditional doctor's bag—contained soap and paper towels. We used them to wash hands in the home before touching the patient. The water often came from an outdoor pump. The bag held a thermometer on which we were to use the elaborate cleansing technique. There was probably also a BP cuff and stethoscope. Aseptic technique was a major part of this class. One afternoon, we washed our hands and then they were cultured on Petri dishes. In a few days, ugly colonies of bacteria were revealed—even after washing! By then, preaching aseptic technique was preaching to the choir!

One of our assignments was to present a public education event. I chose to hold a dorm session about birth control methods. The group was nice-sized and informal. With models borrowed from the Health Department, I expounded upon methods from least to most effective. No one could wish for a more engaged audience of college women. Interestingly there were many aside questions about anatomical relationships and the physiology of menstruation. They were not nursing students and, though probably experts in their fields, what they did not know about my topic could have filled a book. I had to admit, I enjoyed the educational process. I learned not to assume that someone who was accomplished and affluent knew more than my illiterate patients. Both needed to be approached with dignity, respect and acceptance. I had to grow enough to reach any level. Passing your water, peeing, urinating, voiding, dropping a tear (Irish). I had to learn them all.

Another of our assignments was played out at Lincoln High School—then the segregated black high school. Many of the female students there had weight problems. Though obese, their nutritional status was poor. Their diet reflected their culture—high in pork fat and salt; and their low income—high in starch. Betty and I started a club for teen girls who wanted to lose weight. I don't remember the club's official name. Between Betty and me, short-speak was The Fats Club. The UF campus was large and we had walked everywhere for three years. Betty and I were thin—one hundred twenty pounds or less. We were white. Our impact was questionable in our abbreviated time with them. We brought healthy snacks and showed movies. I learned to run a projector. We led outdoor exercises—two skinny white girls running around with two hundred plus pound black teens. Quite a picture!

In the lecture section of Public Health, we were assigned to present information about governmental programs available to help our patients. Aid to Dependent Children and Social Security were a few. At that time, nurses also functioned as social workers. One group, concerned with the somewhat dry content and drowsy afternoon meeting time, created a rural family called the 'Taters. There were Ma & Po Tater, Sweet Tater, Tater Tot, etc. Each character had a problem which could be solved with a referral.

Throughout this course, our section instructor, Virgie Pafford, dispensed jewels of wisdom. She used common sense and was realistic. When she made a home visit with me, she, like Miss Hilliard, was an impressive role model with the patient. We found one new mother chewing her infant's nails to trim them. There was a screen with holes, flies on the bottle, children unsupervised and barefoot in the sandy yard. In the car, I could list the problems but threw my hands up, unsure where to start.

Virgie was clear that no one could ever hope to fix the entire situation. With the mom's history, chewing the baby's nails was probably better than using a sharp instrument. She had instructed the mom about getting the screen fixed to prevent potentially fatal, fly-borne diarrhea in the infant. She made a referral for continued observation and care to the REAL public health nurse. Virgie's approach helped me to recognize that people are imperfect and always will be. There is a continuum. She managed to remove the pressure to be the perfect nurse who fixes things. It was professional serenity—not indifference. In later years, I would need to tap into that concept.

After graduation, I learned of a subsequent group's very bright Public Health nursing student who was abducted and raped. Only after the fact, did I realize that going into the boonies to provide health care to the less fortunate carried attendant risk.

Gerontology

While studying Public Health, we were required to take a two-credit course in Gerontology taught by the Assistant Dean of Nursing, Lois Knowles. Gerontology was in its infancy and the concept of a long, happy, active life post-retirement had not yet arrived. I imagined Miss Knowles as one of Joseph Mengele's medical assistants at Auschwitz bent on performing human experimentation. On a few instances, we visited a local nursing home to interview old and debilitated patients. To get them to "perform" for her interaction demonstrations, she bribed them with bananas. It reminded me of performing circus monkeys. I saw no love there at all. The last thing I ever wanted to be was a gerontology nurse. Older folks were fine but to group them together and treat them like monkeys—no!

Graduation with a Bachelor of Science in Nursing had certainly fulfilled my parents' mandate for a college degree. Socially and academically, my world view had broadened. I had enjoyed the anonymity of a large campus and interacting with a diverse group of students and faculty. Except for becoming engaged, my mood was not entirely celebratory. I felt every bit the Bull Shit Nurse who now faced the grave responsibility of caring for not just one (as in school) but many patients. My concerns were concrete. Exactly what did I know how to do? Could I do it safely and efficiently? I was shy of risk. The familiar Shands would be a good place to try my wings.

Endnotes

1. Elise Fitzpatrick and Nicholson Eastman, Zabriskie's Obstetrics for Nurses, 10th Edition (Philadelphia: J.B. Lippincott, 1960).
2. Reva, Rubin. "Puerperal Change," Nursing Outlook (December 1961): 753-755.

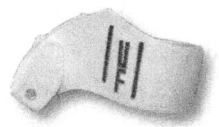

CHAPTER THREE
Grown Up Nurse: 1967-1972

Graduate Nurse (GN) to Registered Nurse (RN)

Intermezzo. That was the musical theme and title of one of my favorite 1930s Ingrid Bergman movies. It marked her introduction from Sweden to the American public. Now my *time between* GN and RN was my introduction to the world of REAL nursing. My heart soared to have finally arrived. I was afraid of the giant responsibility. Though Danny and I had become engaged during my short visit home, I had committed to returning to the University of Florida's Shands Teaching Hospital as a Nurse I on the OB unit.

My mantra was *study, study, study*—fearful that I wouldn't pass Boards in October. The State Board of Nursing Exam was held in a rundown Jacksonville hotel over two days. Tests were in segments reflecting the various nursing specialties—Med-Surg, OB, etc. Once passed, GN became RN. Not Great Nurse and Real Nut as I dubbed them, they were actually: Graduate Nurse and Registered Nurse. It could take a month or more to get the State Board results.

I had moved to an apartment with three other girls—all still in school, none in nursing. Danny, my fiancé, drove up from St. Pete on weekends. The apartment was just down the road from the hospital, so I walked to and from work—often at night—years before the Gainesville Ripper killed four women in that area. Orientation was unit-specific and took less than a week. UF grad, Pat Dobson, oriented me. I was instantly a team leader on the evening shift but rotated monthly from evenings to nights.

At the time, state-owned Shands' units were decentralized. The ultimate nursing authority was the Dean of the College of Nursing—never on the unit. Reporting to her was the Maternal-Infant Section chairman, Professor Jen Wilson, who turned up occasionally with students. Reporting to Jen was Audrey Urquhart, our Nurse III. Equivalent in status to the Nurse III was the Unit manager who ordered supplies and supervised unit secretaries. Each floor had the same structure, formed a decade before at the Health Center's inception. Dean Smith wanted nursing freed from the traditional concerns of unit maintenance and transcription. The goal was high-quality care with nurses fully occupied only with patient care issues, not extrinsics. Sometimes it worked. Sometimes it did not.

Being a part of the university community meant that Shands' RN's were usually married to students. Once hubby graduated, the nurse moved on with him. Or, like me, once the RN married, she would move. While Shands' RN echelon was transient, the LPN's and NA's were local, had tenure, and were not easily influenced or intimidated by young whippersnapper RN's. They were expert at evasive maneuvers. Moonlighting or extra shifts were common since there was no central nursing pool. Some could be found, particularly during the night shift, asleep in the rooms. I mention it not to disparage them, though I believe that when you are paid to work—work! But certain social and organizational dynamics were afoot for which I was totally unprepared. Technically, I would be their boss, but time was on their side.

The Medical Program paralleled nursing. Dr. Harry Prystowsky was the ultimate OB/GYN authority. He was the physician/professor/director of the OB/GYN group. Prystowsky presided over Grand Rounds monthly on Saturday morning. His underlings trembled at the thought. Prystowsky directed a four-year Residency program with at least one resident in each year's slot and a plethora of med students fulfilling their obligatory OB-GYN rotation. Not all med students enjoyed OB/GYN. Each was worked to the bone with long hours and lots of "scut" work, necessary but mundane—like doing a urinalysis or spinning an H&H (hematocrit & hemoglobin). Residents and med students made regular rounds as a group every morning when med students reported a summary of their patient's progress. To be prepared, the students arrived early, waking their patients at an ungodly hour just to have their stories straight for the resident. The comfort or convenience of the patient was not a consideration.

I was blessed to be working the evening or night shift, only tangentially involved in rounding at the end of my shift. But med students stymied one aspect of my professional growth. They were to start all IV's. They were to insert all naso-gastric (NG) tubes. Part of their training entailed inserting them in each other—they said to manufacture empathy. Consequently, working in the same hospital where I had been schooled meant that I would not learn to perform either procedure. Lung-sounds and heart sounds were also in their domain. But hanging and timing IV's—that was mine. In the wee hours of the night I stealthily slipped into four bed wards to hang IV's illuminated by my flashlight. Trying not to disturb the patients' sleep, sometimes I was confronted in the murky darkness by wide white eyes in dark faces. I don't know which of us—patient or nurse—was more startled.

We practiced Team Nursing with the RN (GN—me) leading a team of LPN's and Nursing Assistants. There were three wings—each with a team on the evening shift—consolidated into one large team on the night shift. The Team Leader made the assignments, passed meds, hung IV's and performed treatments (like wound care) unless there was an LPN or RN on the team to whom that could be delegated. The nursing station was huge with a wrap-around desk in front to greet the public. It looked out on the intersection of the three wings. A huge supply cart stocked with IV tubing, dressings and other supplies was adjacent. There was not an individual patient charge system. Supplies disappeared from the cart in a fast-moving stream. With so many disciplines using it, there were no good controls. A central metal table graced the middle of the nursing station where Team Leaders had their IV bottles lined up and labeled in the order in which they would be hung. Along the wall was a refrigerator where fragile meds were kept until they were ready to administer. Next to the refrigerator was a wall of shelved multi-dose med bottles and small patient-med cubicles. We poured our own oral meds and injections for the shift according to their designated hours. Except for dead night, there were so many distractions! I worried that I might draw up the wrong medicine. So, I arrived a half-hour early to get a head start on my meds before I had any other responsibilities. There were rumblings from above—Nurse II and Nurse III. According to wage and hour laws, my tactic was not permissible. But the law was not enforced. I would rather violate wage and hour laws than inadvertently kill someone. End of shift was the same when I stayed to finish my charts. I was gung ho and just wanted to . . . do good. The notion that I should be able to complete a heavy workload, involving human interaction and foibles, within a set time-frame with an assembly line approach seemed ludicrous. I was convinced that being unconcerned with uncompensated overtime was a hallmark of true professionalism. In my first RN position, I was new and slow. I had never or rarely practiced in nursing school what was being asked of me now. To do the job correctly, I needed time. Another more adept person could have been more of a wiz. *I* needed more time.

Luckily, during my brief orientation, I was assigned to GYN surgical preps (enema & shave) the evening before surgery. The following night I provided the same patient's post-op care. This taught me in a way that my classes had not about surgical nursing and management of complications—paralytic ileus (paralyzed bowel), infection, and dehiscence (incision opens). It probably saved my life on the State Board Exams in October.

Finally a nurse, I was happy as a clam, my only wish—roller skates to speed me from room to room! The responsibility weighed heavily. One evening, the other two nurses were off the floor for something and I was the only nurse remaining on the entire unit. They were away only a few minutes, but I felt the onerous responsibility. Standing in the hall outside the desk, I alternated looking East, North and West, watching for a light or a call from an NA about some unknown disaster. On the four-to-midnight shift, the other two Team Leaders were GN's like me. Not the best orientation in the world for us nor a safe situation for our patients. Yet, in numbers, there was strength. We supported each other.

On the midnight shift, another RN was the team-leader. I team-led on her off days. To me, she was old—probably in her fifties. Old for a college town. Of course, she had years of experience. A diploma school grad, the high point of her night was transcribing doctor's orders in her beautiful and legible script. She also loved the chart check done on this shift. All very sedentary occupations. It was I who ran around between patients, administering meds and IV's, and doing treatments. This woman gave life to one of Dean Smith's lectures. The Dean believed that diploma school students were used for service to the extent that, once graduated, they moved as far away from the bedside as possible—choosing management or education. The Dean claimed that, though diploma grads might doubt it, UF produced nurses engaged in direct patient care. Seeing the diploma school mentality in the midnight shift nurse was believing it.

An interesting member of the night crew was a tall, black, thirtyish nursing assistant named Mrs. Thompson. She was a lovely person and a lovely person with whom to work. Shy and deferential to a degree with which I was not comfortable—she was the other extreme from the long-term employees who sought to do as little as possible. She had unfailing confidence in me when I had none in myself. She asked what to do and then did it. When she smiled, a beautiful set of gold capped teeth emerged with a central star and moon the only glimpses of white enamel beneath.

For several nights, I assigned Mrs. Thompson the care (bedpans, repositioning, vital signs and cat bath) of a thirty something black woman post caesarian section. The woman's incision had dehisced. Now she had a large open abdominal wound which I irrigated and packed. After several nights, one other staff member asked me if I knew that the patient, while pregnant, had been in a juke joint knife brawl. Mrs. Thompson's husband had been her victim. I was dumbfounded. Not once had Mrs. Thompson mentioned the incident nor had she asked to be relieved of the assignment. From all accounts, she had been giving her usual excellent care. When I pulled her aside, she confirmed the report. Of course, I relieved her from future care of the woman out of concern for both. But Mrs. Thompson's smiling discussion of the situation was as dispassionate as talking about the weather. It revealed a disconnect between cultures that I wondered if I would ever bridge.

At Shands, patients were moved from room to room at the drop of the hat. A woman developed an infection and needed to be moved to a room alone. A baby died, and the mother was moved to a section without new mothers. Labor patients were moved to post-partum. Each patient was moved *in* her bed. Nurses pushed the very heavy, patient-occupied beds to their new destination, navigating halls and doorways while young male med students and residents looked on. I was very strong. My fiancé was a traditional gentleman. It was important to him to open doors for me. That meant that I had to wait, stifling my impatience, until he walked over to my side of the car to open the door. It felt disingenuous. At work, I was superwoman. On my own time I was a fading violet. Go figure!

The night shift occasionally ordered food delivery to buffer the three to four a.m. doldrums that invaded before the mad scramble to prepare for morning rounds. I usually selected candy from the basement machines. Once, the staff asked if I wanted to order-out a chicken sandwich when they did. Sounded good to me. When the food arrived, they handed me a soft white bread sandwich. Inside the bread was a fried chicken leg complete with bone. Another cultural discovery!

I have mentioned the problems of planned pregnancy or the lack thereof in the population that we served. Black and white—all poor. An exception: the occasional professor's wife with a private MD. Children begat children. Women in their thirties were mothers of many.

When I was team leader, a mature woman was admitted with pre-eclampsia, then went into labor. She was a gravida **twenty**! I was scared to death she would drop the baby before I rolled her to L&D. Later I discovered that a uterus pregnant twenty times is a tired uterus with not much "squeeze" left in it. She delivered the next day.

Some pregnant mothers were admitted with gonorrhea or syphilis. Untreated, gonorrhea would, in addition to causing great abdominal pain, scar their tubes and predispose to infertility or tubal pregnancy. Gonorrhea could blind a newborn and syphilis could be passed on to him, too. Usually the father was not in the picture.

Given the repetition of these situations over a four-year residency, it was easy to understand how our residents could become jaded and cynical. They tended to be gruff and poorly communicative. Some were very large. All were white. They could be intimidating to poorly educated, predominantly black women. Heck, they intimidated *me*! On rounds they casually informed a patient that they would place an Intra-Uterine-Device (IUD) before discharge to prevent pregnancy. There were medical reasons to avoid another pregnancy which could exacerbate uncontrolled hypertension or diabetes. Some women opted for a caesarian section (C-section) followed immediately by a hysterectomy—dangerous and bloody when performed post-partum. With a history of repeated pregnancies and without intervention, many women would return in nine months. If the mother *did* have male support—physical, financial, or emotional—she would feel compelled to give in to a *roll in the hay* long before it was safe—regardless of medical advice to the contrary.

From the perspective of age, I appreciate how disheartening and depressing these women's situations were. At the time, all I was able to identify was a knowledge deficit. When the residents made rounds and *informed* (not *explained*) what they would do to prevent pregnancy, it was obvious that they might as well have been speaking Greek to the women. I made it my business to return to the patients afterward to speak with them as another woman. The challenge was to use basic words, familiar objects. The uterus was a womb. The vagina was a birth canal. A straw could be an IUD. I tried to make it a discussion and to engage however many patients were in the room. Probably the best that I achieved was defusing some fear. I discovered that I liked reinterpreting all the medical jargon (gobbledygook) into something understandable. How different this was from my public health assignment to teach birth control methods to college co-eds! Yet how much the same.

The months rolled on toward my wedding date in February. I became adept at hanging IV's. At that time, they were in glass bottles with rubber stoppers through which we jabbed a spike with a drip-chamber and turned the bottle upside down to hang it. There were no pumps, no filters, no alarms for blockage or infiltration. I carried a sliding calculator which converted the ordered number of cc.'s per hour to the number of drops per minute. In the wee hours, flashlight in hand, I trans-illuminated the drip-chambers to count the drops.

Night shift also required GYN expertise. A major operation called an exenteration was performed at our teaching hospital. Not exoneration but exenteration. It was a last-ditch attempt to cure uterine cancer. The uterus, tubes and ovaries were removed. Because the cancer had spread, the bladder and colon were removed too. It was radical surgery, taking hours to perform. Bowel surgery, by its nature, can result in an infected incision with dehiscence—more so with poor nutritional status or a faulty immune response. Exenteration resulted in an open abdominal wound, colostomy bag and urostomy (bladder removal) bag attached to the abdominal wall, and a very debilitated patient. At the time, there was no enterostomal therapist or wound care nurse. A pharmacist who happened to have an ostomy consulted. There were two types of bags and the name of the game was to get a seal. I frequently failed miserably. The patient's gas would fill the bag and pull it off the abdomen, creating a mess. There were no bags with vents—we punctured the bag with a needle—a serious no-no I later discovered—to release the gas. That made the odor constant. Eventually, it leaked. There were no odor-proof bags, no face-plates with convexity to counter poor stoma placement. I can only imagine how the patient must have felt contending with it all. It seemed a fate worse than death.

GYN wounds like this, as well as a plentiful number of dehisced caesarian sections, gave me plenty of wound care practice. Irrigations with peroxide followed by saline-moistened packing were de rigueur for most wounds. One enterprising resident had me pour honey into an open abdominal wound in the era before wound gel and calcium alginate. Thanks to venereal disease, injections were plentiful. And since many mothers had difficulty urinating after a vaginal delivery, there was plenty of practice catheterizing patients. At first, I had difficulty deciding the gauge of catheter (straight, not indwelling) to choose for my tray. Catheter trays were metal, not disposable. They were wrapped in linen and autoclaved. Catheter (Foley or straight Robinson) and drainage bag were added separately. To avoid patient discomfort, I chose a twelve (tiny lumen) and then was stuck securing it as it drained . . . and drained . . . and drained . . . . I learned, through the school of hard knocks, to elevate the bed before catheterizing, minimizing back strain while I held cath in place as it drained . . . and drained . . . and drained. I did not learn to pass an NG tube or to start an IV thanks to the med students. Lacking those skills would be an impediment once out of the protective cocoon of the university setting.

Marriage and Work at a Community Hospital

Amazingly, I continued to grow and thrive as a nurse throughout the fall of 1967 despite our impending nuptials. I still craved roller skates to keep up with the frenetic pace of a teaching hospital where vital signs could be ordered every fifteen minutes, and everyone had some sort of complication. As my February wedding date approached, I resigned and returned home to St. Petersburg after the holidays. Following a brief honeymoon to Florida attractions, it was time to apply for a job. I desperately wanted OB, aware that many hospitals required basic Med-Surg experience before working on their OB unit.

St. Anthony's had just completed building a massive new addition to the west, parallel to the hospital in which I'd worked and volunteered. The west building was large, roomy and spacious—primitive by today's standards—but homey— *and* completely air conditioned. *Ahh the small things!* The Maternity Unit was on the third floor of the new building which connected directly to the old on each floor.

The OB unit was new, but the nurses were not. I interviewed with Head Nurse, Sister Mary Bede, a Jamaican Franciscan nun, educated in England as a nurse-midwife. Positive and energetic, I suspect that she had been charged with replacing the former long-time head nurse and transforming the old crowd of nurses into a more modern and enlightened group. Her enthusiasm translated neither to the old timers nor to the medical staff. Young blood, I fit her need as did some other new grads arriving within a few months. Sister Bede addressed me by my new name with a Jamaican lilt—Mrs. New´-ton.

For the first few months of my employment, post-partum and nursery were briefly on what would become the GYN end of 3 West. Later, it moved to its permanent spot on 3 NW. The main nurses' station was out front near the elevators. The post-partum section was behind it with the nursery in the middle. Windows lined two sides of the nursery but none to the outside and sunlight. Sunlight is useful to new babies with post-delivery jaundice—a common but potentially dangerous situation. There were twelve post-partum rooms, most semi-private, a handful of private rooms and one four bed ward. Jutting off the east side of the circular configuration of post-partum rooms was the horse-shoe-shaped labor and delivery unit. Any working nurse would tell you that it was designed poorly. Obviously, the architects of the spanking new building had not consulted the folks who would work there.

Labor and Delivery

The entrance to L&D (Labor & Delivery) was just off the elevators and to the right of the main nurses' station. Beyond was a hall of eight small labor rooms with adjoining bathrooms. The beds in L&D were high with side rails like adult cribs. A tiny abbreviated nurses' station to the left of the entrance contained a well-stocked, locked narcotics box, phones, and the labor and delivery log. Ever-the-secretary, it was the nurse's task to log, in beautiful script, each patient who had been in labor with the eventual outcome, time of birth, weight of infant, etc. The older nurses coveted the job. Fine by me.

Two prep rooms were designed to admit patients. The prep entailed shaving all pubic and perineal hair. An enema—high, hot and hell of a lot (otherwise known as a triple H)—was administered before taking the patient to her labor room. The prep room shower was seldom used unless a woman arrived obviously filthy. Over time, the prep rooms were abandoned, and the preps were simply completed in the labor room.

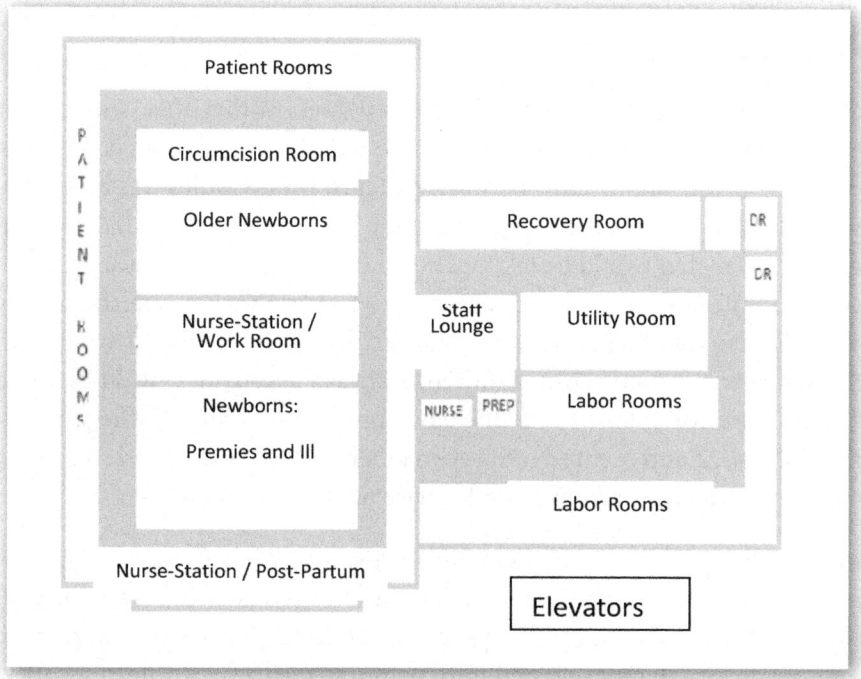

Figure 8 *The layout of 3 NW.*

The distance between the mini nurse station and the labor rooms presented real safety issues since there was usually just one nurse in L&D. Births numbered one hundred or fewer per month. Several women could be laboring at once. Many labors were prolonged more than twenty-four hours—primarily due to early and frequent administration of Demerol (a narcotic), which slowed labor.

When the birth was imminent, the private physician was seldom present—though there was a sleep room for physicians. He was phoned by the nurse. The patient was rolled by stretcher to one of two functioning delivery rooms. A nurse anesthetist was summoned from her sleep room. After delivery, the baby was taken to the nursery while the woman was carted back to the recovery room in the part of the U parallel to the labor rooms.

Across from the recovery room was a utility room. There all the delivery instruments and the Kelly pad (black rubber, placed under the delivering patient, channeling blood, amniotic fluid and maternal feces away from the patient into a floor bucket.) were scrubbed by the nurse while she monitored the recovering patient. Lomie Crawford, a very sharp African American nursing assistant close to my age, would occasionally be "in the back" to assist. On *very* good days, there would be another RN. The RN or Lomie—not the housekeeper—wet mopped the delivery room floor post-delivery with Vesphene solution. Everything was "Vesphenized." Vesphene was anti-microbial holy water. The solution in concentrate form was pumped into a bucket of water. It burned on skin contact.

Mrs. Riddles, an older African American woman with a New York accent was the housekeeper assigned to L&D on the day shift. She cleaned the halls and the floors of the labor rooms between patients. Mrs. Riddles was quiet and kept to herself, but I enjoyed her. She taught me how to wield a mean delivery room mop in a way that would be fast and conserve energy. Every day, part of her job entailed watering the mats at the entrance to L&D with a watering can full of Vesphene, an alkaline germicide solution. The idea was that it would sanitize the shoes of folks entering. Amused, I always asked Mrs. Riddles when her flowers were going to sprout. One day, I brought in a huge tissue paper flower on a long stick and secured it to the mat before Mrs. Riddles arrived. That certainly evoked a laugh from the otherwise taciturn lady!

Most of the RN's were in their mid-forties to fifties. Old enough to be my mother. They had worked there forever and were resistant to anything different. "We tried that, but . . ." They were all diploma grads. Rules were inviolate. They held in contempt two and four-year grads with very little clinical experience—experience that they had *in spades*. War stories abounded about nursing school—working in Central Supply Room (CSR); sharpening reusable needles; scrubbing instruments before sterilizing them; slaving away as surgical scrub nurses. I had none of these experiences. I had been educated quite differently from my working-nurse role models.

I tired of the old saw that the only reason to have a BSN was to be a manager. From their perspective, here was a young know-it-all nurse aiming to be their boss with none of their school or lifetime experiences. Untrue! I was humbled and insecure at my lack of experience. Working with these women became *my* real initiation, *my* hazing, *my* trial by fire. All I wanted to be was a good nurse— a good Post-Partum and Nursery nurse.

Unfortunately, Sister Mary Bede had other ideas. "Mrs. New´-ton, you are young. You are flexible. You are able to work all three areas—Post Partum, Nursery, *and* Labor and Delivery." Oh boy! I have always felt slow but willing to work at what others seem to do quite easily. I am not a quick thinker. I would be an abomination in the ER. It is simply not a strength. L&D is like an ER—in fact, we snickered at ER personnel whisking laboring moms up in wheelchairs lest they "pop" before arriving at our door. So, it was with trepidation and misgiving that I began to learn L&D—what was mysteriously called *The Back*.

My introduction occurred shortly after I began work at St. Anthony's. The labor nurse was in her late fifties, tall and angular with jerky movements, reminding me of a fear-inspiring high school nun I knew and had tried to avoid. There were one or two patients in labor.

In Gainesville, the patient had remained herself, albeit in episodic pain and with whiffs of nitrous oxide at delivery. Here, staff physicians **believed** in twilight sleep with religious fervor. Most of the women were coached by their doctors to run to the hospital when their water broke or when contractions began. They were promised that they would not feel a thing.

At the time of admission to L&D, these young women—most in their twenties or early thirties—were given 100 mg. of Demerol followed by 50 mg. of Demerol every two hours until they delivered. The obstetrician responsible for the most OB admissions per month demanded an even larger dose—150 mg. and then 75 mg. every two hours. Most were medication virgins and the doses kept them zonked. Heavy analgesia slowed labor. The addition of Lorfan supposedly lessened the effect of respiratory depression in the baby when administered close to delivery.

Not even huge doses of Demerol blunted the experience of the contraction. The third ingredient in the medication cocktail addressed that issue. It was scopolamine (scope)—an amnesic. It not only dried secretions to prep for general anesthesia, but, combined with Demerol, lowered inhibitions. When a contraction arose—literally the muscular uterus would rise in the abdomen—the women awakened and screamed bloody murder. They did what nature intended—sat up and rocked. They called out, "The doctor promised he would put me to sleep." *You are asleep.* Because when everything was over, they had amnesia. At least that was the plan. But speaking with mothers on Post-Partum, I discovered that their memories of labor were often distorted—like what the drug culture called a "bad trip." When a newly hired unit secretary was assigned to orient in labor and delivery on a very active day, the screams were so plentiful and so loud that the new employee simply never returned from lunch.

That first day in L&D, I worked with the older nurse whom I can only describe as cranky. When her patient woke with a contraction, grabbed hold of the bars, sat up and began to rock, scream and cry, this nurse placed her hand flat on the patient's sternum and pushed her back down, flat—probably the worst position for a laboring mom, compressing the major blood vessels behind the uterus. The nurse retorted, "Well if you didn't want this pain, why did you get pregnant?"—or words to that effect. I was flabbergasted. "She won't remember it anyway."

Fortunately, this nurse was soon transferred off the unit. She was replaced with a rotund fiftyish diploma school nurse from Maine named Miss Steele. Steele had tons of experience but a decided limp. If a nurse worked with her, she was the legs and action while Steele stayed by the phone calling doctors, nurse anesthetists, etc.

One of my first days, at change of shift, the evening nurse, Lucy Graham, a pretty, fortyish nurse with a syrupy southern drawl, creamy complexion, dark hair and red lipstick arrived in L&D to take report. Simultaneously, a laboring mother was wheeled in. "Newton, would you take her to the prep room, prep her and give her an enema?" she asked. Old guard nurses called each other by last name only—military style—tough. Flattered at her apparent confidence in me, I did as she asked, giving the patient a peri-prep (leaving hair on the pubic bone as at Shands) and a Fleets enema. When Lucy returned to inspect, she scowled. "You gave her a *Fleets*? What's all this hair on the pubic bone?" That was when I learned the meaning of a triple H enema—which Lucy said she would administer—disgusted with this useless BSN. I ended my shift not for the first time feeling just that—a bull shit nurse. I was an outsider among these folks who should be my colleagues. I worked very hard for their acceptance. No job was beneath me— emptying the trash, lifting the soiled linen bag into the laundry chute, mopping the floor, scrubbing the instruments. Each time I was burned, I learned from it and made corrections. I aimed to be above reproach.

My previous mention of twilight sleep did not describe the mechanics. At UF, we had used disposable needles and syringes. Here, the hospital had recently changed from reusable to disposable needles but still used glass syringes. That was fortunate because of the way twilight sleep was drawn up. Demerol came in a large multi-dose vial, a bottle with a 30 cc. capacity and a rubber stopper for access. Lorfan was in a smaller glass ampoule which had to be cracked open with a wrist snap. Scopolamine, however, came in tiny tablets in a little bottle. To draw up the medication, the nurse dropped the Scope pill from the bottle into the plunger-less syringe. The glass plunger was re-inserted and used to grind the pill to powder. Then the Demerol was drawn up followed by Lorfan. Before drawing up any medication from a closed vial, you must draw up the number of cc.'s of air you plan to withdraw. The air is injected into the vial, then the med is pulled into the syringe. If that is not done, a vacuum occurs and whatever is in the syringe is drawn into the multi-dose bottle. Imagine how much Scopolamine could have been in the dregs of that Demerol bottle. Today's nurses would find the whole procedure unfathomable—thankfully!

Each obstetrician was a character. There were no women obstetricians on staff. At Shands, interns, residents and med students had been ever-present. No worries. Here, the situation was completely different—a private hospital catering to private patients; private doctors on whom it depended for admissions. Here, nurses managed the labor, phoning in physician updates. When the patient was ready, the doctor was called in from—wherever. One of them went fishing on his boat. His wife literally raised a flag if we called requesting his presence. In 1968 there were no cell phones. One doctor routinely rode on his motorcycle already dressed in road-dirty scrubs. (Nurses' scrubs were clean every day.) Over-weight, huffing and puffing up the stairs, Dr. Harley arrived

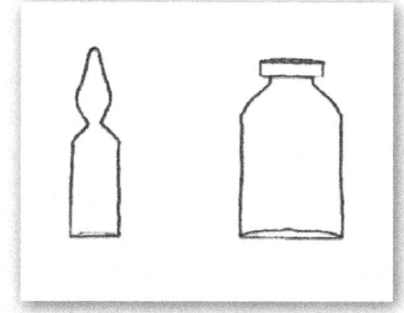

Figure 9 *(L-R) Ampoule & Vial*

in the delivery room. Another doctor was sure to be on the golf course or at its nineteenth hole.

Some nurses are smug about knowing when someone will give birth—and, for that matter, when someone will die. Nothing but bravado. You can sense the general rhythm—as in gauging when to jump in while playing childhood jump-rope. But what if the end girl unexpectedly drops the rope or loses rhythm? The same is true with labor. Predictions about the actual time of delivery are guesswork at best. Calling the MD in too early or too late—either way—blame the nurse.

When to call the doctor was a conundrum. When I was hired, only doctors were permitted to perform vaginal exams to directly monitor the cervical dilation and station (the relationship of the infant's head to the ischial spines of the mother's pelvis.) We nurses with less sanctified hands had to do it through the rectum. Another example of Fred and Ginger—backwards and in high heels. We felt with a single finger through several layers of muscle and connective tissue while the docs felt it directly with two fingers in the vagina. The result, apart from supreme maternal discomfort, was that we spread fecal material to the perineum and the doctors plugged it right on up the vagina. Oh, it wasn't that blatant—we all took precautions to keep the perineum clean. But, microscopically, it was probably true.

Puerperal fever deaths had been common in the nineteenth century when doctors did not wash their hands going from one patient to the next, taking pride in their blood-smeared gowns. Better aseptic technique in the 1920s and antibiotic development in the 1940s made hospital deliveries safe.

Learning styles vary. Some people are visual, some are auditory, and some are tactile. I am visual, not tactile, so interpreting rectal and vaginal exams was a rough one for me. Once Sister Mary Bede had obtained permission (I have no idea how) for nurses to perform vaginal exams, I literally developed a *feel* for it. With my two fingers inserted in the vagina, I visualized the cervix, vagina and pelvis. I became pretty accurate. There was one doctor who—no matter the nurse—always debated her findings. If she said the patient was three cm. dilated, then he would say no she was four. If the nurse said she was four, he'd say she was three. No rhyme or reason. He simply had to have the upper hand, the last word. The actual numbers really didn't matter. What mattered was the nurse's ability to pace the labor performing vaginal exams, timing contractions and noting behavioral changes.

If you imagine a woman laboring with IV and fetal monitor in place, you are wrong. None of these were in use. The fetal monitor was the nurse, armed with a device called a fetoscope which made her look like a unicorn. It was a stethoscope attached to a metal strip which fit over the nurse's head. It conducted sound via her skull bones and through the tubes to her ears. With her head, she pushed the bell into place on the maternal abdomen and listened. Depending upon the baby's position, it could be easy . . . or not. The sounds were faint, rapid and sometimes difficult to hear. I worked hard to keep a poker face to avoid alarming a mother simply because I had difficulty hearing. The fetal heartbeat and maternal blood pressure were monitored throughout labor.

Sometimes, a breech birth was in the making—baby-bottom first. I had become so adept at vaginal exams that I was a little too cocky. Convinced that I felt a scrotum on one woman's baby, I announced to the mother that it was a boy. At delivery, I discovered that the *girl's* vulva had simply been swollen from pounding against the cervix with each contraction. At the time, no routine ultrasound alerted the parent to the baby's sex.

There was a real problem with breech babies. The actual delivery was very tricky. With normal, head first (vertex) deliveries, once the head is out, after suctioning, the baby can take in oxygen. He no longer depends solely upon the cord for it. Fortunate. Because the cord is compressed between the baby and the pelvis on the way out. Imagine a breech birth—the head is inside; the buttock is outside, and the cord is compressed by soft tissue and pelvic bone. The head—still inside—is the largest part of the baby's body. The shoulders are the second largest. There are only a few minutes to rectify the situation. In the days before modern obstetrics, a baby stuck in this position could spell death not only for him but for his mother. In modern obstetrics, a breech birth can be delivered by Caesarian section. But, in the 1960s, the risk/benefit ratio was believed to make a routine section inadvisable. Now C-sections are much more common. Then every doctor's worst nightmare was getting the breech stuck—half in and half out.

Versions of breech delivery include—frank breech (buttocks first), single or double-footling (feet first) and other variations. Close to the end of my tenure at St. Anthony's, I was confronted with one. On the evening shift, an older nurse, Carol Benedict, and I were working labor and delivery. Lomie Crawford, the Nursing Assistant, was also there—unusually good staffing for an evening. I was the team-leader. No patients were in labor. Other days it could be raining patients.

A white, mildly obese woman in her mid-thirties was wheeled up from the ER through our swinging door with haste. Her water had broken. She was in active labor. I suspect there had been previous pregnancies. Most important—she was unregistered. She had no prenatal care, making it a high-risk pregnancy. The on-call doctor would be hers. In this instance he was literally on the golf course. The situation was unusual because any unregistered patients appearing in the ER in early labor were shuttled over to the public hospital, Bayfront. It connected directly to All Children's—appropriate for high risk cases.

The patient was several centimeters dilated when I first checked her and contractions were minutes apart. She estimated that she was less than nine months along. Carol and I medicated her and called the doctor who promised to hustle. We took her straight from prep over to the delivery room. The nurse anesthetist sat at the head of the table unwilling to administer anesthesia until the doctor was present. With each strong contraction, the presenting part—the buttocks—inched further and further down. I didn't break the table to put her legs in stirrups. Instead I donned sterile gloves and placed a sterile pad just under her buttocks. The patient's expressions of discomfort increasingly worried the anesthetist who asked me if she should administer gas. I told her it was a breech and that she needed to use her own judgment. Carol was at my side preparing to receive the baby. I watched the vulva bulge further and further. With the next contraction, the tip of the buttocks emerged. Someone had to do something, or the baby would die within minutes.

I remembered a diagram in a maternity nursing text which I still studied religiously. It showed the obstetrician's hand entering the vagina underneath the emerging baby, his finger placed in the baby's mouth to guide the head out and under the pubis. That is exactly what I did. Fortunately, it was a small baby—maybe six pounds. I forgot one element of the maneuver. I forgot to wrap a towel around the buttocks and lower trunk. What happened next was the result. During the next contraction the baby emerged. The legs which had been straight with feet against the ears in a pike position, flipped down and out. I felt it. That was when the mother experienced a 1° tear.

Carol became the pediatric nurse, drying the baby, wrapping him and putting antibiotic ointment in his eyes. But he was still attached to mom via umbilical cord. The placenta was still in mom. Its presence could become the source of massive bleeding. We waited. I massaged the fundus (top of uterus) to encourage it to contract, hoping to squeeze the placenta off the uterine wall and out. We put the still attached baby on her abdomen, thinking that it would stimulate oxytocin and involution. Still no doctor. Still no doctor. In the cold delivery room, the baby needed the incubator to keep it warm while adjusting to the world. The practice of using a knitted cap to cover the head which is the area of greatest heat loss had not yet arrived. Finally, I clamped and cut the cord which had long since stopped pulsating, freeing Carol to tend to the baby in the incubator.

The mother was mildly sedated after her admission—Demerol and a few whiffs of nitrous oxide. Finally, the doctor, whom I will call Joe Cool arrived, and commanded the anesthetist to "put her under." We put the patient in stirrups and broke the table. Inspecting the perineum, he gave me an approving nod that she had only experienced a 1° laceration. Usual obstetric practice was to cut a midline or medial-lateral episiotomy before birth essentially giving the patient a 2-3° laceration (albeit with smoother and easier-to-repair edges) a few minutes before the delivery of the presenting part. Later, my legs shook outside the delivery room when Lomie congratulated me on what she knew enough to realize could have been a disastrous situation.

Why had I been hesitant to cut the cord? Because, *legally*, the one who cut the cord was the one who delivered the baby. Technically, that was me. But the doctor "covered" for me and took credit. In those days, many old guard nurses expected that the doctor would "cover" for them with this and many other issues. I had no such illusions observing that, for many physicians, the mantra CYOA would have been descriptive. A subtext of this predicament is the question of who should be reimbursed for the actual delivery episode in the peri-natal care continuum. Their "cover" did not just benefit the nurse.

Joe Cool was part of a triumvirate. One of his partners, slightly younger, was a veteran of WWII in the Pacific. He was BIG, fair and Nordic and could have been the white version of the Buccaneers' defensive tackle Warren Sapp. He had huge hands but was supremely gentle with his vaginal exams. He acted goofy on a personal level but was a treasure trove of medical information. You had to ask him. He was not a show-off. He was quietly intelligent and well-read. One evening, a very obese woman was in labor and medicated. She began grunting with contractions but wildly resisted my attempts to separate her legs to check her progress. Fortunately, this doctor was asleep in the Doctors Room. I called him sheepishly and apologized that I really wasn't sure just how far along the patient was. The doctor, with my help and the leverage of his height, separated her legs far enough to see a sweet little head crowning, parting her vulva. Together we sped her to the delivery room.

Joe Cool's other partner I will just call Dr. Saint—which he was not. This guy had practiced as a GP before completing his residency in OB at Bayfront. I call him Saint because he made a great show of flaunting his Catholicity, wearing his scapular and medals prominently so all could see rather than under his clothes like most people. Whenever something happened that he didn't like, he flew in a tantrum down to the hospital nun-administrator. He made sure everyone knew how tight he was with the hierarchy. His temper was atrocious and had us all stepping on glass. I did that *literally* one day in the delivery room when his barked orders rattled me. I reached into the cabinet for an ampoule of Pitocin stored in a light, open plastic box. When I removed the ampoule, the whole box of fifty came crashing to the ground. They crunched under my shoes when I rushed to get what he wanted next. From behind his mask, he asked calmly, "Do I make you nervous?" Understatement! Compared to his partners, this man was short in stature with small hands. His vaginal exams were rough—poking and prodding—an extension of his personality. Some nurses dubbed it small man syndrome.

It is worth mentioning here that the doctors in the late sixties' St. Petersburg were upper class. No, they weren't the Firestones or other reclusive multimillionaires living in the mansions of Park Street. But they were the crème de la crème of society. Most of them lived in posh Snell Isle or Pinellas Point areas. Probably fifty percent of the yearly debutants were physicians' daughters. The doctors belonged to the Yacht club and/or any of the variety of country clubs. They were wealthy. They were educated. Their wives were constantly in the social pages for Junior League, Queen of Hearts Ball, and a variety of charitable fundraisers. Who were we nurses? Blue collar stiffs who had no time, even if interested, to achieve charitable notoriety. The bottom line was that the balance of power was heavily weighted in their direction—men, socially prominent and influential, well-educated and—most of all—the source of hospital revenue. Is it any wonder that they were courted and treated like kings?

Perpetually discontent, doctors didn't agree with that assessment. At that time, they began to build hospitals of their own. Palms, Ed White, Sun Bay and Hubert Rutland were originally built with physician investment, giving them a stake in how the hospital was run—or so they thought. Years later that pipedream was laid to rest and they sold to major hospital chains.

Concomitantly, it was an era of civil unrest. The Civil Rights Movement emerged. In 1966, Joe Waller, later known as Omali Yeshitela of the Uhuru movement, tore a painting which he believed badly depicted African Americans from the wall of St. Petersburg City Hall. Civil disobedience. The 1968 garbage men's (African American) strike featured marches for better wages and better working conditions. There were riots in town. St. Anthony's was just north of an African American enclave called Jamestown. It was before the Interstate was built, separating Jamestown from the hospital with an elevated wall of roadway. Employees were drilled on what to do in case of a riot—keep patients away from windows, bring them into the hall. Contingency plans were made to bus us to work from St. Paul's should the danger escalate. In February 1968 during the week-long teachers' strike, the school system bussed-in what my striking mother called scabs (teacher replacements—usually socially prominent wives of professional men).

Until then, there were fewer than a handful of African American nurses at the hospital—working invisibly in Pharmacy or CSR. Most blacks worked in housekeeping. But now, post-civil rights legislation, more African Americans became aids and LPN's. During the racial unrest, some of the white staff feared black staff allied with militants in their private lives. Whites were now befuddled about what to respectfully call them. Negro had formerly been a term of respect. Now Black was coming into use but a co-worker friend balked that she was not black but coffee with cream. Lomie Crawford, the nursing assistant whom I remember fondly was a tall and imposing African American woman who could threaten with a hard, intimidating stare. I liked Lomie.

I mention social issues because of the contrasts. We nurses, not well-paid (albeit better than the sanitation workers) believed that we could not ethically strike. What? Abandon the patients? It could not be done. So, while physicians navigated from their high society pedestals; racial unrest threatened; the Viet Nam War raged on; and protests escalated, we nurses simply carried on. We took whatever ball was thrown our way and dealt with it regardless of race or social class. We got the job done. We were women and the possibility that we deserved anything better had not dawned on us.

Remember the doctor who always equivocated about dilation? I learned plenty from him—in all the wrong ways. Dr. Nearsighted was a tall, graying older man, his face screwed up in a perpetual squint. He was extremely myopic but not pleasantly like the cartoon character Mr. McGoo. We earnestly prayed that the babies he circumcised emerged from the circumcision room with all that they should. He performed very clumsy episiotomies. Once he tried to tell me that it was Rh-negative, not Rh-positive babies whose Rh-negative mothers needed RhoGAM. [1] In short, I would never trust him with my baby or my life. Yet his bedside manner with post-partum mothers was smooth as silk. While many other doctors ran in and ran out for the post-partum checkup, he leisurely sat assuming a paternal air while chatting with his patients at length. I recognized, and wished consumers did too, that bedside manner is no indicator of wisdom or clinical expertise.

One day while I worked on post-partum, the L&D nurses cared for a laboring patient with an unusual amount of vaginal bleeding. They phoned Dr. Nearsighted and, as expected, he minimized their concern. Standing their ground, they declared that they would do no more vaginal exams and that he needed to come in and monitor his patient. It went over like a lead balloon. Why were the nurses concerned? A small amount of vaginal bleeding is expected—particularly when the cervix begins to dilate, and the mucous plug is released. The nurses in question knew this. They knew normal labor. And they knew that this bleeding was not normal.

There were two possibilities—both ominous. One was the possibility of an abruptio placenta, meaning that with each contraction, the placenta separated from the uterine wall, causing mother to hemorrhage and the fetus to have less oxygen. The other possibility was placenta previa, meaning that the placenta emerges first when it has been implanted in the lower part of the uterus. Think big blood vessels for child and mother. In labor, as the cervix (which is the shape of a doughnut) begins to flatten (efface) and dilate, the placenta sitting on it is dislodged. Abruption. In case of a previa, you do not do vaginal exams! Today, the problem is identified early on ultrasound and handled accordingly—usually C-section—because the baby cannot be delivered vaginally *through* the placenta. In the sixties, there was no routine ultrasound. A skilled practitioner could pick up evidence such as the fetal position and the location of the uterine souffle (sound of blood coursing to the placenta). There *is* a problem when experienced labor nurses say there is a problem.

The doctor arrived, minimizing the nurses' concerns even as he flipped the covers to see bright red blood on the patient's puddle pad. Infinitely wise, he donned his glove, stuck his large fingers up the vagina and discovered first hand that it was, indeed, placenta previa which he had perforated with his finger. Then the hustle began in earnest because the labor area was not yet set up to perform C-sections. The patient was whisked down the elevator in her labor bed in a frenzied rush to the second floor OR for an emergency C-section. I don't remember the baby's condition. In the recovery room, the mom bled again going into shock. She returned to surgery for a hysterectomy—future pregnancy denied.

As if that story about Dr. Nearsighted were not enough, there is another. I worked another evening shift with one of my favorite people, Sadie Burton. A Kentuckian, Sadie was a very experienced L&D nurse in her thirties. Sadie was tiny with freckles, and a very whimsical sense of humor. Unless the Head Nurse specifically assigned me to be team leader in L&D, I always deferred to Sadie's expertise. On this evening, early in the shift, we admitted one of Dr. Nearsighted's patients. The dark-haired woman with brown eyes and a good tan was pretty and slim with a huge belly. Her labor had begun a month ahead of her due date. Her soldier husband was in Viet Nam. Labor progressed. Sadie asked me to go to dinner first. Hopefully, we could both get our evening meal in before the delivery. Wage and hour laws pushed us to take one half-hour break and one fifteen-minute coffee break regardless of unit activity—even if we didn't want to. Management was strict on that. If I thought no one would notice, I would be contrary.

When I returned from the cafeteria, Sadie was in the delivery room with Dr. Nearsighted. He was yelling (not unusual): Where was another bulb syringe? Where was another incubator? As if three kids who had lived together in their mother's womb for months could not share! God bless Sadie. She tried to deal with him and to deal with the fact that what the doctor had thought would be twins had, in fact, become triplets. He was losing it. The mother was not a factor at this point—she was anesthetized. We needed to anesthetize the doctor. I took care of the three premature handsome dark-haired, round headed little baby boys and transported them to the newborn nursery. They were approximately three pounds each and adorable, but their condition was tenuous. Nursery Nurse, Tommy (Florence Thompson) learning of the delivery, had called the most important person to her—the priest. Only then did she call the pediatrician. She had already placed Miraculous Medals and Sacred Heart scapulars sealed in autoclaved formula bottles in each of the Isolettes which were heating. When I called our head nurse to warn her that the next shift might need more help, she told me to stay in the nursery with the babies and to take care of Tommy. One of those beautiful babies died within forty-eight hours but the other two survived. Happily, through the Red Cross, the father was relieved of duty in Viet Nam to deal with his unexpectedly large family.

The last story about Dr. Nearsighted occurred on Thanksgiving Day. A young primigravida (a woman in her first pregnancy) was wheeled in shortly after noon in active labor. The woman *had* been instructed not to eat or drink anything after labor began to prevent aspiration when she was anesthetized. Ignoring those instructions, she and her family had their big Thanksgiving dinner *DESPITE* her contractions.

On admission, her water had broken, and labor progressed at a merry clip. She was already at least five (out of ten) centimeters dilated at a plus station. We called the doctor to inform him that she was progressing quickly and asked/ advised, "You don't want to give her an enema at this point, do you?" Maybe we should not have asked. "High, hot and hell of a lot," was his reply. We had already medicated her. During her perineal prep she managed to vomit that sumptuous Thanksgiving dinner complete with cranberry sauce all over herself, the bed and me. She had very few results from the triple H. The doctor arrived. Her labor progressed. She was drunkenly transferred from labor bed to gurney for transport to delivery.

Once she was anesthetized and up in stirrups, Dr. Nearsighted, who had inflicted that triple H enema, sat gowned and gloved, near her perineum. With the baby's descent, out gushed the results of the enema—all over said doctor. A small measure of poetic justice, it brought a smile to my face under the mask.

L&D could be very busy or amazingly quiet. There were some shifts with no one in labor. We used them to clean and restock. But, sometimes the cupboards were full and equipment sparkled. During those shifts, to pass the time, I matched literary quotes or music to objects or procedures found in obstetrics. For example, lochia (post-partum uterine bleeding like a very heavy period) became post-natal drip. The drip part was because if you couldn't find a new mother in her bed, you could usually follow the bloody trail to the bathroom. The narcotics box became "I have a place where dreams are born, and time is never planned" from Peter Pan. About the Kelly Pad—the rubber malodorous chute placed under the buttocks in delivery—"the smell of blood is there still, and all the perfumes of Arabia cannot sweeten . . . " a quote from Macbeth.

Early in my L&D tenure, I was assigned to be alone in the back. Initially L&D was empty but, mid-morning, a woman with intact membranes (water had not broken) arrived in active labor. She was a multigravida. In the prep room, I shaved her and was preparing an enema. Sister Mary Bede arrived to relieve me for that mandatory coffee break. She would finish up the prep. Remember, she was an England-trained nurse midwife. I rarely escaped to the basement cafeteria for coffee, preferring just to use the bathroom in the nurses' lounge. Coffee and cigarettes, essential to many, were not my thing at all.

In the bathroom, suddenly, I heard the usually soft-spoken Sister Mary Bede calling loud as a chanticleer with anxious authority, "Mrs. New´-ton, Mrs. New´-ton, come quick." I returned to the prep room to find Sister's hand up the woman's vagina. Sister Bede explained that she had been ready to administer the enema when, with a contraction, the woman's membranes ruptured. Because the head was not engaged in the pelvis, the cord had prolapsed, slipping down the vagina ahead of the baby. With each contraction, the cord was pinched against the pelvis by the descending head—asphyxiating the baby before birth. Sister was performing a maneuver to prevent cord compression by preventing further engagement of the head into the pelvis with each contraction.

Sister directed me to call the woman's doctor. Then she sent me for portable oxygen for the mother. To give the baby his best chance, the woman could not be sedated, in-spite of increasingly strong contractions. By that time, I had found the anesthetist who assumed position at the head of the bed to administer that oxygen via a mask. The huge, crib-shaped bed was pushed out into the hall by the three of us aiming toward the much larger delivery room down the hall and around the corner.

In that very poorly laid out L&D, my role was to get this, do that. Young and quick on my feet, I had alerted Post-Partum to nab any obstetrician who was making rounds. Tension was palpable. In walked the previously mentioned Dr. Joe Cool. No matter the mayhem afoot, he always kept a cool head. With Perry Como-like smoothness, he always said, "Don't worry about a thing. Everything will be okay." He was the most skilled obstetrician we had. Joe decided that he was going to deliver the baby right there in the hall, in the bed. "Sister, would you please take your hand out of the vagina?" he asked politely as though it were the most common thing in the world for her to be doing. Just then, the patient's obese obstetrician, the one who rode his motorcycle in scrub attire, came huffing and puffing around the corner. "It's alright, Harley," said Joe Cool. "I got it. You assist." Fortunately, the labor moved quickly, and the mother cooperated as best she could. Just as the head crowned, there was so much tension on the cord that it broke. Harley gasped. But Joe Cool said, "Don't worry about a thing," as he grabbed and clamped, quickly delivering the baby. It was fine. Had I been alone in that situation, I would not have known what to do. Now I did.

Nursery

The newborn nursery was my special joy. I loved to work there. Loved those babies! Newly-wed, I was sure that whatever I learned among them would have future personal application.

Babies were wonderful albeit noisy at feeding time. At the beginning of a nursery shift, an extensive hand and arm scrub was required. As in the rest of the OB unit, the uniform was a white scrub dress furnished by the hospital (no pants allowed—unlady-like). In the nursery or post-partum, we were required to wear a hairnet—flattening our hair and making us look like cafeteria workers. Only the frilly handkerchief in our breast pocket was missing! Nurses also wore caps. Bobby pins tangled in the nets. God forbid if there was a pregnant mom with ante-partum problems! The fetoscope was placed under the cap and tangled in the hairnet! In L&D we wore paper shower caps. Believe me, if looking gorgeous is a high priority, nursing is not the profession of choice!

At any given time, there were eight to twelve babies in the nursery. After their mother's discharge, some infants remained there—usually because of complications like prematurity or birth defects. Less stable babies were kept to the south of the mini nurse station. Stable infants more than twenty-four hours old were to the north of the station. Mothers' rooms ringed the periphery separated by the hall.

After an infant was delivered, it was brought, swaddled, to the nursery and placed in an incubator, a metal box on wheels with glass windows on front and lid. At the extreme right end of the box was a trough of sterile distilled water sitting over a light bulb. The heat of the bulb warmed the box and vaporized the water—helping to loosen any remaining respiratory secretions. It was possible to attach oxygen if needed. Vents were opened to prevent high oxygen concentrations from blinding the baby. Sicker or premature infants were placed in higher and larger Plexiglas boxes called Isolettes. Isolettes had two ports on each side which could be used for the nurse's arms when providing care. Ports were closed when not in use. Isolettes were warm, could have oxygen and the baby was completely visible. Radiant warmers hadn't yet arrived. Apparently, only RN's were capable of cleaning Isolettes after use—or so the hospital thought. Vesphene of course! When cleaning Isolettes or mopping the delivery room floor, I thought of Dean Smith. The UF program might not have been a diploma school, but now I was immersed in my own version of a diploma school.

Nursery was the domain of the nurse and aid assigned to it. Only when babies were brought to their mothers for feeding did interaction occur with mothers who were learning to feed their infants. No on-demand feeding here. Probably only ten percent of moms breastfed. They were usually the affluent, better educated women. No matter—breast or bottle—all babies received only water for the first twenty-four hours—supposedly to assess their ability to swallow without aspiration. Their moms having been well-medicated during labor, many of the newborns were sluggish and had problems getting their swallowing together. Sometimes they choked or had an episode of apnea (not breathing)—so the water was fed by the nurse. Later, when the babies went out to their moms, they usually returned with very little missing from the bottle. We fed them more. We helped them in ways that mom didn't know how. That made us feel good about ourselves, but I was aware then that it did not always achieve the same for the mother. I spent a lot of time coaching mothers. I was torn, aware of my responsibility to observe the preemies and newborns in the nursery. There was no such thing as rooming-in. The well babies over twenty-four hours old were in Plexiglas bassinettes on wheels with a cabinet of supplies (diapers, blankets, A&D Ointment, cotton balls) underneath. Yet they were *carried* out to the moms in our arms at feeding time.

When I received a newborn from the delivery room, I performed a cursory assessment. He had already been weighed. My task was to clean him and measure his length. Each newborn kit had a disposable paper measuring tape. I grasped the baby's ankles with one hand holding the tape and suspended him head down to measure. Newborns tend to ball-up in the familiar position which served them well for nine months, so holding them this way for a few seconds yielded accuracy. More than once, a new father or grandmother came to the window only to look on in horror at the ubiquitous procedure. The windows made *every*thing done in the nursery visible to *every*one. Several times, if the baby still had a little blood on his head from the delivery, the dad became woozy. He had not been a part of the labor and delivery and did not see it contextually. Several dads fainted in the Recovery Room—possibly out of relief or, possibly, out of shock at rejoining a wife who looked as though she had been through a war.

The permanent Nursery Nurse on evenings, Tommy Thompson, had been there so long that her babies had babies—and *their* mothers remembered her. If I worked Nursery, it was usually in the daytime where my co-conspirator was a very short stubby thirtyish aid from Fall River Massachusetts named Shirley Ainsworth. Newton and Ainsworth to the old guard—and to each other. Ainsworth was wonderful with basic care of the well babies. I trusted her completely. She had a sharp eye and would alert me if one of them looked dusky. What would I do? Stimulate it by rubbing its back; suction it with a bulb syringe; if needed, employ some oxygen. It was not unusual but could be a potentially serious event. Ainsworth would do anything, keeping the place going if I were busy with a preemie or helping a doctor in the circumcision room. But there was one thing she would _not_ do—handle a dead baby. I wasn't crazy about the idea either and was a little afraid. Death had not been a nursing school experience and, except for that morgue visit, barely a topic.

One day, a very tiny two-pound preemie not expected to live—didn't. The protocol was that the infant should be washed and swaddled; one of his two armbands was removed and pinned to the outer blanket. "That's *your* job," Shirley was quick to assert. I did it. The skin was shiny and cool. Later in the week when I prepared a whole chicken for my husband's dinner, the coolness, and size reminded me of that baby—as has every bone-in-place chicken since. It was policy for an ER orderly to take the swaddled body down to the morgue. Several years later, that policy was scratched. An orderly had become hysterical when his package emitted a sound, not realizing that air in lungs and stomach can be forced out with pressure and position change and pass by the vocal cords. Carrying the deceased to the morgue became another task for the RN only.

I finally learned to pass a naso-gastric tube on a preemie in the nursery. Preemies were either too weak to suck or lacked the sucking reflex. We had special red preemie nipples requiring less effort to suck and we used them when babies were able. We also stuffed preemie nipples with a cotton ball for use as pacifier. But those tiny babies, already thin, needed nutrition to gain strength. They were fed in small quantities through a tube passed through the nose into their stomach. This type of tube had been reserved only for med students in Gainesville, so it was a first for me. Believe me, I read up on it in my pediatric text at home. I can't remember who walked me through it with the first baby, but I became adept at it. After assuring that it was not in the trachea rather than the esophagus—potentially fatal—the tube was taped in-place on the infant's cheek, negating the need to repeat the process often.

I loved those little preemies with the round heads and bug eyes. One of the aids, Ginny, fondly referred to them as roaches. They were ugly to her but beautiful to me. They had personalities all their own and were in the nursery for long enough to really get to know them. Actually, we felt they were ours since already discharged mothers came no more than once a day—often less. The rule of thumb was that the preemie should grow to five or six pounds before discharge—depending upon the skill and reliability of the mother.

Occasionally, a birth defect presented itself. An obvious one—initially traumatic but with long-term promise—was hare-lip and/or cleft-palate. The hare-lip was a disfiguring lip gap which could extend up through the nose. Cleft-palate posed a more life-threatening concern. With communication between the roof of the mouth and the baby's nasal passages, swallowing and getting the formula down into the stomach where it belonged rather than back out the nose or into the lungs became an issue.

There were two types of adaptive nipples for this birth defect. One was a regular but slightly stiffer elongated nipple with a round ended flap over one side. The flap was placed on the top of the baby's mouth where the palate ought to be, the actual nipple beneath it. The other type was an elongated nipple with an extra bulge at its base. It looked like a duck. The bulge, during sucking, occluded the opening in the palate. Choosing the nipple was a matter of trial and error. Different babies adapted differently, so in these cases, we nurses took the responsibility of feeding the baby until it was safe, and we could teach the mother. Eventually each of these deformities could be repaired surgically and would be fine. Horror often was the first reaction of parents whose perfect baby balloon had been burst. One mom was an exception. Then I noticed her handsome husband who had a very thin white scar above one bow of his lip.

Within days of my St. Anthony's employment, a baby with a birth defect was delivered. The boy, Daniel, was full-term with spina bifida and a meningomyelocele. Spina bifida is a neural tube defect which occurs early in pregnancy. The spine and skin do not close. An opening in the spine could lead to infection. With a meningomyelocele, the spinal cord protrudes through the opening in a sack which looks like a bubble on the infant's back. The newborn's mother's name was Daniella. Danny remained in the nursery after Daniella's discharge. She returned daily to hold and feed him. Waiting for the neurosurgeon to close his back, I spent considerable time talking with her. As for Danny, we nurses loved him and felt he was ours, too. It was before All Children's opened, so the corrective procedure was performed at our hospital. Then we waited for what could follow—hydrocephaly (common name: "water on the brain"). We watched for the "sunset eyes" appearance and took daily head circumference measurements. I don't remember if Danny did develop hydrocephaly but, if he did, a shunt draining the fluid from the brain's ventricle into the abdominal cavity would have been placed.

Twenty years later, walking my dog in a previously unexplored neighborhood, I noticed a twenty-something kid in a wheelchair working on his car. I thought nothing of it. Unexpectedly, a middle-aged woman sprinted from his house yelling, "Danny, Danny, this was your nurse." It was Daniella. Danny, a normal teen, could have cared less. He was normal in every way except for being paraplegic. But I was touched that after all those years, Daniella had remembered.

Every morning around eight, multiple pediatricians descended upon the nursery for their initial assessments and daily follow-up with moms. It was like mini-rounds. I accompanied them when possible. One of the pediatricians, Dr. Ed Cole, was politically active and, years later, became mayor of St. Petersburg. Another, Dr. John Cordes, was an affable southern gentleman, always in a pleasant mood and very sharp on his assessments. One day while he assessed a newborn with an unusually shaped head, I made the general comment, "I think he has *FLK* syndrome (nursery-nurse-speak for *Funny Looking Kid*). Dr. Cordes laughed and said yes, the head was odd. He chalked it up to birth trauma and molding.

Annoyed that I had made such a weak case, I was certain that it was more than molding. How could I articulate it? During labor, the cranial bones mold to the shape of the vagina—thus, the elongated head. The trauma of the head acting as a cervical battering ram during labor can lead to soft tissue trauma and swelling of the presenting part. That swelling is known as caput succedaneum. For the same reason, babies can develop little "horn buds" which are really hematomas.

That night I returned to my pediatric text scouring for information. Aha! The next morning when Dr. Cordes arrived, I pronounced that the misshapen head looked like craniosynostosis, premature knitting of the cranial bones which does not allow brain growth. Hmmm. He said—let's take an x-ray. Sure enough, the baby had craniosynostosis which was surgically repaired.

I learned from this situation to respect my intuition and to articulate specifically and scientifically. Communication is the essence of nursing. Until these experiences with doctors, I had not understood how *many* modes of communication nurses need in our repertoire. Patients have their own culture and educational levels. Nurses are completely different. Doctors are different still. Though my goal became learning the language and hot buttons of my target audience, I was a long way from proficiency!

I have mentioned Florence (Tommy) Thompson, the multigenerational evening nursery nurse. She looked like an older Martha Raye (WWII-era USO comedienne) with steel-grey well-styled hair (netted of course), a matronly figure and a very large red lip-sticked mouth. As a Catholic diploma school grad, one of her fondest memories from school was cleaning the priest's canary bird cage. Even after so many years of nursery nursing, she remained intensely sincere and worried herself to death over each and every one of her charges.

Commonly, hospitals have a thirty-minute over-lap of shifts so that the on-coming shift can receive report about their patients' conditions and care. At the time, each nursery baby had a card in the Kardex with that information. The very tight-lipped and humorous night nurse, Shirley Aunspaugh, always gave pithy and terse reports. Reporting off to Tommy was another matter. As succinct as I wanted to be, Tommy felt the need to give me her report about the *previous* evening as I reviewed what had happened just *today*. By custom, the person giving report sat at the desk flipping through the Kardex. Tommy, receiving report, stood at my left, taking notes. She called me Newton and was the only one who seemed able to make that brusque, military form of address sound like a term of endearment. She was totally guileless and believed that everyone else—me included—was as sincere and well-meaning as she. That said, sometimes it was all I could do to suppress my giggles as she dramatically described how she had coached this mother or that during the previous evening.

You would think breast feeding would just come naturally but it doesn't. Inserting what might be an inverted nipple on a tightly engorged breast into the baby's mouth while not smothering him takes a certain amount of savoir faire and coaching while stimulating the baby's rooting and sucking reflexes. Tommy was the coach extraordinaire! During report, she elaborated on the previous night's coaching, literally manhandling her own very ample breasts to demonstrate, all the while making facial grimaces, using those large Martha Raye lips. Needless to say, if report lasted less than thirty minutes it was a miracle. But the show was priceless.

One of the pediatricians who had probably been middle-aged when Tommy began working in the nursery was feeble but still practicing. At one time, he had been the only pediatrician in St. Petersburg. Like Tommy, his babies were having babies or, perhaps, their babies were having babies.

One of his newborns developed a case of erythroblastosis fetalis (hemolytic disease of the newborn). Erythroblastosis occurs when an Rh-negative mother's antibodies attack the Rh-positive baby's red blood cells. With a profusion of dead red blood cells (bilirubin), the newborn's bilirubin levels become elevated and his skin appears jaundiced (yellow). High levels of bilirubin can cause brain damage. All babies experience mild jaundice on the days after delivery. That is normal. But the situation is compounded with erythroblastosis. Ultraviolet light can break down the bilirubin. But, alas, our nursery had no outside windows. Commercial Bili-lights, a cradle of fluorescent lights over a bassinette, were on the market but our maintenance department designed and built several less expensive versions. The infant was placed under the lights, naked except for eye patches. The bilirubin was monitored daily. If all went well, the baby was discharged with the mother who would be told to keep him undressed near a window. If the bilirubin was still high, the baby would remain in the nursery for monitoring.

In the case of a skyrocketing bilirubin, the last choice was something called an exchange transfusion. In an exchange transfusion, baby's blood is drained in small quantities, alternating with an infusion of his blood type without the Rh factor. All the baby's blood is not replaced but enough is exchanged to bring bilirubin levels down. This entire procedure might not even be performed now due to the development and wide-spread use of RhoGAM (see previous end note) in the late sixties. But at the time, I was aware of the exchange transfusion being performed several times.

When I assisted, the exchange was performed on this elderly pediatrician's baby. I took the baby to the delivery room, placing him under the bright light above the delivery table. There was a sterile tray of instruments which I opened beside the table. Both the doctor and I were dressed as though for surgery. There was a plastic trough in the shape of a baby with Velcro wrist and ankle restraints. This freed me to be able to assist. The bag of blood was hung. The doctor, shaking, cut down the umbilical cord and inserted the fine catheter. He proceeded to draw blood out, alternating with replacing it. I must have been monitoring the baby but all I remember is the doctor's shaking hands. The baby—miraculously survived. Not long after that, the doctor retired.

CPR was being introduced then. I was excited to attend an educational program about infant CPR. It entailed using an Ambu bag (large compressible bulb with oxygen mask) and fingertip chest compressions. Little did I know that, within a few weeks, I would use it.

It was evening. Earlier in the day, a premature infant had been delivered and was presently in an Isolette. His condition was poor. He weighed not quite two pounds. All Children's Hospital was new, up and running. But many of the obstetricians at that time did not believe in extraordinary measures for tiny babies. They feared that rescue would result in long term impairment. They took to heart the admonition, "Let nature be your teacher."[2] Nature did not make mistakes. So, it was "sink or swim" in our nursery for the preemies delivered by these docs. At the time, the pediatricians did not press the point. We saved many as small as two pounds but that was pushing it. It wasn't just the weight. What mattered was the preemie's ability to manufacture surfactant in the lungs to keep the alveoli from collapsing.

Throughout the first part of my shift, the infant's condition continued to deteriorate—duskier, gasping breaths. The pediatrician had not seen the baby but had promised to come in at dinnertime. I skipped dinner. Suddenly—no breaths. I whipped out the Ambu bag with the tiniest face mask we had. After a few puffs, it was clear that I could not get a good seal—his face was too small for the mask. My stethoscope found no heartbeat. I flipped open the Plexiglas hood, placed my lips around his nose and mouth and began to administer small puffs of air—the oxygen near me—and I began to compress his sternum rhythmically with two fingers.

Just then, Dr. Welty, a tall, lean, graying partner of Dr. Cole arrived. I kept going but prayed to God that, since the doctor had arrived, something not in my bag of tricks could be done. He approached the Isolette, asked me to stop, and examined the baby. It was no use. He seemed moved by the fact that I had attempted resuscitation and asked me to accompany him to the mother's room. When we arrived, the dad held her hand. Dr. Welty expressed his sorrow that the baby had been too immature to live. He said that this nurse (pointing to me) did everything she could to keep him alive—"even giving him breaths." Though they half-expected the result, the couple cried. I returned to the nursery.

Never did I offer them an opportunity to see their baby—a fact for which I am retrospectively sorry. If there was any comforting to do, the post-partum nurses did it. I returned to the nursery to bathe, wrap and identify my lost baby. I was numb. I could not believe that the woman who had not wanted to touch a dead baby a short time before had now performed mouth-to-mouth on one. My pride in having overcome my fear was surpassed only by my sorrow for that lost baby.

Post-Partum

So far, my experiences have been treated by section of the maternity unit. Actually, the experiences were integrated. Some days I worked Nursery, some days Post-Partum, and some days Labor and Delivery. It was especially nice if I could follow up with my labor patients on Post-Partum but that did not always happen. Besides, the post-partum patients, thanks to twilight sleep, usually did not remember their labor or they had snatches of grotesquely inaccurate memories.

Nursery and Post-Partum were my favorites. I enjoyed introducing new moms to their babies, helping them to feel confident about their care. Because visiting hours were short—afternoon and evening—without family or significant other, the women were all ours. Generally, they were not charity cases or unwed teens. They were usually white middle-class married women. If they had not necessarily planned their pregnancy or had mixed feelings, they were usually pleased—occasionally ambivalent—to be mothers. Most were just a few years older than I. Some had been my high school classmates. Night clothes from their packed suitcases looked more like fancy honeymoon attire—not always the best choice when dealing with the heavy post-partum lochia. Bedside flower bouquets were scattered with baby's breath flowers—pink carnations for girls, blue for boys. New moms were treated like queens by their families and by us for the miracle they had produced. We served soft drinks in a glass on a tray with a doily. We were, in turn, the recipients of box after box of candy upon their discharges. One of my colleagues who prided herself on shiny shoes, neat uniform and cap had the annoying habit of punching chocolates with her fingertip to discover the filling before choosing.

Teaching mothers was a marginal but enjoyable part of the job. Essential was the life and death issue of monitoring their fundus, episiotomy and lochia. That was the reason for their three-day stays (five if a C-section). We monitored for hemorrhage and infection of either their uterus or suture line—episiotomy or C-section. A bowel movement before discharge was mandatory. I called it being "paid up." They were ordered stool softeners and, if no defecation by day two, received a cathartic. Some episiotomies or tears extended to the rectum or were darn near it. That was behind the concern about stools. Enemas were contraindicated.

A check of the fundus, lochia and episiotomy was performed each shift or more often if there was a concern. The fundus is the top of the uterus. After delivery, it could be palpated at the level of the navel. The process of it shrinking to the level of the pubic bone is called involution. If the uterus didn't contract down on the huge blood vessels that once supplied the baby, there could be a serious post-partum hemorrhage. It was more likely to occur within the first forty-eight hours post-partum but, for one of our mothers, it occurred at home thanks to retained placental fragments. Massaging the fundus stimulated the uterus to contract. Primigravidas didn't mind the massage. Multigravidas found the stimulation painful—but their sluggish uteruses needed it most. Putting the baby to breast could have potentially accomplished the same.

Since most mothers did not breast feed at that time, managing breast engorgement between the second and third day post-partum, became an issue. The breasts would already have been producing colostrum, the "first milk"—yellow in color. For the newborn it contains many nutrients, confers immunity and acts as a laxative to help pass meconium. After delivery, maternal breasts became tight with massive blood supply and milk—painful rocks if action were not taken. Some doctors ordered a medication to prevent lactation which worked—so, so. Some did not and insisted that their patients be fitted with a breast binder. That time-honored form of torture was a cotton rectangular cloth sheet with straps. The sheet was tightly pulled over the breast by the nurse and pinned in place down the front with up to fifteen large safety pins (no Velcro® then). It totally flattened the breast—like the Flappers of the 1920s. It was not comfortable. One of the nurses creatively discovered a partial solution. Before pulling the binder tightly across the woman's chest, she cut an extra-long sanitary pad in half, placing half under each breast. Procedure completed, the woman had a supportive "uplift." The binder was so tight, it was a wonder she could breathe! It might seem sensible to the uninitiated to simply empty the breast by expressing the milk—but that only stimulates the production of more—in spades! Breast milk is governed by the law of supply and demand.

Lochia was inspected for amount, color and odor. Like amniotic fluid, the normal odor was salty, semen-like. Anything else could herald infection. The amount diminished each day and the color changed from sanguineous (bloody) to sero-sanguineous (lighter/thinner) to brownish. Fundus and lochia checks in relation to days post-partum gave a particularly accurate picture about involution and infection. Immediately after delivery, lochia was copious. More often than not, the first trip to the bathroom resulted in a bloody trail. Of course, the housekeepers did not clean the trail, the nurse did.

When the mother lay on her side, by slightly separating the buttocks, I could visualize the episiotomy. Unlike at Shands where med students and residents new to episiotomies did not always have a satisfactory result (it came apart), these obstetricians had beaucoup practice and I don't recall any problems—except with Dr. Nearsighted's patients.

Post-partum routine was standardized. On the day shift, after breakfast, the moms were led down to the sitz bath room as it became available. The tub was a shortened version of a white porcelain floor tub. The woman undressed and squatted down so that her feet and legs were outside the tub and her entire lower torso was inside it, covered with warm running water. Care had to be taken that the water was just the right temperature. There was a numbered dial, but we were encouraged to test it with an immersible thermometer. While the woman was "sitzing" to promote episiotomy healing, we returned to her room in pairs, made the bed and tidied-up. When the moms returned, their babies were carried out for feeding. The entire procedure was repeated in the evening. No one was qualified to clean the dirty sitz bath after each use—except the nurse or aid. It involved very rigorous scrubbing of all surface areas with Bon Ami, followed by a Vesphene soak and rinse. The concern was legitimate. If not cleaned properly, the shared tub would be an excellent mode of spreading puerperal fever to every mother on the floor. Cultures of the tub and of the newborn nursery were taken episodically to evaluate the success of our efforts.

Not surprisingly, an occasional woman experienced signs and symptoms of a urinary tract infection—burning with urination, frequency and fever. At Shands, the symptoms had been addressed with a urine culture and sensitivity (C&S) to identify the specific micro-organism and to discover the specific anti-biotics to which it was sensitive. Obtaining the specimen involved an elaborate prep of wiping and separating the vulva, discarding the first voided urine and then "clean" catching the rest. With a perineum exuding lochia at the speed of light, it was an awesome and often not very effective undertaking. At St. Anthony's, a culture was rarely ordered by the physician. Instead he would order a low level antibacterial (sulfa) which usually did the trick. It might have been an early version of cost containment. It might have been a practical solution by reality-based, seasoned obstetricians. After a while I stopped asking, "Do you want a culture?"

In the evenings, after visiting hours, the priest from Pastoral Care brought Communion to any Catholic in the hospital who wanted it. The priest was a Franciscan Friar wearing the iconic brown hooded-robe and sandals. Someone accompanied him, ringing a small dinner bell to alert people to the presence of the Blessed Sacrament. When she heard the bell, Tommy, sincerely devout, would drop to her knees in the nursery. One evening, something happened on post-partum which furnished humor for days. An RN and Dr. Saint were performing incision care on Post-Partum. The wire mesh dressing basket held suture removal kits and copious gauze dressings. When they left the room, the Saint took the lead followed by the RN carrying the dressing basket. At the familiar ring of the communion bell, the Saint abruptly and ostentatiously dropped to his knees. The unsuspecting, Protestant nurse continued, promptly tripping and falling over him—basket, sterile supplies and all. Neither was hurt. To an outsider, that might not seem very funny but to those who had suffered through the man's pompous piety, it was uproarious!

I mentioned the Head Nurse, Sister Mary Bede, at the beginning of this section. She had replaced a head nurse of more than twenty years. The woman's name practically evoked genuflection by her former staff. Later, Sister Mary Bede was transferred and was replaced by another Franciscan nun, Sister Rose Marie. But everyone knew the *REAL* (unofficial) Head Nurse—an LPN by the name of Mrs. Goodrich. Goodrich was sixty if not more, with a short, manly cut—white hair, tinted red. She had the appearance of a battleship, thick around the middle, Boston-accented cigarette voice, and no hesitancy to make her needs known. Her posture was excellent—head held high. Goodrich intimidated me. Her powerful and prestigious niche was ordering all unit supplies. She minutely reviewed each object with the supply room guys before accepting them. Those fellows must have dreaded her reviews. According to Goodrich, charting should follow a certain format and that format only. To her, higher education was for those with ideas of grandeur. She took pride in her bed making—particular, down to the placement of the sheet's hem. She wasn't shy about voicing her belief that modern young nurses clearly graduated clueless.

I discovered that she had attended a diploma nursing school in the 1930s but was required to drop out because she married. Chastity had been a requirement for nursing students then. Because of WWII, a nursing shortage developed as RN's joined the military. The concept of an LPN was born. <u>L</u>icensed <u>P</u>ractical <u>N</u>urses receive one year of training—usually through a vocational school. Goodrich became an LPN, working in a Massachusetts mental hospital. She was married with adult children. I had the impression that she ran the marital ship as well as ours. She was scary.

One afternoon, a post-partum patient was unable to urinate. We had an order to catheterize her as needed. I was Team Leader working with, among others, the unofficial Head Nurse. It had been a while since I had catheterized a patient and I was not yet accustomed to the pre-boxed packages that were used here unlike Shands' metal autoclaved tray. I asked Goodrich to do something else while I catheterized the woman. "Oh, I can do that for you, Newton," said

Goodrich. "No, I need to do it," said I. Sure enough, after preparing everything, while placing the Robinson straight catheter onto the sterile field, I contaminated it. (At least I recognized it.) I grabbed another. Undoubtedly the whole procedure took longer than it should have.

At the end of shift, Goodrich waited for me at the front desk. "Newton, I could have done that cath," she said with tears in her eyes. At that moment, I was able to see beyond my own feelings of inadequacy. I had wanted to do it as a grown-up nurse. I had wanted to hone my skills without necessarily advertising how inadequate I felt. Instead, Mrs. Goodrich worried that I doubted her ability. Once that sunk in, I was able to assure Mrs. Goodrich that, yes, I knew that she was much more adept at it than I. But I needed practice. Finally, I think she believed me. And, finally, I began to see that the bluster and braggadocio of the older nurses stemmed from their own insecurities. From that moment, I quietly transitioned from a youthful outsider isolated by my education to their colleague and friend.

Not long after that incident, a former Army nurse in her fifties was hired to work post-partum. She had a BSN (the third one of us in a four hundred plus bed hospital) and bragged repeatedly about it—unlike me. I did anything and everything to live it down. The eyes of diploma school nurses rolled at her braggadocio. One day she obtained a urine specimen from a patient for urinalysis. The container was a clear plastic cup with a rim which precariously supported a thin cardboard lid. The BSN genius placed the specimen in the Lamson tube and sent it to the lab via the Lamson Pneumatic Tube System. I would hate to have been the lab clerk who received that wet surprise! It didn't take long for the small but mighty Director of Nursing, Miss McCann, to charge up to the unit demanding to know who had performed that stunt. A few days later, that nurse was gone. As a very embarrassed member of the BSN minority, I realized, as I always had really, that higher education is no substitute for humility—or common sense.

Though eventually I could make a bed and clean a sitz with the best of them, another of my strengths emerged and was clear to fellow staff members before it was clear to me. I was able to therapeutically communicate with patients. I not only enjoyed it but related well with them. I could pick up on their knowledge deficits or emotional issues. Some team members preferred not to deal with it. Issues were repetitive to some degree—*why does my baby make that noise, have those pimples, wiggle and cry when he goes to nurse? How can I feed him, burp him, change him? How do I know when to pick him up?* Other issues were not—emotional reactions to infant loss or the loss of the baby they thought they would have. It was supposed to be a boy (or dad will desert us). It was supposed to be healthy. It was supposed to be a Gerber baby. I had an ability to listen *and* teach—to the extent that, when there was a problem, the staff directed me to the patient rather than involve themselves. At least they identified, rather than ignored the issue. In labor, a nurse-friend would say, "You go support the patient. If she needs an IV push, I'll give it." We both understood that IV pushes were my nemesis. Interpersonal relations were not her strength. We employed a fair distribution of work based upon skill sets.

How did I arrive at my skill? The obvious was having had the wonderful role model of Miss Hilliard. At first, all I did was mimic her. WWMHD? (<u>What</u> <u>Would</u> <u>Miss</u> <u>Hilliard</u> <u>Do</u>?) If I *hadn't* been sharpening needles and scrubbing floors in nursing school, I *had* been honing interpersonal skills—at least as they related to patients. But surprisingly, right under my nose on St. Anthony's maternity unit, there was an unwitting role model. He was the overweight physician responsible for half of our admissions. He was the Dr. Harley who had come in huffing and puffing for the prolapsed cord. His patients, like him, were often rotund. We guessed that he had a difficult time preaching against excessive weight gain considering his own obvious girth. Many of his patients were less affluent because his price for pregnancy and delivery was considerably less than his colleagues. The affordable price could have been because he was not a board-certified obstetrician but an anesthesiologist who still occasionally moonlighted giving anesthesia in surgery.

Relatively shy by nature, I quietly observed, noticing how this physician interacted, not just with his patients, but also with husbands and prospective grand-parents. On the face of it, this guy seemed very common but gradually I realized that he had a very sharp mind. He read people—as they say—like a book. From body language and spoken words, he divined who the person was, what she wanted and what was important to her. Like a chameleon, he became her comrade in arms, her best buddy who thought just like she did. Today he was liberal; tomorrow, with another person, he was conservative. His purpose was to manipulate his audience to accept whatever he had to say. It was as though he slipped into their skin, absorbed their core, slipped out and used what he had learned. In a lesser man, it would have been obvious, even tacky. But he was extremely clever. What he wanted to accomplish was usually related to their welfare or to complying with hospital policy. He morphed so easily that I wondered if he had any core beliefs of his own. (He was also the doctor who had offered to let me practice starting IV's on him—proving that he didn't mind pain by clamping his own forearm with an Allis clamp.)

Observing this man's successful interactions, I employed his methods on a small scale. Hospital policy denied family entry to L&D. To the prospective grand-mother becoming a pest at the post-partum desk, repeatedly asking about her laboring daughter, I remarked, "I know it is difficult for you not to be with her. I imagine you may be remembering your own labor. What was it like?" Often the answer was that it wasn't so bad or that she had been testy with folks around her. After reassuring that her daughter was fine, I would affirm that "You know what she is going through . . . a rite of passage for a woman . . . etc." I would acknowledge her need and her expertise while maintaining "the rules" which I was required to enforce. I manipulated but was not entirely proud of it.

One day, I was alerted to a post-partum mother of a stillborn who was crying. The staff asked me to talk with her. I wanted to do this as much as I had wanted to bathe and wrap that dead baby. What scared me? That I would be engulfed by unimaginable grief and pain? I don't know. But I was afraid. I steeled myself to go in, forming a plan to plant myself to avoid looking as though I would run away or engage in superficial conversation. I should appear open, leaning to-ward her, arms not crossed, accepting of whatever she had to say. The plan was hatched like lightening but still I was afraid. I sat there as she cried and talked, everything about me open and accepting and concerned. I hoped that she did not notice that my left hand—the one away from her—had slipped down to the back of my thigh. I pinched my thigh until it hurt—a distraction from the emotional pain which engulfed that room.

Post-Partum was rigidly heavy on rules. Because the desk was out there in front of the elevators and waiting room, post-partum nurses were "enforcers." They interpreted the rules to families keeping vigil for labor patients; families who wanted to go back to the nursery to see the newborns; pregnant women who wanted to tour the facility. Visiting hours were strict—no exceptions. I sometimes found myself enforcing the rules with an imperious attitude. Then, figuratively, I would turn around, slap myself, and ask, "Where did that come from?" *We* faced these patients and families every day. But every day it was the first time for *them*.

Why the need for exaggerated control? Anti-hospital reformers and idealists would have answered that rigidity was inherent in all hospitals. But why? In a society which believed nurses were physician handmaids, we carried most of the ball in what truly was a life or death game. Educationally, probably none of us were prepared to make the decisions which we were forced to make in place of physician. To face the nebulous challenges head-on every day, we needed constants, there had to be a steadying framework, a rudder to grasp. Though the rules were bathed in patient-safety rationale, they were as much for us as for them.

An innocuous *rule* was typified by the exchange between Sister Mary Bede and me one afternoon early in my employment. While I carried a lunch tray out of a patient room, Sister Bede appeared at the nurse's station. She asked, "Mrs. New´-ton, where is your dignity?" "Pardon me, Sister?" I asked, thinking that I had misunderstood. "Where is your dignity?" Puzzled and unthinking, I shot back earnestly, "Sister, I have no dignity." Chuckling, she replied, "No, your cap. Where is your cap?" I had forgotten it at home. "Bring it tomorrow," she smilingly reprimanded. So, my cap, my hierarchical symbol, was my dignity. I didn't tell her that the day before, in full battle regalia, I had answered a patient's call light and asked if I could help. "A bedpan," she had said. When I moved to oblige, she responded, "Oh no. You're the dietitian." My balloon deflated, her response had made the impressiveness of my *dignity* dubious.

A quaint example of *the rules* is one at which both Sadie and I would smile today. I was working in L&D and Sadie, for some ridiculous reason, was on Post-Partum. Sadie was an excellent L&D nurse and my strength was post-partum. Things were slow in labor when Sadie arrived in a dither and, with her beautiful Kentucky accent, complained, "Newton, I have to give an injection to this patient and the husband won't leave the room. Will you handle it?" Holding the labeled syringe, she was obviously frustrated. I said, "Sure." While Sadie monitored my patient, I entered the semi-private room where husband was at bedside. I drew the curtain between roommates, slightly pushed back the covers to reveal a bit of the patient's buttock and administered the injection—all the while talking with patient and spouse. If he had impregnated her, he had seen her before.

Sadie was satisfied that the injection had been given and charted. But why had she demurred? Aware of Sadie's Kentucky origins, I smiled to myself thinking that it had been the sensibilities of a good Southern woman—like putting mint in your julep. Beyond regional color, this was how nurses had been taught for years throughout the United States. Following maxims without thought had been responsible for many problems in nursing. *To protect the privacy of the individual, one must expel her significant other?* It was a black and white world view, not shades of grey, closed to alternatives. Sadie had been victimized by this school of thought as much as had her patient. But change was just around the corner.

Changing Times

Have I mentioned that it was the late 1960s? Twiggy was in, skirts were up and the TV show *Laugh In* was hot. In 1968, Martin Luther King and Robert Kennedy assassinations left the country in shock. Man first set foot on the moon. Post WWII baby boomers were adults. The Viet Nam War and the draft escalated with the 1968 Tet Offensive. Clean cut young men, going off to war in gung ho John Wayne, *True Grit* style, returned (or did not) disillusioned, greasy-haired, mustachioed hippies marching in Viet Nam Veterans Against the War (VVAW) protests. Many of us believed that the older generation had sent the younger generation off to fight, be wounded, maimed, or die for a questionable cause in which they had no stake. It shook baby boomers' confidence in authority. We stopped placing blind faith in THE ESTABLISHMENT.

In 1969, close to half a million hippies converged in Woodstock, New York for a four-day festival of sex, drugs and rock and roll. *Hair*, the rock opera, became the anthem of youth. Black Panthers mirrored racial discontent. Unlike the fifties, sixties' demonstrations were not always peaceful. *Don't trust anyone over thirty* was the mantra. *Pig* meant cop. Bob Dylan sang, "*The times they are a changin'.*" And they were . . .

My conservative, Catholic, straight-laced hospital was changing, too, due, not in small part, to the infusion of young nurses. While I became seasoned, I remained the only nurse on OB with a bachelor's degree. But I had been joined by other young two and three-year grads.

In the community, among the ranks of new and prospective mothers, there was a movement afoot which eventually changed the delivery of maternal–infant care. Locally it began with a chapter of the International Childbirth Association (ICEA). The ICEA championed the "natural childbirth" methods of Dr. Grantly Dick-Read,[3] a British obstetrician who wrote *Childbirth Without Fear* and lectured in the U.S. during the 1950s. He believed that education to combat fear of the unknown combined with relaxation using deep-breathing would foster an easier and quicker childbirth without medication. At almost the same time, Ferdinand Lamaze,[4] a French obstetrician, used Pavlovian conditioning to prep the mother to react to contractions in a specific way. The result was the same if not better. The Lamaze method in this country was popularized by Elizabeth Bing, a physical therapist.

A commendable goal for both methods was to avoid the possible adverse physical effects of twilight sleep and anesthetics on the baby. I've mentioned how **very** much narcotic (Demerol) was typically administered during labor and how sluggish the babies were for hours afterward. Another goal of natural childbirth was to provide a positive birthing experience and to speed maternal infant bonding. The down side of these developing movements: they tended to set the gold standard for success as taking *no medications at all*. If the mom failed at this, was she not beginning the relationship as a failure—arguably much worse than delayed bonding?

I attended a local ICEA meeting at the behest of a mother who read me as quasi-sympathetic. Discussions centered on how natural childbirth and breast feeding were thwarted at every turn by uncaring hospital staff (not just at our hospital). These were lay people. They were zealots. At the time, I thought they oversimplified, envisioning evil behind every health care professional. It *did* open my eyes to how we could appear to the uneducated public. Their premise was that, if medical people stepped out of childbirth, everything would be fine. At this point in my story, the fallacy of that argument should be clear. In the hospital, we used the medical model of ruling out pathology—not to stymie their childbearing experience but to save their lives and the lives of their babies, I thought.

If my reaction to the zealots was mixed, the effect that any mention of natural childbirth had on the obstetricians was apoplexy. One was a man not previously mentioned whom I will call Charleroi. He was a father of many, on the cusp of retirement. When it was his turn to take weekend call, he admitted multiple women on Saturday for induction. If he had to be on weekend call, then he might as well be busy. Our method was not the well-regulated IV induction via Pitocin. Our patients generally did not have an IV line. IV analgesics were administered directly into the vein by needle. Instead, to induce labor, Buccal Pitocin was administered. They were like little Chiclets™ placed in the buccal space between the gum above the molars and the lip. They dissolved there and liberated the oxytocic to contract the uterus. Each half-hour we added more Chiclets™ until significant labor began. Once the fetal membranes bulged from a dilating cervix, the obstetrician vaginally inserted what looked like a long plastic crochet hook and painlessly snagged the fetal membranes, "breaking the water." Then the head descended, becoming a better dilating wedge. But rupturing membranes was only performed when the head was engaged in the pelvis, preventing prolapsed cord.

Back to the obstetrician, Charleroi. Once his multiple patients were in labor and had been administered twilight sleep, he sat at the small nurse-station in the labor area chewing the fat with the nurses. While we entertained him, his patients were not being helped. This father of many floored me one day during a delivery when, speaking of natural childbirth, he pronounced: "If a father saw his baby being born he would never want to have sex with his wife again." My jaw dropped behind my mask as I bit back the caustic comment: *Sure hasn't stopped you!*

Another doctor persisted in calling the La Leche League, the support group for breast feeding mothers, the La Leaky League, poking fun at mothers whose bras needed pads to absorb the occasional premature milk let-down. Still another obstetrician commented that, if dads were allowed in labor, there would be another epidemic of puerperal fever. As though dads were contaminated, and obstetricians were not! It was the obstetricians who went from examining one woman to another.

The issue, at base, was control. Perhaps sensing the winds of change, they feared that, awake and aware, women would realize how little the obstetrician was present. If husbands—we thought in terms of husbands, not significant other, or mother, or older children—were in the room, they would also see and hear—not just the wife but staff and obstetrician. Just maybe the birth process would revolve around the needs of the mother rather than the obstetrician. Times were changing. The tide was turning.

I suspect that, when I was hired, Sister Mary Bede already had been charged with making changes. Change might also have been a natural outcome of the changing face of the maternity staff. Change evolved.

The Red Cross had always sponsored prenatal classes on a quarterly basis at St. Anthony's with a handful of prospective parents in attendance. Classes were taught by a Red Cross RN volunteer. The childbirth course was a canned one with guidelines undoubtedly set up nationally by the Red Cross. Eager to observe what our prospective patients were taught, two of the younger nurses and I audited it. We were dismayed. The most memorable part was a recording of different baby cries ostensibly because of hunger or a wet diaper—as though parents' anticipated child's cry would sound identical. Participants practiced bathing a very stiff baby doll—a parody of what bathing a living, breathing, wriggling infant would entail. Reporting back to Sister Mary Bede, we questioned, "What about the concerns that we see new parents have which are going unanswered in the class?" "What is normal for a new baby and what is not?" What happens to the mothers' body during labor and delivery and what is recovery like afterward?" Working with mothers every day, we were attuned to the parents' concerns in a way that the elderly Red Cross nurse-instructor was not.

I don't know how Sister graciously—because Sister Bede was always gracious—removed this lady from the classes. However she accomplished it, she encouraged the three of us to develop our own series of five classes based on what the expectant parents wanted to know. We engaged obstetricians and pediatricians to speak to some topics and covered the rest ourselves. I am sure a great part of our success was the delicious cookies furnished by our now deceased but long remembered cook, Mrs. Pryor. Initially the class was free, with just a handful of participants but, over time, attendance mushroomed to close to one hundred. We charged a small amount, believing that by charging we implied that it was worth something. I am certain the hospital never made money on the classes, but they were a source of terrific community PR. It brought people in. The obstetricians and pediatricians considered this their moment to shine and to garner a little free publicity in an era when it was unseemly and unethical for physicians to advertise. The classes gave us a leg up on trust when the actual day of admission arrived.

Wiedenbach's *Family-Centered Maternity Nursing*,[5] one of the texts which I had used at UF, provided a conceptual framework through which the *family* was considered the unit of care—not just the mother or just the baby—but the family. Rooming-in was one element of the family-centered approach. Rooming-in allowed the mother to keep the baby at bedside for as much as she was able, to change the diapers, to wash, to take the temperature, to feed—all under the nurse's watchful guidance. With rooming-in, the goal was to do everything possible to make the mom an expert, rather than to snicker at her ineptitude behind closed nursery doors. Post-partum and nursery nurses shared responsibility for teaching. Fathers were included as much as possible and visiting hours did not exist for them. They could come any time.

The second element of a family-centered approach was allowing fathers or, in their absence, a supportive other to be present not just in the labor room but also in delivery.

Shortly before my tenure at St. Anthony's ended, rooming-in was introduced making St. Anthony's the first in Pinellas County. First it was rooming in; later dads in labor; and, much later, dads in delivery. Imagine the enormous pressure this evoked from disgruntled physicians. We depended on them for our business!

It was an enormous cultural challenge for all of us. Yet it was accomplished.

Before Sister Bede was transferred to another assignment, she bequeathed us a small treasure from her native Jamaica (I like to think) or maybe England. It was dubbed the Mother-Craft Room. It was a large former nursery on the south wing where we kept our teaching models, diagrams, baby dolls, and, yes, knitted uterus. My mother-in-law, Leola Newton, knit a fire engine red uterus from instructions I found in a publication. It had a long, thick cervix which could dilate and efface. I made a primitive-looking fetus doll with placenta and cord. In the afternoon before public visiting hours, we brought new moms to Mother-Craft. Using a real baby, we demonstrated bath and cord care and entertained discussion.

A little more than two years after I had begun to work at St. Anthony's, I resigned. My husband had completed his preliminary work at the junior college and had been accepted into the College of Engineering in Gainesville. Had it not been for that, I would have been content to spend the rest of my life at St. Anthony's. I was not the same person I had been when I started. I had a wealth of experience and did not think twice about performing a myriad of procedures that I had felt "iffy" about. I had my own war stories. I felt sincere affection for the people with whom I had worked. There were positive changes, of which I had been a part. Change had led to better and more patient/family-centered care. I had earned the respect of my colleagues. I was still learning but had come a long way.

My evolution had occurred partially because of the security of being in a very content and happy marriage. I felt grounded at home. No worries. We would move to Gainesville where Danny would begin school and I would continue to support us until he graduated and worked in his own profession. Then kids, even if it meant twilight sleep (ugh!).

Back at Shands

My old OB-GYN unit at Shands had changed little. We still wore caps and, thankfully, still addressed each other by our first names. With my experience, I was hired by Jen Wilson, the College of Nursing Maternity Section Chairman, to be Nurse II of Post-Partum / Nursery—a step up from my previous Nurse I position. In the Nurse II position, I would have twenty-four/seven responsibility for my unit. My counterpart was Maria Rooney, Nurse II of GYN. The Nurse III, Harriet Daniels, was present only briefly before she began graduate school. Then Maria and I were left to fill her shoes—which we could not.

I previously mentioned that there was no Director of Nursing, no centralized staffing—so we were it. Unfortunately, this meant that, with three shifts to staff around the clock, staffing was a huge part of our job. Without a centralized hospital staffing pool, it was a big issue because we were forced to replace people who had called in sick with our own staff's overtime. Use them too much, and *they* got sick. Some counted on overtime and wanted more. But the folks who worked more than their forty hours were likely to have poor performance or to be found quietly nodding off in a nook or cranny of the unit. Maria and I, if we could not find someone, were duty-bound to work an extra shift for the missing person. Part of the job was being called twenty-four/seven for a staffing problem, a death, a need to transfer patients. It seemed no one could think for herself. Maybe I or someone before me made them afraid to. On-call meant being close to a land line. There were no cell phones. A large unit beeper was used on rare occasions when we were not close to a phone—like when attending a football game.

I was never cut out to be a manager. This job made me realize it. The staff was never happy. I never created a schedule everyone accepted. To "take control" I rearranged everything in the newborn nursery—I am sure much to Bessie's consternation. Yes, Bessie who had called us Frick and Frack still worked there. Bessie was a kind person who took it well. But later I recognized that my approach was like a dog peeing on a lamp post to claim it as his own. Later in my career, I watched new managers do the same thing. I should have asked Bessie and her associates how *they* would like to order *their* nursery.

Harriet Daniels, the short-tenured (in my time) Nurse III was an African American Floridian who had earned her bachelor's degree in nursing from Florida A&M, an African American institution. She was all spit and polish with sparkling white, modest uniforms, a traditional cap and shiny white shoes. She was very much a traditionalist. She suffered no fools and was not one herself. She arrived early in the morning before change of shift to assure that the night shift chores had been completed—emptying trash, laundry, cleaning the utility room, etc. If they had not, she would figuratively nab the person responsible and set her to task. She knew her staff—transient white new-grad nurses, permanent and predominantly black LPN's and aids. To all her staff, she communicated that she had her hand on the pulse of the unit and that things had *better* go as they should. Most white people, particularly at that time, could never hope to emulate her approach which was, indeed, effective. Certainly not this wimpy white woman!

Harriet recounted a night when an aid had called in sick for her shift. Harriet, suspicious and aware of the aid's location, took it upon herself to make a "sick call." When she arrived, the woman was on her hands and knees scrubbing the floor. "If you're well enough to scrub the floor, you're well enough to man your shift. Now let's go!" she had said. The aid worked her shift. Everyone knew not to mess with Miss Harriet. At St. Anthony's, the nuns had left notes. Here, Harriet was confrontational.

In Harriet's absence, Maria and I could not possibly approach her style of management. It showed. Maria was much better at it than I. She graduated from UF after I did, and her only work experience was on that unit. Her area was GYN, but she was pregnant—so the other parts of the unit were also of personal interest. Maria was a trooper. We lived in the same mobile home park. Her husband was enrolled in UF College of Law and she was their support. Maria had very prominent scoliosis. As her pregnancy progressed, the lordosis of pregnancy put a significant strain on her back which looked like a question mark. It made working in late pregnancy difficult. But she did it!

Maria and I often rode together to work, discussing issues of the day. In 1970, *Roe v. Wade* was filed in Texas. It would be reviewed by the Supreme Court in 1973. Maria was progressive about abortion, believing it a woman's right. I, with my Catholic background, believed it was murder. Both of us were aware of the history of criminal backstreet abortions and their ultimate loss of life—not just of baby but sometimes of mother. We also knew that most of the criminal abortions were chosen by married women—not promiscuous teens as abortion foes claimed.

The times were revolutionary—particularly in and around the college. Hare Krishnas dressed in robes, chanting and walking the streets of Gainesville and the University. There was an honest-to-goodness counter-culture hippie commune in Micanopy, a rural community just south of Gainesville. There, pregnant women cavalierly delivered at home. Placentas were consumed or planted under a sapling. No thought was given to potential complications of delivering without medical personnel. One baby delivered there was brought to our nursery with severe jaundice. The possibilities of any complications had never crossed the parents' consciousness.

Early in my tenure as Nurse II, I was asked to report to the floor's examining room where I found a graduate student's sari-clad Indian wife. The woman was an out-patient. I was asked to help her undress and get up in stirrups in lithotomy position (on her back, with legs mechanically separated by two "stirrups"). When the doctor returned, he held a large syringe with which he proceeded to artificially inseminate her. He tilted the table head down into Trendelenburg position, directing me to stay with her like this for ten minutes then let her re-dress and leave. I was amazed by what had taken place. It was my first encounter with infertility problems and artificial insemination. Later, the resident confided that an anonymous donor's sperm were mixed with the husband's semen so that there would be a very slim chance that the paternity would be his.

One morning I arrived on the unit to find a twelve-year-old girl. That wasn't surprising. How many times had I seen children that age admitted with PID (pelvic inflammatory disease—gonorrhea) or a pregnancy? This one was different—a nulligravida (never pregnant), very childlike, behaving younger than her years. She had been admitted the evening before with acute abdominal pain. Unaware, she had been having menstrual periods for some time. The problem was that she had not just an intact hymen but a thick, fibrous membrane totally occluding her vagina. Uterine lining, shed monthly, had built-up and backed-up into her peritoneum, creating acute pain. The evening before, the residents and their professor had taken her to the operating room to surgically incise the membrane, allowing for flow of debris. Her vagina had required vaginoplasty. It had been packed with gauze while the girl was still under anesthesia. Now the resident directed me to be his chaperone while he removed the packing and introduced what looked like the plastic barrel of a syringe to keep the vagina open.

The resident's heart was in the right place. He was disturbed by what had happened to the girl. But clearly his professors had not provided the psycho-social background or guidance that he needed in this situation. By nature, he was what southerners might call a pushy New Yorker. He had short man syndrome (like Dr. Saint in St. Petersburg) with a short, stocky build and short, jerky movements. He tried to be gentle, but children are sensitive to underlying tone.

Once again, not directly involved with the patient, I knew nothing about her but was literally grabbed to be a chaperone. To avoid accusations of molestation or rape, the nurse is traditionally present when a male doctor performs any form of physical exam, particularly a vaginal exam. Interestingly, the reverse is not true.

Both parents had been with the child, but the mom had left for breakfast in the cafeteria. Dad was on the girl's left near the head of the bed. The resident explained his plan. He sat on the bed to the girl's right at thigh level. When he began to remove the packing, the child wiggled, kicked and screamed. The dad was forced to restrain his daughter's upper extremities while I held her knees. The doctor was in kicking range. When he inserted the plastic syringe-sized tube, the girl went ballistic! I was not prepared to deal with this. The child didn't relate to me, a stranger, but to her father. I was struck with the image of this innocent pre-pubescent child—unaware of the intricacies of what it meant to be a woman, to be a sexual being, to share her mysterious changes with other women, to share herself with her first lover. Now, her first experience with having her period, with vaginal intrusion was a grizzled man with a New York accent while her father (another man) restrained her. The experience would probably haunt her for the rest of her life, impacting her every sexual relationship. Retrospectively, her mother, not her father, should have been present. Had the resident given me fair warning rather than grabbing me as he would have grabbed a utensil, I could have had an opportunity to know the girl better and to possibly explain, in her terms, what would happen.

A Birth and Added Responsibility

When Maria delivered her baby, Brian, at Shands, she used the Lamaze method that she and her husband had practiced. Some of her early labor was spent in our kitchen playing cards. Brian was born with a huge crop of black lanugo, downy hair often present in newborns. It later yielded to blonde hair. While Maria was on maternity leave, I covered all three areas (Post-Partum, Nursery & GYN), working to fill-in when staff called in sick. I made no sick calls like Harriet. Involving myself with GYN, I was struck by some of its horrors. This was not your small community hospital GYN unit filled with mid-life hysterectomies. People were sent to Shands from all over the state as a last-ditch effort to salvage a situation beyond most doctors' abilities. Usually the problem was cancer—ovarian, uterine, cervical or vulvar. I was not conversant in the jargon of staging and grading then. But I knew that the women we treated had extensive disease.

The OB-GYN residents, guided by faculty, performed radical surgery the likes of which I have not seen since. I have mentioned exenterations (removal of bowel, uterus, ovaries, tubes and bladder). Frequently the women became massively infected and were placed in isolation. Care was given—gowned, gloved and masked. The exudates smelled like cheese going sour. On one occasion, I packed an abdominal wound. The woman's knees were bent and slightly spread. I realized that I could look into her abdomen and out through her pelvis to the bed between her legs. She was not much more than a skeleton. One of the women in her mid-thirties was a former prostitute. Cervical cancer risk is higher in women with multiple sexual partners. Miraculously she survived drastic surgery, was discharged home only to return later to have her vagina reconstructed (so she could ply her trade?).

Several women had vulvectomies—the removal of inner and sometimes outer labia (genital folds) due to cancer. The incision could extend up to the pubic bone. These incisions often became infected with open gaping wounds. The immobility which followed predisposed DVT's (blood clots) to form in their legs. Some traveled to their lungs, forming a life-threatening PE (pulmonary embolus). Every morning on rounds, the OB-GYN's had the med students calculating the fluid and electrolyte needs of obviously failing patients. One day I asked Tony, one of the residents, why they prolonged the agony for these women. What was the point of maintaining their fluid and electrolyte balance when the hope for cure or even relief was nil? It bothered him, too, but the students and residents were learning skills that would be valuable to them later in their careers when they would use them to help patients who *could* be saved.

At the time, Shands was a state-run hospital dependent upon the legislature for funding. By the end of the budget year, items were in short supply. With so many students, faculty, residents and staff traversing the department daily, things tended to disappear. When water pitchers vanished, we used emesis (kidney shaped) basins to provide bedside ice water. Tiny German roaches crawled all over everything, including bedside tables. A dead mouse/rat was found inside the premature nursery closet (Not my nursery—one run by the pediatric department). Theoretically, the Unit Manager dealt with the problems. They were hospital-wide problems with seven different Unit Managers and seven different Nurse III's applying band-aids separately. Someone way above my pay level must have recognized the value of centralization. The position of Director of Nursing was created. *HE* was Julian Cicatello. As a manager, I had little time to reap the benefit of his arrival.

So far in my nursing life, I had become seasoned as a professional at St. Anthony's. Skills were polished; confidence gained. Employment as a Nurse II at Shands was an opportunity to discover how ill-suited I was for management. Just as in adolescence, I was unconscious of the forces shaping me and was only peripherally aware of the societal forces continuing to mold me. The Viet Nam War with its erosion of confidence in authority, the hippie movement, women's liberation, and the movement for racial equality—all extrinsic—subliminally formed the nurse whom I was becoming.

Endnotes

1. **Rh⁻** mothers lack the Rhesus factor as part of their blood type. Pregnancy with an **Rh⁺** baby leads to co-mingling of maternal and infant blood. Lacking the factor, she develops Rh antibodies. Each subsequent pregnancy with an **Rh⁺** baby creates a stronger immune response resulting in the fetus' or infant's grave illness (erythroblastosis fetalis / hydrops fetalis) or death. RhoGAM, given after delivery, prevents that problem with subsequent pregnancies. RhoGAM was new and very expensive.

2. William Wordsworth, "The Tables Turned," *Lyrical Ballads* (London: J. & A. Arch, 1798).

3. Grantly Dick-Read, *Childbirth Without Fear* (New York: Harper, 1943).

4. Marjorie Karmel, *Thank You Dr. Lamaze* (University of Michigan: Lippincott, 1959).

5. Ernestine Wiedenbach, *Family Centered Maternity Nursing* (New York: Putnam, 1958).

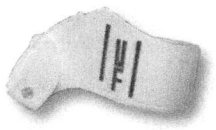

CHAPTER FOUR
Life Altering Change: 1972-1976

Death

A little more than a year after our arrival in Gainesville, my husband, Danny, was diagnosed with glioblastoma multiforme, an incurable brain cancer. He lived three months after surgery. Danny's illness and death profoundly impacted me and my subsequent nursing career choices. Our experience was personal. The belief that, in marriage, two become one had been the truth for us. His illness was my illness. His death was mine.

Shock or numbness cannot begin to describe the feeling of being run over by a Mack truck. I walked, talked, and functioned as a nurse (poorly)—but I was in no way present to the moment. During his illness, I had dealt with his medical symptoms as they arose—nausea, impaction, incontinence, double vision, aphasia. I dealt with them in a constant state of surprise, seeking advice from my sister-in-law. Though a nurse, I knew nothing of Med-Surg or neurology. This was my husband! His death when we were home alone together was unbearable. I found myself clawing at the air trying to pull his spirit back into his body. The solace was that, with his surgeon's blessing, he had not experienced the agony of a death with med students balancing his electrolytes and keeping him alive forever at Shands.

My grief became one of my most valuable life lessons, understood only in retrospect. With a month's Leave of Absence (LOA) I found myself re-ordering my life, cleaning and reordering the kitchen cabinets—making them mine. I constantly struggled between wanting to keep things the same versus making them work in my new life. Despite very supportive staff—Bessie had given me a small bell to put at Danny's bedside so he could call me, brother and sister-in-law, and friends, I was, at core, alone with my grief. Maybe more so in a youthful college environment where death of peers was an anomaly and few people had experience with death or bereavement. I grieved for the husband whom I had adored and who was my heart and soul; for myself and for a life that would never be; for the children we wanted but would never have; for the guy who made me feel protected and safe; for the man who understood "men things": cars, plumbing, carpentry; for the total emptiness of being alone. I considered ramming my car into the I-75 overpass concrete supports on Archer Road. What stopped me? Who would take care of our dog and cat?—Simultaneously enough and pathetic!

Returning to work, I was in another world. I requested and was given a step-down to team leader without a salary change thanks to Jen Wilson. That was good. Had it not been for that and his life insurance, I would never have been able to pay off Danny's bill for a week in the hospital for brain surgery. I dealt with patients' questions innocently asked. *Do you have a baby? What does your husband want?* Each was a knife through my heart.

It was a period of merely working—not with enthusiasm—just working. My friend, Maria, planned to leave in the spring to study for her master's degree in nursing. She asked if I wanted to go to grad school with her. Fortunately, we had been required to take the Graduate Record Exam (GRE) before graduation. That prerequisite was not an issue. Honestly, I absolutely did not care what I did—so, why not? It really didn't matter. We both applied for federal nurse-traineeships and qualified. Traineeships were scholarships designed to underwrite providing the workforce with more nurses with graduate degrees. Masters-prepared nurses were needed in nursing education as more programs opened. They were also needed as nurse-specialists and managers in hospitals. Aware that management was simply not my cup of tea, I chose the nursing educator track.

Grad School—A Welcome and Needed Retreat

Thanks to the traineeship, I did not work. All my attention went into that year of classes and clinical experience. Jen Wilson was our primary professor—a truly lovely lady. Miss Hilliard was now an adjunct professor working toward her PhD. She would later initiate and direct UF's graduate level nurse mid-wifery program. Still, we were lucky to have her as an instructor for several classes. I took some educational psychology courses and a course about the Junior College. Both nursing professors invited us to their homes for classes or just to chat. They were open, loving and giving—great role models. Our mothers in nursing!

Our Maternity section was small and several of our fellow students came straight from their bachelors' programs. They lacked the experience that Maria and I brought to class. As the television character Monk would say, it was a blessing and a curse. It was a blessing because we could add a touch of realism. It was a curse because our experiences were not always the best example of how things should be.

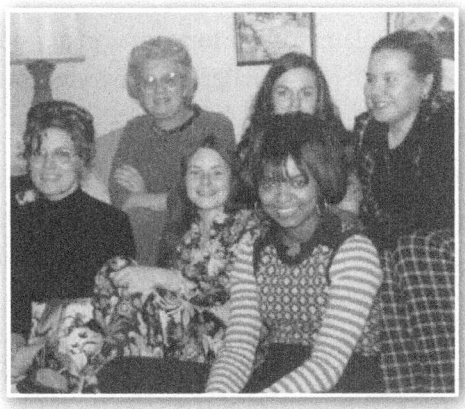

Figure 10 *Our Maternal infant Graduate Students Meet at Miss Wilson's Home. Miss Wilson, our professor, is back left. My friend, Maria Rooney, is in front of her. Anne and Lynne are to Miss Wilson's left. Tanya and Bernadine are to Maria's left. From the outfits, clearly, this was the "Age of Aquarius."*

A major thrust at the College of Nursing at that time was the Nursing History. I have hinted at the divide between actual nursing and the so-called "ivory tower." For close to a century, nurses had essentially followed physicians' orders without particularly problem solving—not much different from being a short-order cook! If that were all that nurses were or did, it would hardly justify a nursing program in an institution of higher learning. Incorporating components of physiology, sociology and psychology contributed to academic legitimacy. But a systematic, science-based approach to nursing would further legitimize it as an academic pursuit. Nursing educators borrowed from their allied discipline—Medicine. Doctors assessed, diagnosed and then wrote orders. Eventually, their "science" morphed into SOAP (Subjective, Objective, Analysis, Plan) charting. SOAP allowed all health team members reading the chart to understand the patient's problem and progress, and the doctor's direction. Older physicians might not have SOAP-ed, but medical students had used the method for a few years.

Nursing began to parallel the medical model. At about this time, not only were nursing histories (like medical history but unique to nursing) implemented but a very convoluted method of making nursing diagnoses was devised.

As an undergraduate, l had used the Nursing Care Plan to identify a problem and write approaches. For example:

Potential Post-Operative Infection: Monitor for signs and symptoms: Fever, purulent exudate, erythema.

A care plan worked for a practicing nurse. It was simple and forthright. Even then, I silently wondered if anyone would read them. Hospital nursing was not a sit down to read job. It was constant motion and making decisions on the fly.

In graduate school, the push was for nursing histories—ok. But nursing diagnosis was evolving into statements like: *Alteration in fluid and electrolyte balance due to polyhydramnios.* Then there would be the behavioral objectives: *Upon completion of her labor and delivery the patient will . . . .* Frankly, I never warmed up to either the diagnoses or to the behavioral objectives. They hogtied the nurse while expecting her to function. It was a pedantic exercise. To my thinking, if used at all, it should be as an instructive method for students. For those in practice, the peculiar jargon created interdisciplinary chuckles. It was helpful to no one. If the physician's process were as convoluted, the patient would die before his first order was written! My practical realism collided with popular academic thinking. But, having been through the wringer of loss, the nursing history and diagnosis were the least of my problems.

We concentrated on small aspects of care, and completed studies, following mother-baby units in their homes as well as in the hospital. Later in the year, I taught a lecture to the undergraduate students as part of the educator track. I remember my first lecture to an amphitheater-sized room. All nerves, my knees trembled out of sight, standing behind a solid bar-like table. Extremely nearsighted, I opted *not* to wear my glasses. The student group blurred like an impressionist painting, making the situation less scary. Don't ask me the topic of my great erudition. Suffice it to say I survived.

I mentored some undergrads, accompanying them for their clinical experiences, coaching when needed. At this point, the bachelor's students regarded me as a fellow student and were less guarded in their discussions than with the *REAL* instructors. One junior nursing student felt torn between being a nurse or becoming a zookeeper. Her passion was snakes. Nursing v. snakes seemed an oxymoron. I encouraged her, in a non-judgmental way, to follow her passion.

My most valuable non-nursing course was taught by Dr. William Purkey, a perceptual psychologist in Educational Foundations. He was a magnetic speaker, rooted in the belief that people (students/patients) view the world through personal and cultural filters. Their behavior is based upon their perceptions. What seems illogical to one person makes sense to another. "How do we know that this is not a classroom but a jail cell?" he would loudly demand, challenging our perceptions. What made us think it was a classroom? No bars on the windows, a blackboard, etc., we would answer. His point was to challenge our own perceptions to be able to enter another's perceptual field. That was the only way to issue positive invitations to change, to grow. Another of his famous quotes was: "There are no free lunches. You pay for everything you get. If you choose to go left, you cannot go right. If you choose to go right, you cannot go left." A modern Robert Frost,[1] he believed that to every action there are consequences—both desired and undesired. Beware the undesired consequences!

Grad school was a retreat of sorts. It was a blessing to me at a point when I needed to ponder and reorder my world gone topsy-turvy. It was an opportunity to read extensively and to research the literature about topics of interest.

While studying, I was struck by the masculine imprint imposed upon women by male obstetricians. For example, the Greek root word for uterus is *hyster*— also for hysterics. The *mons veneris* literally means *mountain of Venus*. Excellent *Playboy* fodder! I imagined the snickers. Female body parts were named after the men who had discovered them. For example, Dr. Montgomery described the small pimple-like crinkles around the nipple (*Montgomery's* tubercles) as "a host of miniature nipples scattered over a milky way." The *Fallopian tubes* were named after Gabrielis *Fallopius* who described them. The *Graafian follicles* of the ovary were named after the Dutch scientist, Reinier *De Graff*. Men were like ancient moon walkers, naming female topography after themselves! When a woman miscarried, the cause could be an incompetent cervix—at a time when *incompetent* is the last thing a woman needs to hear about herself. Freidan's *Feminine Mystique*[2] was popular at the time. The subtle emergence of feminism was felt even by those of us who eschewed "bra burning radicals."

Simultaneously I discovered what life as a widow meant. If I wanted to hang a picture, I had to hang it. If a drain needed cleared, I had to clear it or call a plumber. If a bill needed paid, I had to pay it. These were all tasks that tradition and our marriage had dictated Danny would do. Man things. No different from all the widows and single women before me, I was learning to do it all. Rather than feel sorry for myself—I had done plenty of that—I bucked myself up singing the latest hit by Helen Reddy in my discordant voice. Why not? Who would hear?

I Am Woman
. . . Oh yes, I am wise
But its wisdom born of pain.
Yes, I've paid the price
But look how much I gained.
If I have to, I can do anything.
I am strong.
I am invincible. I am woman. [3]

The more I sang it, perhaps the more convinced I would become.

Part of grad school involved studying the Lamaze approach to childbirth in addition to family-centered maternity nursing. Shands already permitted the husband or significant other to be present for labor and delivery. Modified rooming in was offered. But Shands' clientele were primarily poor coming from the outlying rural areas. With a few exceptions, middle-class town folk and some professors' wives delivered in the city hospital called Alachua General Hospital (AGH). It offered more privacy and less confusion than Shands. Until a few years before, AGH had provided segregated maternity care—blacks treated in a basement unit while whites received care upstairs.

Alachua General was the St. Anthony's of Gainesville—at least the St. Anthony's which I had first encountered. AGH was a city hospital run by a Board of Directors who did what they could to satisfy the obstetricians who brought them business. The obstetricians still lived in the dark ages—at least I thought so.

Having converted to the *religion* of prepared childbirth and family-centered nursing, as militant as a reformed smoker, I was easy pickings for a group of zealots aimed at marching dads into labor and delivery at AGH. In the middle of my graduate year, some of these folks decided to storm the Bastille (AGH) by addressing their concerns at a public board meeting. Of course, they tipped off the local media. I sat with that group as the meeting rolled on interminably. Finally, an opportunity to speak about family-centeredness arrived. I didn't speak but served as their resident medical professional. After the meeting adjourned, I experienced fifteen seconds of fame when I was interviewed for television. Later in the month, I and some lay militants, attended a hospital luncheon with the obstetricians, arranged to placate us after our appearance at the board meeting. The luncheon did not go well. If the obstetricians had been opposed to dads in labor before, now they were entrenched. Later still, Miss Hilliard shared in her soft way that she thought my having attended these meetings had been a mistake and that it was much better for change to come from within. She believed that we had probably set the cause back. She was right.

That fiasco was not my last encounter with Alachua General. Assigned to take a recorded prenatal history, I chose a pregnant neighbor. Her husband was a student in the College of Architecture. Cindy worked at the VA as a dental assistant. They were both far from their supportive family up north. It was their first pregnancy. Delighted to be pregnant, she was due in approximately two months. Cindy was a very pretty, dark-haired young woman in her early twenties—hopeful and happy—except for one gnawing concern. Before she was aware that she was pregnant, she had been prescribed an antibiotic. She downplayed her concern about its potential effects on the baby, but her misgiving was ever-present like a tiny mole hill in a verdant lawn.

With the couple, I attended Miss Wilson's Lamaze class and we practiced together. One night, Cindy's husband knocked on my door. Her water had broken. Though in good labor, a self-conscious neatnik, she had just showered. They asked if I would come with them to Alachua General where she was registered. We sped into the night—the couple in the front bucket seats; me straddling the floor hump in the back, timing contractions and giving short breathing commands. We landed in the emergency room and were escorted directly to L&D. I introduced myself as an RN graduate student who had worked L&D. Amazingly, I was admitted—but her husband was not.

Labor progressed swiftly. Cindy was five centimeters dilated when admitted—great for a primigravida! That Lamaze method put laboring moms in a much better place than their twilight sleep sisters! Cindy's doctor was called in and, before you knew it, we were in the delivery room. I coached at her side. Cognizant of being in an enemy camp of sorts, I did whatever I could to avoid getting in the way or interfering with doctor's or nurses' directions—no major missteps by this UF affiliate!

Cindy's legs in stirrups, the table was broken. The doctor, gloved, inserted his fingers for a vaginal exam. Though he was masked, I noticed a change. Cindy did not. Sharply, he directed the anesthetist, "Put her under." Only after his patient was asleep did he divulge that the baby was anencephalic. The baby's head was presenting. He had felt nothing but soft tissue. No skull. The doctor chose general anesthesia because he could not deal then with her inevitable response. He needed to get through the delivery. The child was perfect in every way—except that one major one. Dainty arms and legs. Pink. She breathed. She cried. They hustled her off to the nursery.

The physician disappeared. He returned as we transferred Cindy to the recovery room and asked me to help him to break the news to her husband in the waiting room. The dad, in shock, held his composure. We three returned to the recovery room and Cindy. The upset obstetrician had called his wife to ask her how to proceed. He blurted formally, "Cindy, your baby has a birth defect that is incompatible with life," and continued to describe the problem. Then he left, shaken. Cindy, in shock, holding her husband's hand looked to me, asking hopefully, "But, if they can fix it, will she live?" I tried as best I could to deliver the news again that it could not be fixed, and that living was impossible.

I don't believe Cindy ever saw her baby before she died. People seemed to want to protect her from the sight and I was not as strong an advocate for her as I could have been. She named her daughter Nichol. Later, she gave me a charm of the word LOVE. On it was engraved "Nichol." I still have it.

Enveloped in that little nuclear family as I had been, the loss of Nichol was a stunning blow to me, too. I was rocked by the loss and felt great empathy for the family. As always, I turned the situation over in my mind asking how I could have served her better—been more supportive. I was glad that I had "walked" with her through it and furnished some support. Cindy and I spent many postpartum days talking about the loss. Surprisingly, I discovered that I was not tempted to avoid it. I was no longer the nurse who had to pinch her thigh to be able to stay in the room. The truth surfaced slowly. With my husband's death I had experienced the most painful loss I could ever imagine. I never had to fear anything hurting me as much. It was as though I had been inoculated by grief and, while retaining a deep sense of it, I never had to fear it again.

Graduation day arrived before I knew it. This time there actually *was* a graduation. Not a pinning or a capping or a taking of the Nightingale pledge—but a cap and gown, campus-wide graduation in the Florida Gymnasium. Shortly before, I had been inducted into Sigma Theta Tau, the national invitational honor society. I absolutely would not miss graduation! Closure is important— particularly in times of transition. Maria and I marched in our black caps and gowns. With our master's degree, we wore an apricot velvet hood (symbol of nursing) with a satin orange and blue lining (UF colors).

A seminal year of my life closed. I still keenly felt Danny's loss. Maria and family would return to Punta Gorda. In-laws Marian and Dave remained in Gainesville.

A whole new world of nursing education had opened, and I was diving in head first. Remembering my nursing colleagues at St. Anthony's, I winced at what some could interpret as degree-overload. To them a BSN had been overload! I just felt lucky—lucky to have stumbled upon the nurse traineeship which allowed me to spend that year of retreat; lucky to have been exposed to diverse ideas; lucky to have had the time to mull them over, to distill them and to make them mine. I hoped to be able to use my knowledge for the betterment of nursing and of our patients. Grad school had programmed me to continue to learn throughout my career, using the scholarly skills which I had been taught. Every subsequent day of nursing practice would be an extension of my academic career.

Filled with desire to be to nursing students what Miss Hilliard had been to me, I was eager to teach. The University of South Florida in Tampa would open their College of Nursing in the fall. I decided to apply for a faculty position. Meanwhile, my former nursing school pal, Mary Kay Habgood, an instructor at St. Petersburg Junior College, would be on maternity leave soon. Aware of my plan to return to St. Petersburg, she suggested me as a substitute instructor for the last weeks of her clinical group.

Substitute Teaching

I remember very little of those first few weeks of being a clinical instructor at Palms of Pasadena Hospital. Mary Kay had taught Med-Surg. There I was— with a master's degree *in maternal infant nursing*. There I was—the person who eschewed her limited undergraduate experience in Med-Surg nursing. To my credit, I *had* learned much at Shands about GYN nursing, postoperative nursing and wound care. I understood hospital structure, nursing hierarchy and how to be a guest in a hospital which was not mine.

I arrived early before the students, collaborated with the charge nurse to make assignments, and assisted the students to perform new procedures throughout the morning. The post-conference preceded lunch. I was thrown for a loop when a student was assigned to a young man dying of a glioblastoma. His wife was present. While encouraging the student(s) to also consider her and her feelings, I was aware enough to try to avoid projecting my personal experience onto theirs.

An initially nerve-racking conundrum presented when one student's patient required an NG tube. I had never passed an NG tube on an adult. Shands had reserved that pleasure for med students. But I had passed them on babies. That was a plus. Fortunately, the students had been recently exposed to the basics. We survived it together. So did the patient. The only hitch was his deviated septum. There were several NG tubes to pass during these last few weeks of their senior term as well as other procedures like injections and catheterizations. The total experience was a good one.

Before I was hired to finish the term during Mary Kay's maternity leave, I had, of course, interviewed with Almeda Martin, the Director of the Nursing Program at SPJC. She was a lovely and gracious woman in her early sixties. *Cosmopolitan* comes to mind. Classy dresser. Her figure was typical of her age—trim, a little thick around the middle. Her hair which should have been grey was colored blonde and worn page-boy style. She had been DON of Lenox Hospital in New York City. A diploma grad from Philadelphia School of Nursing, she had both her bachelor's and master's degrees from Hunter College. With her upper-class New York accent, she sounded a little like those 1930s movies about the well-to-do. I could picture her in the *Philadelphia Story*. But, unlike Katherine Hepburn, she was diminutive. Her gracious and hospitable personality belied a very sharp mind. She had been instrumental in getting NLN accreditation for the program.

Almeda and I clicked. She was very welcoming and, at the end of my brief Med-Surg sojourn at Palms, she asked if I would return as the OB instructor come fall. I apologized that I could not commit because I anticipated an interview with the USF Dean. Almeda graciously understood but was anxious to finalize her faculty for the fall. It was May. At the end of May, I interviewed with the founding USF Dean, Gwen MacDonald. She reminded me very much of Polly Barton, my pediatric professor—large, imposing, and stern. It was difficult to divine her thoughts. She impassively informed me that I "would hear." When I did not hear by the end of June (USF's first class began in September), I was concerned. If I waited long enough, I could have no job at all. A bird in the hand was worth two in the bush. At the end of June, I called Almeda Martin. If her position was still open, I would be very happy to accept it. In July, USF called. I had been accepted there, too. But it was too late. I was now an SPJC Nursing instructor. I had made the commitment and would keep it.

I was ambivalent—not in resolve—but in enthusiasm. I had originally sought a university position in which time would be divided between teaching, research, clinical practice and community outreach. It had been the ideal preached at UF. In that atmosphere, I could stay current, continue learning, and apply my new-found knowledge to educating nurses and the public. At SPJC, there was only teaching—in volume. In addition to lectures on Mondays, I would have two groups of fifteen students in the clinical setting four days per week. After a few weeks, they would rotate and then I would have two new groups, then they would rotate again. I was the only maternal infant faculty that first year, developing and presenting my own maternity lectures as well as some broader nursing lectures. In one three-and-a-half-month term, I would see eighty students through clinical. Volume, volume, volume. There would be two months' vacation each summer. That was attractive at first. Little did I foresee how necessary those months would be to recuperate. The plus side of working at SPJC was that there would not be the daily commute to Tampa that USF would have required. The first USF faculty included only nine nurses. In addition to forming the curriculum, they were charged with earning accreditation for the program in two to three years. In retrospect, I probably made the right choice.

Back in the Saddle Again

During that summer between terms, I arranged to work temporarily on my old unit at St. Anthony's where I had maintained contact with friends who worked there. One of them, Judy, who worked L&D evenings, shared an interesting experience. Judy was a very direct, straight-forward, Tampa-born Hispanic nurse. Former military, she had little patience with interpersonal relations. She excelled at starting IV's and monitoring labor. If you looked past her diffidence, she was actually a very nice person and a supportive friend. We played tennis every Sunday for years at what we jokingly called the Church of St. Fossil (Fossil Park).

One evening, Judy worked alone in L&D. Remember how awkwardly L&D had been designed. The only phone in labor was at the entrance in the small nurse-station which housed the narcotics box. That evening, the newly married teen daughter of a hospital department head was admitted. At the time, Sister Gladys was the administrator. She, the department head, and the teenage father all waited nervously in the large waiting room by the front desk while the girl labored. Judy had prepped and medicated the patient (twilight sleep). Labor progressed quickly for a primigravida. It was time to repeat the medication. Judy returned to the nurse-station to draw up the medications and to phone the doctor, alerting him to the rapid progress. Narcotics boxes are locked with two different keys. Using a narcotic required keying in, keying out, logging the medicine out and only then drawing it up. Time consuming. Narcotics are counted at the beginning of each shift and the count must be reconciled with the log.

Returning to her patient, Judy found the room and the bed empty. It was a stationary high bed with high, footboard to headboard side rails like a child's crib. A sound came from the adjoining bathroom. There sat the patient on the toilet, wiping her perineum with toilet paper—while the cord dangled from it. Confused by twilight sleep, the patient had interpreted the pressure of the head on her rectum as a bowel movement and scaled the side rails. The baby had "delivered itself" in the toilet while Judy was at the nurse-station. Fortunately for the baby, the toilet water softened the descent. The newborn had slid down and up with his head above the water. He was breathing. No phone was nearby for Judy to summon help. With a commanding voice acquired in the military, Judy exhorted the woman to get back to bed while protecting the baby still connected to mom by the cord. Finally, the doctor arrived, facilitating delivery of the placenta.

Although under the influence of twilight sleep, the teenager remembered enough. In the recovery room, she chirped to her teen husband that she had the baby in the toilet. Much to Judy's chagrin, he promptly blurted the news to the department head and administrator in the lobby. Judy returned home that night and "had a stiff one." After years of use, the L&D unit was miraculously upgraded. A phone and narcotics box was placed in an alcove in the middle of the labor room hall. Also, I suspect, staffing was re-examined. Sometimes it takes personal impact to make things happen.

Sadie was now the OB Head Nurse and she asked me to take her place while she vacationed for a week or two. Suddenly, I was a manager again. But the backup system of nursing hierarchy on which I could rely for support was absolutely cushy compared to Shands. So, I consented. In my absence, new people had been hired. The unofficial Head Nurse, Mrs. Goodrich, had retired after a heart attack. C-sections were now performed on the unit in the larger delivery room. RNs from each shift had been taught to scrub in. Family-centered maternity nursing reigned supreme on post-partum but, more importantly, dads were tentatively beginning to be included in L&D—but only a few.

After Sadie returned from vacation, the summer passed uneventfully. It was as though I had never left. I felt very comfortable there. Though some dads were included in labor and in delivery, reviews were mixed. Some fainted. Some "got in the way." None were prepared for what they would face despite the still on-going very popular basic childbirth class.

SPJC Maternal Infant Instructor

The previous "OB" instructor, Bernie, had not specialized in maternal infant nursing. She believed that a nurse is a nurse is a nurse. There was a very scant content outline. In the one-week prep before the students arrived, I re-wrote the syllabus and learning experiences. I negotiated times for the students to be on the unit with Bayfront Medical Center, the Public Health Department and a few doctors' offices, meeting at their facilities.

Bernie warned me that I would need tennis shoes to cover the entire unit at Bayfront where students were in labor, delivery, post-partum and nursery. The units stretched the entire length of the building. She was right. I purchased a pair of conductive tennis shoes so that I could run from one end to the other without stopping to don conductive booties in delivery. Conductive shoes prevent sparks which would ignite flammable gasses. I whittled my clinical group down from thirteen to ten or eleven by rotating two to three students per day outside the hospital to obstetricians' offices or public health prenatal clinics. It made each clinical day more manageable and increased the time I was able to spend with each student. It was still a large group to handle in three different departments. Considering how green these second-term freshmen were, I constantly prayed that they would not kill anyone while I was not standing over them.

The SPJC curriculum was theoretically two years but many students wisely spread it out to more by finishing their non-nursing courses before entering the nursing program. Anatomy and physiology as well as microbiology were stumbling blocks on the road to nurse-hood. The nursing program admitted eighty in each class. There was pressure from the community—SPJC was a community college—to graduate as many as possible to ameliorate the nursing shortage. Not all who applied and were admitted were academically or intellectually qualified courtesy of affirmative action and quotas. If an African American student failed or was suspended, inevitably the NAACP weighed in. We were forced to monitor and document students who did not achieve a minimum standard of safety. That monitoring came at the expense of bright, safe students who could have profited from a little more instructor time. Though it was in our best interest to produce nurses to fill community needs, it also behooved us to graduate safe and competent nurses.

Much of the "weeding out" occurred in the first two semesters of the freshman year. That was where maternity nursing was placed—in the second semester. During the previous term, the students had learned basic nursing skills—much of them in our department learning lab. They had been introduced to live patients (usually geriatric) at the VA Medical Center or Palms Hospital where they made beds, gave baths and took vital signs. They had not yet administered oral or injectable medications or considered basic pathophysiology.

The composition of the student body at the junior college was not what I had expected. At UF, undergraduate nursing students had been predominantly kids just out of high school. Not here. Here it was a wicked mix of all flavors. There were new high school grads, yes, but there were also mature—even sixty plus year old—learners. Some had other careers but had decided to change them. One was a math teacher with a graduate degree. One was a successful realtor. One was a mermaid at Weeki Wachee. There were several women contemplating divorce. They sought a profession to finance the divorce and to support them and their children. Several men considered our program a stepping stone toward becoming nurse anesthetists. Several students were LPN's going through the motions to become RNs. Some LPN's believed that they were already functioning as RN's—might as well be paid as one. Challenging them to expand their thought process proved its own challenge. Instructors viewed LPN re-treads with cynicism. RN represented more than the procedures you could perform or the salary you would make. It represented the informed judgment that you used.

I have previously mentioned nursing's academic struggle to define its science. What made it different from medicine? How could it parallel or mimic medicine? UF might have been obsessed with the nursing history, but SPJC was no slouch in the nursing theory department. Its curriculum was based on Faye Abdellah's *Twenty-One Nursing Problems*.[4] Abdellah, a prominent nursing scholar, identified *twenty-one nursing problems* which supposedly covered the entirety of nursing care. The problems were subdivided into categories: physical, interpersonal and common elements of care. Typical problems were: maintain oxygen to all body cells; identify and accept positive and negative expressions, feelings and reactions; maintain good hygiene and physical comfort.

Each of the four semesters was assigned its own problems while course titles followed the medical model (OB, Pedes, Psych, Med-Surg). My maternal infant area was nowhere to be found in the problems—or maybe everywhere. I was assigned maintenance of elimination. Breast feeding and birthing magically became elimination. That incomprehensible allusion is what happens when an artificial construct dictates a curriculum. I suspect Almeda was its source; but undoubtedly sometime in the past the faculty had agreed. Almeda was a great believer in faculty *consensus*.

I took it with good humor but choked a little reading student papers on breast feeding required to relate to the elimination theme. To the students, I was supportive of the construct. Privately, I felt it was a waste of time. *Spit it out. Tell it like it is. Be direct,* I wanted to say. Implying that the twenty-one problems were something which they would encounter as graduates, when they absolutely would not, could confuse and distract the students. *Let's give them a vocabulary which their fellow professionals (respiratory, speech, occupational and physical therapists, dietitians, physicians) would understand,* I thought.

Almeda was also enchanted with the *Logos Model of the Nursing Process.* Each term, students took a patient situation and diagramed it out on a poster—always referring to one of the *Twenty-One Nursing Problems.* In my section when it was due, it was required to confront maternity issues of elimination. The Logos Model was composed of a series of rectangles within rectangles pointing to other rectangles. The basic process was: assess, analyze, diagnose, intervene, evaluate. The objective was to teach critical thinking. I doubt students made the connection.

The eighty students in our section learned medication administration and, crucially, injections. Their education began in the learning lab where the resident instructor was Betty Dutter, RN, a motherly but wily woman who had worked there for years. Some called her Mother Dutter. Students watched a programmed instruction with films. There were vials filled with plain water to be drawn up. Students injected the water into metal basins filled with sponge and covered with a latex glove. Surprisingly, it *did* approximate the feel of an injection—way better than my cadaver had! In second session, students rotated through three instructors—two Med-Surg; one maternity. The Med-Surg faculty felt that they did not have enough opportunities for injection experiences. So, I was co-opted into doing that also. Fortunately, Bayfront's staff was very responsive. Aware that I was looking for injections, they were quick to offer.

The lecture content for the entire three groups together was about pathophysiology and my newly dubbed specialty of "elimination" which included the GI tract and the female reproductive system. One of my lectures concerned birth control choices and their effectiveness. Going from the most effective to the least effective, I opened class by pronouncing that the most effective method was an aspirin held between the knees. The group of eighty students laughed uproariously. After class, a tiny eighteen-year-old student named Vicky approached me shyly to ask if I had been joking—or not. I was reminded that, though many of the students were world-wise, all were not.

Concerned that all students might not have the opportunity to witness a delivery, Bernie had used a short film produced by the military. It didn't waste time with labor but confronted the viewer with a bare perineum, up close and personal, during a bloody delivery—in technicolor. Not my style. It was out of context and could lead students who had never witnessed a delivery to consider it a gruesome event to be *endured* by patient and onlooker.

I chose a different film, *All My Babies,* a black and white film which is now preserved in the Library of Congress as culturally, historically and aesthetically significant. It was produced by the Georgia Department of Public Health in 1953 to train granny-midwives. Set in a rural black community, it contrasts the labors and deliveries of a woman who had prenatal care with one who had not. Home labors and deliveries were presented contextually. The film illustrated the importance of support throughout labor as well as clean technique. African American spirituals provided background music. At the end, the granny-midwife says in her sleepy southern drawl, glancing at a wall of baby pictures, "Why, honey, I'm proud of all my babies." This was a good beginning, cueing students to consider the entire experience. No matter how many times I showed the movie, there were tears in my eyes as I rewound the film. I wanted my students to love maternity as I did—not to define it as a technical feat.

The Nursing Department was housed on the first floor of the Social Arts building. I had toured it for its grand opening many years before when I had met then college president, Dr. Michael Bennett. The nursing department housed a large auditorium, rotated between its four sections. Betty Dutter had her learning lab. There was a small conference room, used for classes and faculty meetings. Most instruction, other than full group lectures and learning lab, occurred at area health facilities.

Mary Kay was my office-mate in an airy windowed office overlooking the parking lot and Fifth Avenue. She continued to teach fourth session, supervising her students at Palms. Mary Kay was a logical thinker who balanced my more visceral responses. With laid back humor, she reminded me of Carol Burnett.

The first year, my section-mates were seasoned instructors, Pat Rice and Roseanne Hutter. The next two years they were replaced by Jan Whitman and Gail Baughman who had offices down the hall. Gail was a very tall, slim, blonde from the Great Lakes area. Jan was short with short sandy blonde hair, wire framed glasses, and the self-contained manner and diminutive voice of a nun. Jan and Gail were my age. They were both from the north. Particularly Jan, expressed the belief that education and health care in the south was woefully below par. To this Florida grad, that rankled like a pea under my mattress!

But I "stifled" per Archie Bunker's admonition in the then popular television comedy, *All in the Family*. Years later when Jan returned from doctoral studies in the north, she acknowledged that Florida might not be so behind. Here, health professionals hail from all over the country and the world, bringing a rich diversity of people, talents and knowledge. She had found the north a little parochial and in-bred.

Jan and Gail were self-assured and clear in their assessments. I, on the other hand, usually perceived fifty shades of gray. I was odd woman out and not just because of my area of expertise. After the first year or so, Almeda assigned different part-time instructors to assist me to cover the expanse of Bayfront's maternity unit—Jean Wortock and Susan Schaeffer. They were only present part-time and had no real responsibility for student evals. But they were a welcome addition to this frenzied, isolated nurse. Jean, later PhD, became Dean of Nursing when SPJC transitioned to St. Petersburg College.

Mrs. Dutter discovered three of our students cheating on a test in her learning lab. At a meeting with Jan, Gail, Almeda and me, we decided to expel them. We were idealists who could not countenance cheating in nursing. My sessionmates and I were unaware that, earlier in the term, a similar situation had occurred in the first session. Those three instructors, with Almeda, had decided only to suspend the students, not expel them. Mrs. Dutter was aware of both situations—as was Almeda. The first-session students had been white. Ours were black. It didn't take long for the NAACP and heaven knows what other civil rights organizations to descend upon SPJC Administration. The result was that we not only accepted the students back but passed them on to third session. Had we known about the first incident, our actions might not have been the same. But our opinion would stand that nursing is no place for cheaters.

One day, a student submitted an assignment about her post-partum patient. There was not one complete sentence in the paper. Her written English was atrocious. She was a very nice, pleasant and, I believe, intelligent student—the kind of person anyone would want as their nurse. I spoke to her about the paper, confiding that someone in college who planned to communicate with doctors and other professionals needed to be able to write complete sentences.

What she shared amazed me. She had passed college freshman English. Speechless, I saw red. This nice young woman had been cheated by the college. With her paper, I stormed over to the English department director. He read her paper with dismay. Consulting her record, he discovered that she had been in a remedial English class at the college before taking freshman English—and had passed both. She was black. He had not known so many of "them" were getting into the nursing program. In the English Department, if they showed any improvement, they were passed. He expressed concern about interfering with African American cultural language. Really? If I take a French class does it interfere with my English? We all have a certain dialect and use colloquialisms reflecting our family and friends. Teaching an alternative does not change access to that. It just furnishes an alternative. The student had paid to be taught that alternative.

Pinellas County Public Schools, despite the Supreme Court's 1954 ruling in *Brown v. the Board of Education*, had not desegregated until 1971. My mother taught senior English at Northeast High School through most of the seventies. As she described it, socially, desegregation was a nightmare. Behaviors that would not have been tolerated at a segregated black high school went unchallenged due to a fear of reprisal by civil rights groups claiming discrimination. It was good enough to keep the peace; why try to uphold academic standards? That philosophy apparently had continued in college. To me, it was a huge injustice to the black students who needed the tools to succeed—not the assumption that they wouldn't or couldn't. I have known too many bright, sharp, motivated black nurses to believe otherwise. What happened to the student? She dropped out. Did the English Department make any changes? I hope so.

Two women impacted me as a novice instructor. One was Mary Jean Etten, a former nun with a beatific smile who enjoyed wearing clunky jewelry. With a large frame, she could pull it off, looking feminine and modern. I found her to be full of fun and mutual interests. She had both bachelors and master's degrees and worked on her doctorate. She was very motivated, living alone, commuting on weekends to visit her good friend, Sue, in Brooksville. She and Sue, a USF professor, were writing a book on gerontology. [5] Mary Jean taught first session students and she scared the pants off them. They complained to us in second session that she was uncompromisingly demanding. That was difficult to reconcile with the Mary Jean whom I knew. Over time, I realized that students, stressed to succeed, could percieve each instructor as an impediment to attaining that cap—including me!

An extension of Mary Jean's expertise was her interest in hospice. At the time, there was no such thing here in Pinellas County and only a scattered few in the USA. I viewed end-of-life care through my perspective of family-centered maternity care. Sensing a kindred soul, Mary Jean asked me to attend a meeting of a group which would eventually develop The Elisabeth Kübler Ross Hospice. Like the early ICEA meetings I had attended, the meeting was held in a private home. Like the ICEA meeting, people sat around complaining about the horrors of hospital deaths (ICEA: births). Participants were relatively affluent, educated people who demanded more of their deaths (births) than would a person of less affluence. Though I had genuine respect for their concerns, through the perspective of my experiences, I felt that a little less stridence, a little more conciliatory tone might achieve a few more of their goals. I did not pursue involvement but did attend forums which they sponsored with the talented speaker/author, Elisabeth Kübler Ross.

Another instructor was at the other end of the spectrum from Mary Jean in every way. Tiny, sixty-something Vi (Violet) Wilkinson, fourth session psych instructor, was a mighty mouse and a force with whom to be reckoned. An FSU grad, she had been the psychiatric nursing instructor at SPJC for some time. She had short cropped black hair with a few strands of grey and wore rimless glasses. Her very thick drawl was Florida-panhandle-southern. Vi was a no-nonsense kind of gal in all ways—particularly with her well-planned behavioral objectives and learning activities—each with pre-test and post-test. She kept a stash of psych articles culled from nursing journals and made them required reading. Vi's students were so well educated that psych was usually their top scoring test on State Boards. Despite being a tad jealous of that achievement, I felt great admiration for her methods. She was a meticulous educator.

Many SPJC days blur as one. Some incidents stand out.

I watched a good student draw up her first injection when she blurted, "Stop looking at me, you're making me nervous." We both laughed but then I explained that the only thing I could do was look since it was my responsibility to the patient who would receive it—and to my license.

The major purchase I convinced Almeda to make was a life-sized pelvic model with interchangeable uterus and cervix. I used the model to demonstrate the basics of pelvic exam and the relationships of pelvic organs. Usually, I asked students to insert a speculum to see what the doctor would see when he performed a Pap smear. One student was flabbergasted. During her own Pap smear at her doctor's office, she had seen a speculum which looks like a duck's bill. She had assumed that it was used to snip a piece of her cervix for a specimen. Her relief at the new-found revelation that the speculum simply propped open the vagina for swabs was palpable. I used her perception to underscore the valuable role of the nurse as educator.

On another occasion, I coached a student giving her first injection. The patient was bottom-up, facing away from us. For what seemed like an eternity, the student stood over her. She had identified the correct site, using anatomic landmarks. She held the uncapped syringe, using a dart-like motion to repeatedly get as far as the skin—then pulled back before it hit. She was as afraid as I had been so long ago.

Just then, her contemporary entered and spoke to me from behind the curtain. "Mrs. Newton, I've been trying to administer a rectal suppository but when I looked at her anus, all I could see was a giant rose." After all the pushing and pelvic congestion during labor, many women developed massive external hemorrhoids which looked like a thick petaled rose—but this was the first I had heard them called that. Torn between the two students, I directed, "Use plenty of KY-jelly and aim for the middle of the rose." Eventually, both the injection and the suppository were successfully administered.

Another student was a wholesome little redhead who lived in a religious commune and waitressed at the commune's restaurant. Wouldn't you know, I inadvertently assigned her to a post-partum patient who was a witch married to a warlock! They looked very Goth with stringy long black hair and black nail polish. It was a test of acceptance. The student, inwardly shocked, passed with flying colors!

Facing her preconceptions, one of my students was assigned to a woman who had delivered at least two children at St. Anthony's. Now, the patient was admitted to Bayfront for a tubal ligation post-delivery. St. Anthony's, a Catholic hospital, would not perform tubal ligations for religious reasons. The patient was Catholic. I briefed the student on the patient's condition and care. Convinced that the patient must feel terribly guilty about having the tubal ligation, she asked how she should approach her. I said, "She made the choice. Try not to assume how she feels, or tell her how to feel, but ask open ended questions and listen . . . " The student followed through and learned that the patient was relieved that family planning was no longer an issue.

On one of my first clinical days, I assigned three or four students to perform newborn assessments, baths and cord care in the nursery. Afterward, they were to take their baby to its mom for feeding—being sure to check bracelets. Once the nursery students were underway, I dashed out to post-partum and L&D to check on students there. When I returned to the nursery, most of the students were finishing. I asked about their babies' assessments and baths. A slim, quiet student in her forties enigmatically responded, "I didn't think I'd be able to do it," then abruptly left the room. Later I discovered that, in her twenties, she had a stillborn and had not been near a baby or touched one since. This was a wake-up call to me. Students, like patients, were a product of their history. The better I knew them, the more I would be able to individualize my approaches. Unfortunately, with so many students rotating so often, there was precious little time to individualize. But for this one woman, I did try to provide extra time for her to get comfortable with babies, having taken that first step.

At first, I tried to have lunch with the students in the cafeteria. When I joined them, I felt a pall of constraint descend. Belatedly, I realized, they needed time to totally relax without an instructor there to intimidate them. I never *felt* intimidating.

One morning, a nursery aid returned to the nursery from post-partum scandalized because my male student was coaching a mother how to breast feed. Most of the nurses were just fine with male students but it posed more of a challenge for a southern male obstetrician. He became enraged that one of my male students had been coaching an unprepared teenage couple. The student had provided supportive care throughout their labor and—by the way—had done a fine job of it. When the obstetrician arrived for the delivery, he would not allow my student in the delivery room because he was male. On another occasion, when one of my black males was to observe a caesarian section, the same doctor threw an instrument at him. I could have made an issue of it each time. I remembered that, from the hospital's perspective, *doctors fill beds*. Already, we shared OB with the vocational school's LPN program. For a while, *that* had been bumpy. If Bayfront cut us out, our only other recourse—St. Anthony's—did not have the volume of patients needed for my students. Instead, I made it very clear to my male students what a wonderful job they had done and how much of an effort I knew they were making in what had been predominantly a woman's arena. Two years later, one of my male students was an RN employed in the same nursery.

Roe v. Wade had just been decided by the Supreme Court. Doctors' offices began performing first trimester abortions. Second trimester abortions were performed in the hospital—unfortunately in the labor rooms among laboring women. At least they were placed in a private, but not sound-proof room. I did not assign my students to these patients. They had little enough time to experience a normal L&D. Many of my students had religious objections or reservations about abortion. As did I. But my beliefs were beside the point. Whenever the fetus was delivered and was lying in a metal basin in the utility room, I escorted my students through so that they could conceptualize fetal development at x weeks gestation. I thought that would speak for itself.

In the post-conferences on the unit after their morning with patients, we sat in a circle and they shared their highlights—maybe some approaches they found that worked. Once for each group, I brought a metal basin containing a newly delivered placenta and lots of gloves. We peeled the chorion from the amnion to identify them and talk about twinning. We examined the vessels in the cord and the Wharton's jelly around them. We touched the maternal surface. If it felt like sandpaper, we knew that the baby was probably post-mature with interruptions in his placental blood supply—explaining in utero weight loss in over-due (post-mature) babies.

I also told "stories with a point" in post conference about my early experiences on the maternity unit. It helped them to conceptualize approaches to complications like eclampsia, abruptio placenta, placenta previa, prolapsed cord. I was never the hero of these stories—usually the opposite. It was my way of stressing that it doesn't matter if you don't know or are unsure. Learn from your mistakes and don't make them twice. Make every day you work a learning experience.

For three years, I maintained that assembly-line instruction. Before State Boards, I invited graduating students to return for a refresher/review since many complained that this specialized area of nursing had been offered so early in the curriculum that they had trouble remembering it. The OB exam portion of State Boards, if failed, could bar them from that hard-sought "RN."

Increasingly, I realized that the harder I pushed for student experiences (births, baby baths and assessments, catheterizations, injections, evaluation of fundus, episiotomy and lochia, sitz baths, suppositories), the more frequent my migraines. They were predictable on Fridays—the culmination of a week of stress. I would go home to bed Friday afternoon. By Sunday, when I finally felt better, I put off correcting repetitive student care plans until the wee hours. This frenetic pace was no way to live. I missed clinical contact with patients. As instructor, I cued and guided my students allowing them the opportunity to experience what I considered the joy of maternal infant nursing. My only joy was their success.

I was chagrined one day when Almeda asked me if we could make OB a Learning Lab course with manikins and movies! Reading care plans with the inevitable references to elimination for more than four hundred students was boring if not excruciating. Being the gracious hospital guest, smoothing over situations with hospital staff became cumulatively grating. Scrutinizing the high-risk potentially unsafe students, informing a student that she had failed the course—all were unpleasant. I loved the students, loved the faculty, I even loved the hospital. But I did not love my life. I dreamt of alternate ways to use the education that I had been given.

While working temporarily at St. Anthony's between graduate school and SPJC, I had met an evening shift L&D RN named Rosemary Colombo. She was a diploma school grad from New Jersey and the mother of two grade school daughters. Rosemary was a baccalaureate nursing student at USF. She was a highly motivated, forward-thinking nurse. While I taught at the junior college, she was promoted to maternity nurse-educator—a newly created position. She taught staff, patients and the Basic Childbirth course which continued to thrive.

Rosemary met the woman who had taken the maternity position at USF which I had been offered—Jeannette Sasmor. Jeannette taught a continuing education course about developing prepared childbirth classes. Rosemary, Sadie and I trekked across the bay to the USF campus to take it.

The family-centered approach was not going well in St. Anthony's L&D. Physician resistance influenced older nurse resistance by default. Truthfully, even those who were pro dads in L&D worried. Some had experienced inappropriate behavior by the dads. The behavior, for the most part, reflected a knowledge gap or unrealistic expectations.

Incrementally, we plotted to move dads at St. Anthony's to their rightful place. We initiated a pre-requisite class for what the obstetricians termed a *privilege* for the dads. It was an add-on to the *Basic Childbirth Class*. The new labor-specific class was a more intense four-week course, attended by mom and dad in the evening. It was held on mats in the empty physical therapy department. To avoid pre-conceived prejudices against them, we avoided any references to Grantly Dick Read, Lamaze or Elizabeth Bing. Instead it was called the *Prepared Childbirth Class*. Its gravitas was based on having two masters-prepared maternity nurse consultants—Jeannette and me. The tricky part was obtaining the obstetricians' imprimatur by making it seem that they controlled course content. I don't know how Sadie did it, but she obtained their approval. They knew Sadie and me and probably thought we were in their pockets. Extrinsically, patient demand exerted pressure. Our approach represented compromise. Time was marching on.

We began on a very small scale with a group of fewer than five mother/dad couples. Jeanette and I co-taught it and developed it as we went. Guess what? We were teaching Lamaze. We simply didn't call it that. It was operant conditioning with breathing techniques based upon the phase of labor. Comfort measures and positioning were demonstrated; questions were answered, and couples were urged to practice daily between classes. During one class we introduced a Doppler to listen to each couple's fetal heart sounds—a first for several fathers who had not accompanied their wives to prenatal appointments. We toured L&D and explained what happened there. We aimed to make the couples feel at home and confident. I believe we did.

After the first few series of classes, Jeanette dropped out. I continued to teach the classes at night. Then I became the childbirth instructor's educator, teaching some of the maternity unit's RN's to be instructors. I demonstrated through one series, and then observed another series which they taught, providing feedback and encouragement. They did not teach independently until we both agreed they were ready. Happily, one of the RN's whom I taught to be an instructor was the daughter of Dr. Joe Cool. Her mannerisms were very similar to her father and I fully expected her to pop out with, "Don't worry about a thing." Another RN whom I taught was married to an oncologist with whom I worked. Both were great women and excellent instructors. Despite their initial self-doubt, the nurses brought a wealth of labor experience with them. Some OB LPN's also qualified as class assistants. The demand for the classes grew so that, in some months, there were as many as three separate classes held per week. It was a totally delightful experience with a positive impact on expectant parents, the hospital and the nurses themselves.

I had so wanted to be for my nursing students all that Miss Hilliard had been for me. I wanted to set their hearts on fire for maternity. From their feedback in later years, I sometimes succeeded—whether they chose to work in maternity or not. But on a day-to-day basis, I was very discontent repeating: fundus, lochia, episiotomy more than eighty times a term just to be sure that the bare basics were emblazoned on each student's mind to pass the State Board of Nursing Exam.

The fact that St. Anthony's now had a nurse-educator, that the prepared childbirth program was thriving, and that dads were now engaged in labor gave me reason to believe that St. Anthony's was progressively moving with the times. I was most prepared to be a Maternal infant Clinical Nurse Specialist. But Rosemary was doing a great job with that. Part of my master's program had also involved gynecology. So, I thought, *why not throw my hat in the ring. Nothing ventured, nothing gained.* I could not see myself continuing as I had been.

I made an appointment with then Director of Nurses, Pat Ryan. Pat was a rusty haired Bostonian-Irish smoker/drinker who took pride in her shiny white shoes, immaculate white uniform and oblong frilly cap with a thick black velvet band. She was a friend of Sister Gladys, the previously-mentioned Franciscan Administrator. The interview went positively. Miss Ryan posited that, since the GYN census was small, perhaps I would be interested in becoming GYN-*Oncology* Nurse-Specialist.

I had to think about that one. I remembered Danny's bout with cancer and knew how easy it would be to interpret every patient's experience through the window of my own. Then I remembered the case three years earlier at Palms with the woman whose husband had a glioblastoma. The temptation had been to see her experience in light of my own. But, I had quickly recognized that my job was to ask how they were managing and to work from there. At least I would be mindful of my associations and could counter balance them.

Don't get me wrong. I was not one hundred percent convinced about becoming *Oncology* Nurse-Specialist. But I was willing to give it a try. What I was currently doing—teaching basic freshman nursing students en masse—was not working. The teaching part had been good; the mass production and repetitiveness had not. So, I regretfully delivered my notice to Almeda. I would genuinely miss her and my other friends at SPJC.

This chapter of my nursing career had been one of discovery. After Danny's death, I had discovered that I could be independent and alone. I had discovered that the only way to surmount grief is to plow through it, to fully experience it—not to avoid it. It does not destroy. It strengthens. Experiencing patients' grief over any kind of loss was no longer excruciating. I had climbed the mountain and could help others up. I had discovered that I loved teaching but also that teaching topically and repetitively was not for me. I was not sure where the GYN-Oncology Nurse-Specialist role would lead. But a measure of youthful optimism had returned.

Endnotes

1. Robert Frost, "The Road Not Taken," *Immortal Poems of the English Language* edited by Oscar Williams (New York: Washington Square Press, 1965), 504.

2. Betty Friedan, *The Feminine Mystique* (New York: W.W. Norton and Co., 1963).

3. Helen Reddy and Ray Burton, "I Am Woman," *I Am Woman* (Los Angeles: Capitol Records, May 1972).

4. Faye Abdellah, *Patient-Centered Approaches to Nursing* (London: Macmillan, 1960).

5. Sue Saxon and Mary Jean Etten, *Physical Change and Aging: A Guide for the Helping Professions*, Third Edition (U of Michigan: Tiresias Press, 1994).

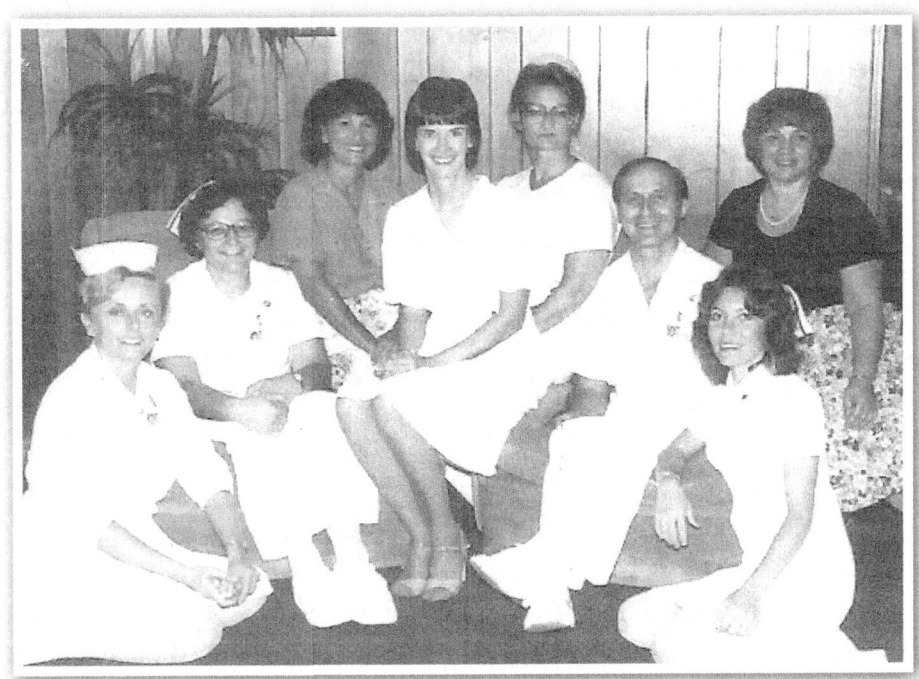

Figure 11 *The Education Department Gathers for Molly's Retirement. Left to Right: Peggy Newton, GYN-Oncology; Dee Dade, Cardio-Pulmonary; Gemma Scardino, Secretary; Dory Snyder Jaworski, PTEC—later Cardio-Pulmonary; Joannie Strayer, ICU; Claude Schmitz, OR–Oncology; Rosemary Colombo, soon to be Director; Christine Bennet Joughin, Enterostomal Therapy.*

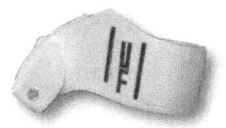

CHAPTER FIVE
Career in Apogee: 1976-1990

USA Bicentennial: Back at St. Anthony's

A surprise awaited when I arrived in June. Instead of working out of the Department of Nursing, I would work in the newly formed Education Department directed by Molly Smeaton, RN.

Close to sixty, Molly was the long-tenured lone hospital educator whom I had known tangentially. I attended a continuing education program she had presented the year before. The subject was Molly's face lift, including a video of the procedure and presentations by Molly and her plastic surgeon. The video was a little grisly—especially when you knew the person whose face was being incised. The surgical result was that Molly permanently looked like invisible clothes pins tugged at her skin from just above her ears. Molly thought it looked fine. Molly was quirky, would do anything to educate, and was not at all cast from the traditional nursing mold. She was a very smart and world-wise cookie. Her children grown, she and her husband spent many days on their large boat. On occasion, Molly asked the department to go out with them for drinks and merriment. On those occasions, Molly wore a bathing suit—and white cotton gloves. Her gloves protected hands with a history of multiple skin cancers on high-risk Scotch-Irish skin.

Molly's assistant director in the education department was Rosemary who continued to be responsible for OB. Later Rosemary's responsibilities became so many that a new OB Educator, Sharon Meece, was hired. Marquette grad Joan Strayer functioned as Nurse-Clinician in Surgical Intensive Care (SICU) and

Recovery. Joannie was like Lucy Ricardo of *I Love Lucy*—full of bustling activity and fun. She was strong, energetic and Nordic in appearance. Joannie was mother of two-year-old Jayson who sucked his fingers while twisting her long, blonde hair.

Another unexpected pleasure was learning that Christine Bennett, one of my former, shy-as-a-mouse nursing students, was off at Emory becoming an enterostomal therapist, an RN specializing in placement and care of colostomy, ileostomy, urostomy and wounds. Upon return, she joined our department. Edna Clifton, a Barry College grad, was Cardio-Pulmonary Clinician. Married to a respiratory therapist, she was extremely knowledgeable about all things cardiac. It was she who held the mandatory CPR instruction for all hospital employees and was very effective in that role.

Last, but not least, was Claude Schmitz. Claude was a Polish-speaking male nurse from Chicago via my high school alma mater, St. Paul's. As a youth, he had joined the Alexian Brothers and graduated from a diploma school. After practicing as a missionary nurse-brother in South America, he had returned to St. Petersburg to care for his ailing grandmother. While working in St. Anthony's OR, he left religious life. Now he was OR Educator working toward his BS at St. Leo's. Claude could be the soul of propriety and uprightness—then go bug-eyed, meaningfully staring at a décolletage that revealed cleavage. Shocked about the high cost of his utilities, he would break out swearing. His repertoire included: (pig-Polish) *toughsky shitsky*; *He* (rude doctor) *puts his pants on one leg at a time just like me*; *Does that threaten you? Assume makes an ass of u and me.* Claude affectionately called me Peginsky. He was like a brother to us all, full of loveable quirks. Additionally, he directed the GU team, orderlies trained to place and irrigate Foley catheters in men. At conservative St. Anthony's, female nurses were not permitted to catheterize male patients.

Clearly the department was going to be large and very sharp. Working with these folks kept me at my sharpest, too. When I had shared my decision to flee academia for the hospital, my mother had been disappointed. To her, it was a step down. With my master's, I had surpassed her educationally (she had a few credits toward her master's) and I had been, in a sense, following in her footsteps by teaching at a college level. Ironically, for the next fourteen years, as a member of St. Anthony's Education Department, I came very close to living that dream situation which I had originally envisioned—a combination of clinical practice, research, education and community service.

Continuing Education Becomes Law

No small part of the decision to create a brand-new education department had been the decision by the Florida State Board of Nursing to require twelve hours of continuing education per year to renew the Florida Nursing License. Until that point in Florida history, the older the nurse, potentially the more antiquated her nursing.

Hospital management recognized that, to keep staff (RN & LPN) licensed and working, contact hours needed to be easily available. One of our charges was providing at least twelve but preferably more contact hours per year. We provided *many* more. We were one of the first state-approved preferred providers in the county. While offering contact hours to our own staff, why not offer them to outside nurses—for a price? Classes attracted revenue—at least to cover advertising and materials costs. But it also marketed us to the community, bringing nurses in the door. It enhanced recruitment. The nursing shortage was real. Nurses from Canada and the Philippines were being recruited by local hospitals.

We took our charge to heart—providing auditorium-filled evening con-ed programs at least once monthly. More than one hundred people attended. The presentations each featured both nurse and doctor speakers. Though we preferred to present courses related to our specialties, some were not.

One of my assigned programs concerned arthritis in which I outlined nursing aspects of care. During the break featuring Mrs. Proctor's cookies, several nurses approached me, praising my delivery and enthusiasm. I must really have done extensive work with arthritis patients. No. I had just researched it. Another unrelated topic for which I took responsibility was *Suicide and Depression*. Again, I was praised for my expertise (assessing suicide risk). No. But, again I had done my research. I discovered that I was able to boil my subject down to basics, using audiovisuals to boost comprehension and retention. An ironic twist followed that suicide presentation. Approximately a month after the psychiatrist presented his portion of the class, his empty boat was found in the bay.

As part of staff development, we encouraged nursing experts from the units to present at the con-ed events. Mona Killough was just such a nurse. A diploma school grad and former nun, Mona pursued her BSN at USF. She was a team leader on our orthopedic unit and co-presented total knee replacement with an orthopedic physician.

Soon, we added more con-ed programs. Reflecting long-range planning, we published a yearly calendar allowing people to plan ahead and register early. Entire courses were usually held at the end of the first shift and repeated in the evening or morning, affording multi-shift access. I developed many courses around my areas of specialization—pain, cancer, chemotherapy, death, GYN, mouth care, breast cancer, care of the body post mortem. The other department members did the same with their specialties. We were uniquely innovative for our geographical area.

For having this new concept of mandatory continuing education thrust upon them, the nurses adapted to it very well and were so very appreciative. Unlike many of my students at the junior college who had absolutely no frame of reference in nursing, these folks had worked in the trenches. They were happy to find applicable information that made sense. We offered so many different topics that they didn't feel forced to attend a class featuring an uninteresting topic merely to accrue the hours.

Though we tried to keep the actual presentation of con-ed classes open and flowing, the State Board had set rigorous requirements to maintain our preferred provider status. Behind the scenes, we religiously adhered to them. For each class, we needed a pre-test, post-test, evaluation (of instructor and environment), behavioral objectives, outline, bibliography, roster and the speaker's résumé or vitae. We followed requirements by the book. These were pre-computer days when paperwork originated via typewriter. We considered the Xerox® machine a boon and having a Selectric, IBM's electric typewriter, a lucky break! Eventually we were rewarded with a secretary.

After many years of offering programs, we provided an all-day seminar for area nurse-educators about developing programs and using A-V equipment creatively—the overhead projector with overlays; synchronized slide–tape presentations; the use of video; writing scripts for video and slide. Neither PowerPoint nor even computers were available then.

Two of my more cherished con-ed programs contained videotaped interviews with two cancer survivors. One was an interview with a grade school teacher, Jane. Jane was a gracious and generous woman who had a mastectomy followed by chemotherapy for Stage IV breast cancer. She had metastases. Jane endured, stayed positive and dealt with the vicissitudes of chemotherapy. She was back to teaching; her hair had grown out and she felt that she was in it for the long haul. The video featured Jane and me in a living room setting, just talking about her experience. To have access to a conversation like this was unusual for the nurses who sometimes avoided getting into emotionally charged issues during the patients' hospitalizations. Hospital nurses were only exposed to cancer patients who were ill and dying. They had no real experience with anything positive about coping and survivorship.

I was prompted to ask another person for an interview because of an unhappy situation on one of the units. A young man in his thirties, a Viet Nam Veteran exposed to Agent Orange, had Hodgkin's Lymphoma and was dying a miserable death. His young wife worked as a secretary in the hospital. Hodgkin's Lymphoma (Disease) is a cancer of the lymphatic glands.

The doctor administered chemo—almost to the very end—in a valiant attempt to cure a very salvageable young man. After he died, the nurses on that unit were disturbed, grousing that they would never have chemotherapy if they had cancer. Alarms went off. Not only were they forming attitudes which could adversely influence their future patient care, but they were excluding potential life-saving treatment for themselves. Even then, Hodgkin's was 80% curable. The person to interview worked as an RN team leader on the unit directly below theirs. Her name was Vivian. She was one of their own.

Vivian was in her fifties and a spit-fire. Svelte, she was immaculate in her starchy whites and cap. Her hair was black as were her eyelashes. She was perky, organized and no-nonsense. A military wife, she had been the equivalent of a four-star general herself, shepherding her large family to ever-changing deployments around the world. Only mid-life had she studied nursing. Vivian had been diagnosed with Hodgkin's Disease several years earlier. She had experienced grueling chemotherapy with bouts of nausea, hair loss and weakness. Her husband thought she would die. But she came through it all—cancer free. Vivian was willing to be taped. I interviewed her in the same living room setting. The tape was shown originally on the unit where that young man had died of the same illness. But it was also used many times over for various programs. I will forever be grateful to both Jane and Vivian for the courage they displayed by "going public" at a time when cancer was shrouded with a veil of mystery and fear.

One of my favorite yearly con-ed courses was about death and dying. For one segment, I created a slide show of literature, music and art through the ages relating to death. We discussed experiences with death, care of the dying and their families. For religious practices relating to death, I invited a minister, priest (from our Pastoral Care Department) and rabbi. Rabbi Luski was awesome, explaining the Jewish perspective of death so well and so convincingly that our predominantly Catholic and Protestant fundamentalist staff left with a very positive view of Judaism. On rare occasion when Rabbi Luski was not available, I asked a friend, Marshall Gootson, to stand in. The students were in awe of his participation in the Chevra Kadisha, a group of Jewish same-sex volunteers who prepare the body of the deceased with ritual cleansing, dressing and prayer.

In-Services: a Component of Quality Assurance

Another type of hospital education did not qualify for contact hours for licensure. In-services had been around since time began. They were usually short classes often, but not always, held on the unit. In-services taught a new procedure, a new way of doing paperwork, or a review required by the state like the fire or disaster procedures or CPR. We were all involved in these on all three shifts—nights and evenings, too. I didn't mind it at all. It was a means of networking with potential con-ed students and discovering what they needed to know. Night and evening staff appreciated our accessibility and willingness to join them.

That points to another reason for founding the Education Department. Administration, now under youthful Administrator, Jim Grobmyer (followed by Dan MacMurray) needed eyes and ears on the ground. Molly reported directly to Administration—and we reported to Molly. If there were concerns, they would be heard.

One fun in-service that I remember concerned fire carries. Fire carries are used to evacuate ill and immobile patients from an area on fire (Signal F). Of course, it is important to save the patient, but it takes practice to do so in a way which will not inactivate a nurse. We educators had all watched a film and practiced on each other. Joannie and I paired up on the evening shift, to demonstrate and practice with staff. We alternated playing the role of patient or nurse, each wearing a scrub suit for modesty. One method involved placing the bed at its lowest level; pulling the patient to the bed edge; kneeling on one leg; pivoting his legs off the bed; and dropping his head and thorax onto a knee before lowering him to the floor on a blanket to drag him to another area. Another involved carrying the patient off from a high bed piggy-back style. We alternated roles and finished the night with many bruises. Joannie was strong. I had a good case of whiplash from her whipping me up off the bed to ride her back. A fire in-service was offered each year—each slightly different from the previous year. Molly was responsible for holding monthly, unannounced fire drills on various shifts.

Disaster was another area for which the Education Department was responsible. In a disaster (Signal D), everyone in the hospital had an assigned role. Designated people remained on their unit; others were dispatched to either the auditorium or to the ER. Nurses from the floors brought IV poles and gurneys. In the auditorium, there was a large closet where folded cots and a medical supply cart were kept—all set-up by first responders. The ER staff triaged incoming patients, sending them either to the auditorium or to the library (then behind the ER). Minor surgery was performed in the back of the auditorium which could be closed off from the front. The convent was the communication hub. During drills, Molly or her designate stood in the auditorium, clipboard in hand, documenting response time for the first responders; how long it took to get the cots in place and the medical cart activated. Did the traffic director do it well? What were the kinks? Several times, rather than a dry run, kids from the local school participated in a county-wide drill. They were raucous—moaning, groaning and carrying on.

Once I convinced my mother to volunteer as a victim on what turned out to be a rainy evening. The county-wide disaster was supposed to be a crashed plane in the Central Plaza parking lot (now the bus station). My mother, in her late 60s and a volunteer, was forced to lie on cold wet gravel waiting for the transport bus to St. Anthony's. I never heard the end of that.

Twice there were REAL disasters. On the evening of January 28, 1980, I taught a prepared childbirth class in the physical therapy department. The class was wrapping up when the intercom pealed: *Signal D.* I excused the class and hustled them out to their cars before reporting to my assigned place—the library and "the nearly dead."

The purpose of triage, performed first at the accident scene and again in the ER, was to decide who could be helped versus who, even if helped, will not live. The ones believed to have a chance are the first to receive care. The library was the place for those not expected to live. I brought mats from my class for the floor. Just as I pushed the library table to the side, Christine, also assigned to the "nearly dead" arrived. She had been called in from home and was scared. So was I—being the elder, hopefully not obviously so. We had no idea what kind of disaster we faced. For Christine's sake as well as my own, I played my inner Sister Beatrice saying that we needed to *take things as they come* and that we were up to the task. We had to be brave. There was a disaster kit in the library with empty water bottles and linen, mouth swabs, etc. We needed to fill the water bottles. If morphine was required, we could get it in the ER. Thankfully, that night, no patients arrived in the library. Later, I discovered that only a few patients had arrived with minor scrapes. The disaster was the collision of the Coast Guard ship Blackthorn with the tanker, Capricorn. The Blackthorn capsized resulting in the deaths of twenty-three crew members. It happened within the vicinity of the Sunshine Skyway. Amazingly, an old, crusty, almost retired surgeon reported immediately to the auditorium where he sutured a few superficial lacerations.

The second REAL disaster occurred four months later. It was early morning and I was across the street at the St. Petersburg Medical Clinic, checking on a patient receiving chemotherapy. She watched television while the IV ran. I looked up to the TV to see the southbound central span of the Sunshine Skyway Bridge destroyed. Missing! A freighter, the Summit Venture, had collided with a support column, sending a large central section of the bridge into Tampa Bay. With it went cars, a truck and a Greyhound bus. One man who survived the fall, Wesley MacIntire, was the only one to arrive at St. Anthony's. After his recovery, he donated a large, framed picture of the Pope in gratitude for his survival and his experience at St. Anthony's.

I was in awe of the well-oiled machine that was St. Anthony's in times like these. Everyone had his or her job. When we each did our part, things went smoothly. Anything could be handled. Individually, we might not feel up to the task but, as part of a larger force, we could handle it.

In the late eighties, there was one person who failed to grasp that concept—a new nun in Pastoral Care. She was new, young and very self-important. She, like me, was assigned to the East Lobby during fire drills. Our purpose there was to lock the elevators and hold them in the lobby to be available to the fire department. We also explained to people at the outside-door that the hospital was closed to them until the situation could be resolved. This role wasn't important enough for the nun who thought she really needed to be at the scene of the fire to provide the emotional support which only she could. One day during a real fire—probably an overheated kitchen hot plate—on the fourth floor, she ditched the lobby and reported to the scene. Already present, our Administrator asked, "Sister, where is your fire station?" She was sternly warned to return to the fire station to which she had been assigned. *Teamwork* and *grandstanding* are oxymorons.

Though the machine was well-oiled, one un-called signal D did not fit the protocol at all. It was in the mid-nineteen eighties at afternoon change of shift. With two-thirds of the total nursing staff present and a hospital full of patients, the hospital received a bomb threat. It was set to go off just after three p.m. Of course, administration contacted police. Apparently, they decided that there was no way in hell to empty the hospital and questioned the threat's legitimacy. The Education Department was enlisted to canvas units for *anything suspicious*. I had no idea what that would be, envisioning a plastic bomb attached under over-bed tables or sticks of dynamite. Nursing expertise is broad, but it doesn't include explosives. We were not to mention why we were opening every drawer in every patient's room. To this day, that mission seems preposterous. Our instinct was to flee. But my peers and I were committed to patient and staff safety. We fulfilled the mission—potential martyrs for the cause. I tried to do it quickly and quietly, calling no attention to myself. Some patients asked me to do this or that for them. I did small things but knew, for their sake, I couldn't permit them to slow me down.

One lady with a new amputation complained of lower extremity phantom limb pain. Quickly, I directed her to rub the same area on her remaining leg. Preposterous as it sounds, there was foundation for contra-lateral stimulation as pain relief in the literature. But I did not have time to expound. As I opened her drawers, looked under her table, and explained rubbing the other leg, she watched me as though I had totally lost my marbles. I did not miss the look but had no time. I rushed to the next room with a stifled hysterical giggle at how I had appeared. The bomb threat proved a hoax—fortunate considering the designated search party.

The department expanded with Joan Stanko—a non-medical person with videotape expertise. Her presence allowed us to videotape small in-services and to show them on the units with portable televisions—not so portable. The large, old-fashioned tube television was heavy. It and the VCR player, also much larger than modern DVD players, were pulled to the units on huge carts—taller than we were. I had graduated from moving beds to moving televisions! Lots of muscle!

I started a series called *Peggy's Petit Pointers*. Loved the alliteration! The pointers were about clinical nursing care or use of equipment. Joan's video equipment room was as large as my kitchen. She had the ability to splice and do voice-overs. The tape was large and industrial grade which could not be played in a home machine. Working with Joan, particularly demonstrating equipment, I became accustomed to lights, camera, action and retakes—as well as writing scripts for videos and a smattering of directing.

One of my more memorable in-services was crafted in response to a growing number of employee back injuries. There had been previous in-services about *proper body mechanics* by the Director of Physical Therapy. She was a very nice person but a very ho hum speaker. To handle it again and to engage all personnel, not just nurses, I wrote a script about Nurses Raggedy Ann and Raggedy Andy—played by Christine and Claude. They were dressed up as their characters—complete with orange yarn hair and painted cheeks. I played television commentator Barbara "Wawa" earnestly introducing the predicament of Raggedy Andy whose back hurt because he was carrying and lifting things improperly. Raggedy Ann pantomimed to him in exaggerated style how to maintain a broad base of support, keep objects close to his center of gravity, how to squat from the hip, not bend from the waist and how to avoid twisting when pulling a patient up in bed. Our humorous approach to an oft-repeated topic met positive reviews.

Another form of in-service offered monthly was Lunch 'n Learn. Nursing and non-nursing staff could bring their trays into a room adjacent to the cafeteria to watch a movie during their lunch break. Usually, they were feel-good movies about interpersonal relations, spirituality, and safety issues.

In 1982, *the Tax Equity and Fiscal Responsibility Act (TEFRA)* changed the way hospitals did business. It was the genesis of *Diagnosis Related Groups (DRGs)* used to determine hospital re-imbursement from Medicare—the bulk of our patients. It was a prospective payment system. Previously, hospitals had billed a fee for services rendered. Now they were reimbursed by diagnosis related group, no matter how many services had been used.

Before DRG's, St. Anthony's had boasted a census of almost four hundred. After *DRGs*, the census was whittled to sometimes less than two hundred. Why? Because doctors were encouraged to discharge patients before the amount of money that had been allotted for their diagnosis had been totally used. *DRGs* not only dictated how much money a given diagnosis was worth, but how many days were allotted for hospitalization. If the patient exceeded the expected days or money allotted, the hospital "ate" the cost of unreimbursed care. No wonder the census—and income—dropped. Suddenly, the hospital was consumed with finding less expensive ways to provide care. Previously staff had regarded providing care as a beneficent endeavor—not a dollars and cents business operation.

Administration wanted to involve the entire hospital community in the business of cutting waste and providing expeditious care. The task fell to the Education Department—specifically to me.

I originated a game based on Monopoly.® For the game, the player was a hospital administrator who drew a patient, a diagnosis and a specific amount of play money. The focus was to consider the actual cost to the hospital of the care that was provided—not the charge to the patient. For example, a CAT scan did not just cost thirty minutes of electricity but millions to buy the machine and salaries of techs who run it. The token represented the patient with a specific disease and money allotment. Beginning with Admission and ending at Discharge, along the way, the patient could land on specific tests, operations, etc. which cost the hospital a specific amount of money to provide or would prolong his stay. He could land in Isolation (originally Jail) and be forced to pick up an activity card set up to represent positive or negative hospital events. A negative event could be that the hospital painted with a subpar paint which wasted money and required more money to repaint. Kathy Quail, who joined our department as ER Nurse-Specialist, played endless games with me to test things out. Surprisingly, it worked fairly well. Some administrators' money remained after their patient was discharged—others were in the red.

I had the boards printed at a map-making company and laminated after we colored them. We held DRG mandatory in-services in the auditorium for all disciplines, trying to mix disciplines at each card table—a housekeeper with a lab person, an EKG tech and an RN. We roamed between card tables, helping where needed and summarizing points. Each table represented a different hospital. Some finished with money remaining; other hospitals did not. It illustrated the value of hospitals banding together (Columbia, HCA, and BayCare) to share expenses and services. It also illustrated the advantage of a diverse patient mix. The process was a good team-building exercise as well as a revelation about hospital finances.

Providing education, we were a creative group, obviously willing to look silly in the interest of promoting staff awareness and education. Rosemary, our Director after Molly retired, engaged a woman from St. Petersburg Junior College to administer the Myers-Briggs Aptitude Test[1] to Education Department members. I had taken it while working at Shands and wondered if I had changed. I had not—and was even more so. Other department members had never taken the test. Test scores are placed on a continuum between four sets of dichotomies:

Extrovert (E)......... Introvert (I);
Sensing(S)........... Intuitive(N);
Thinking(T) .... Feeling (F);
Judging(J) .... Perceptive(P).

Notice that one pole is rational (ESTJ) and one is irrational (INFP). I tested completely irrational! When the consultant explained how our individual traits/strengths combined to make one super functioning department, it clicked. We were very fortunate to have team members who complemented one another. Joannie was a woman of action—she liked to do in-services and preferred someone else to plan them. I was the dreamer, planner and developer but I hated a mechanical repetitious grind. Once we understood our own Myers-Briggs profiles and how they worked synergistically within our group, we became stronger and less apologetic about our weaknesses—more willing to volunteer our strengths.

As a department and individually, we were always involved in professional development—either attending peers' con-ed programs, or intra-departmental education. We did not just provide education and care, but we were intellectually nourished. Outside of work, Claude and I took a Pinellas Technical Education Center (PTEC) class about computers but the information about bits and bytes was not very helpful in an era when personal computers were just beginning to reach the market. Later we took a graduate course on alcoholism, offered at the USF St. Petersburg campus. By then Claude was working on his master's in counseling.

I had an opportunity to present an unusual form of in-service when a new device, the Infusaid Pump was first used in the hospital. A patient with whom I had been working for some time had an Infusaid Pump implanted and was ready for his chemotherapy. The Infusaid Pump delivered chemotherapy continuously in small amounts. The size and shape of a hockey puck, it was implanted on the abdominal wall. The fact that it was totally covered with skin made it less likely to become infected than an external pump. Inside the pump was an expandable gas surrounding a bellows-like inner chamber. The gas naturally strove to expand, exerting pressure on the bellows, forcing the medication out of the container, through a tube to the vascular system. No battery was needed. The pump was calibrated to normal body temperature and the atmospheric pressure at the altitude in which the patient lived. For example, the pump would be calibrated differently for someone living in the Appalachian Mountains than in sea-level St. Pete. In other situations, the pump, loaded with morphine, could be used for pain relief, its catheter placed in the intrathecal space of the spinal cord.

To fill the pump, the skin then diaphragm were punctured with a Huber non-coring needle. Then strong force was required to fill the chamber, compressing the resisting gas. It was not an easy procedure for the doctor. The patient would only feel the needle stick.

Our oncologists had no experience with the pump. This patient was one of theirs. Arrangements were made for a representative from the company to provide a videotape in-service and to answer questions. He arrived but the oncologist did not. I asked questions and viewed the tape—which the rep left with me. When the doctor arrived that evening to fill the pump, I was ready with the videotape. He passed on watching it, insisting that I talk him through it at the bedside. Imagine trying to instruct him while making it appear that he was teaching me. *So, then you palpate the puck for the center, right, Dr?* We managed. The patient thought the doctor taught me well. The scene was repeated in another oncologist's office later when I was summoned to do the same thing.

Our Homes and Our Educators

Over the fourteen years that I worked in the Education Department we had many homes and some revolving members. Initially we were in an approximately ten-by-ten-foot basement room right next to Housekeeping on a corridor terminating with the morgue. In our small room there was a couch and three desks for Claude, Joan, Christine and me. One day, Joan and I were in the office when we heard the most horrific scream coming from the direction of the morgue. We looked at each other and dashed down, throwing open the door to the morgue. There we found the diener collecting specimens from a plainly dead corpse. We never discovered where that scream had come from—he denied hearing it.

As our group enlarged, we moved across the hall, nearer Rosemary & Molly's office and under the old East Building chapel which later became nuclear medicine.

Our office was a large, converted storage/telephone terminal room. We had it painted yellow to bring some cheer into the dank, dark tunnel-like room. The blessing was that there were two cellar windows. Christine and I were set up under one, Claude under the other and Joannie behind us. My mother, newly retired, volunteered for our department. She arrived one day to find Resusci-Annie on the floor near my desk. Annie was blonde. My mother almost had a heart attack thinking that it was her newly deceased daughter.

There was room for a secretary. One summer, our secretary was a young debutante who would resume college in the fall. Her talents lay more in seductive

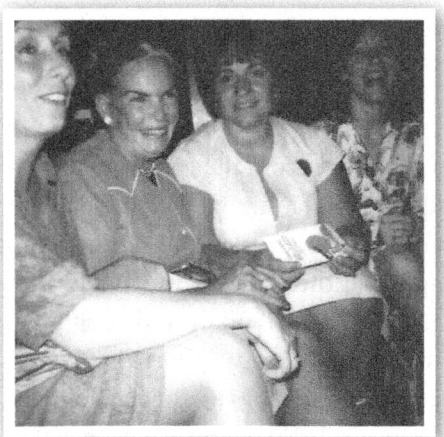

Figure 12 *Molly's Retirement Party. Left to Right: Peggy, Molly, Rosemary and Christine at Arigato.*

dressing than in secretarial skill, but she kept the maintenance men at our beck and call. Though we had several, our longest serving secretary was Anna Collins—fiftyish, married, an Irish-Bostonian and a smoker. Her favorite expression was that she had to *drop a tear* (urinate/smoke). Her patience was short with younger department members, but she was indeed skilled.

After a couple of years, all of us, except Rosemary and Anna, were moved to the second floor of the old Friary across Eleventh Street above the credit union. A former community room on the second floor was used for classes. Individual "cells" were re-made into offices. Outreach Van (mobile bus used for screenings) Director, John Miseroy and RN, Linda Rice, were down the hall.

With the completion of the professional office building (POB) facing Fifth Avenue, we were reunited over there. Rosemary, our department head, collaborated with an Ocala obstetrician, Dr. Doug Hall who had been a resident when I worked at Shands. They originated the *Pregnagym*—structured, supervised exercise classes for pregnant women who wanted to stay in shape for labor and delivery. The *Pregnagym*, later franchised, was located on the first floor of the POB. It was furnished with Nautilus® equipment. To direct the new program, an exercise physiologist and her assistant were added to our department. These two new employees collaborated with the Cardiopulmonary Nurse Specialist to run the *Cardiopulmonary Rehab Program* where participants exercised on the machines while their hearts were monitored.

Rosemary was a mover and a shaker. She very definitely leaned in [2] to the extent that some interpreted as abrasive. Ambitious for our department, she was also personally ambitious. Her talent was utilizing people with diverse expertise.

With the help of each of us with specialties and through beaucoup research, she formulated an *Employee Wellness Program*. It made use of the Outreach bus to offer wellness screenings and counseling—eye, cardiovascular, nutritional, risk assessments—whatever a company wanted to buy to offer its employees. Our competition was Bayfront which had the Times Publishing Company contract. Our largest contract was with Honeywell. At the time, *TEFRA* and *DRGs* hit the hospitals causing depleted re-imbursement, lower census and shorter length of stay. The *Employee Wellness Program* provided additional, balancing revenue and a valuable marketing tool.

I designed some of the handouts used for the wellness programs and learned to perform some of the screening tests including the air puff test (tonometry) for glaucoma. We educators volunteered to man tables in malls, taking blood pressure, testing blood sugar and cholesterol and then counseling. I learned to drive the Outreach bus—no small task—on I-275 and narrow Fourth Street North.

At one point, our department heads were administered a health risk assessment which Rosemary had purchased from a company specializing in risk assessment. Claude and I counseled the department heads about the results and the lifestyle choices which could ameliorate their risks. Most risks would be obvious to anyone—smoking, poor diet, activity choices, or family history. I was tasked with explaining to an African American male department head that, according to the risk assessment tool, his greatest risk of death was homicide!

In the late 80s, we moved to the basement of the newly-built west section of the hospital under the lobby. Adjacent to our department was a series of eight classrooms, some with dividers to make larger or smaller rooms. Rosemary did not come with us. She had moved up to Administration after growing the department exponentially. The *Employee Wellness Program*, *Pregnagym* and *Cardiopulmonary Rehab* folks stayed with her. Her assistant director, Susan Steele, RN was named Education Department Director. Susan, masters-prepared, was a fair-skinned natural blonde in her mid-thirties, a bit self-conscious about her blue-collar family roots. She could be very polished or very blunt. Susan meant well but did not have the maturity or sway with administration to carry the department as had Rosemary or Molly. Her moods were mercurial. Intelligent and savvy, she intuited that, financially, hospitals could no longer afford the luxury of people like us—unless there was a specific, concrete, marketable skill—like wound care nurse. Nothing esoteric or ambiguous. We had a Childbirth Educator. Susan partnered with her and others to learn to become a childbirth educator. She also immersed herself in Christine's expertise as an enterostomal therapist. Susan read the writing on the wall that times were again changing. In a few years she became Bayfront's wound care nurse.

Claude was educator for the GU team—male orderlies who placed and managed Foley catheters in men. Claude had his own portable model of the male genitalia for his classes. Female members of the department teased him mercilessly about his "Wang." Claude assisted one of the urologists to evaluate penile tumescence—determining the penis' ability to form an erection. A man would be admitted to a private room to sleep over-night while Claude monitored a machine outside his door connected to the patient's penis. It graphed the number and strength of erections during sleep. The information contributed to a more specific diagnosis than just "impotence" and could lead to appropriate treatment.

Claude was a good sport. On one occasion, he enlisted the Education Department in an ambitious plan to provide an educational program for another hospital's GU techs. He set us up at stations around a large room, each of us with a male genital model. The stations featured either insertion or irrigation techniques for the visiting students whom we critiqued as they demonstrated. My long-dead father would have died of embarrassment had he realized what I was doing.

Christine Bennett—later, Christine Joughin—had been my student at SPJC and a very fearful, shy one. As enterostomal therapist she blossomed. Initially, she was leery of contacting doctors to request orders. We rehearsed, me playing the part of a grumpy doctor, helping her to choose responses. She was wonderful at enterostomal therapy and, with time and experience, she became even better. Once she told me that she had known that she would bloom in her thirties and indeed that proved true. She succeeded in getting the surgeons to use her to mark the stoma site before surgery to avoid placement in a poor location where it would be difficult to form a seal with the pouch. She insisted on calling the ostomy bags "pouches." A kangaroo became her symbol. She sometimes wore a new brand of pouch filled with water under her uniform—she did not have an ostomy—but she wanted to make sure that the pouch was comfortable and functional for her patients. She became expert in wound care at a moment when development and marketing of wound care products was accelerating. Sharing an office with her was a distinct advantage to me.

GYN-Oncology Nurse-Specialist

When I first arrived in June of 1976, more surprise awaited than the new Education Department. Understanding that my title would be GYN and Oncology Nurse-Specialist, I was surprised to discover that I was only *Women's* Oncology Nurse-Specialist. The *Men's* Oncology Nurse-Specialist would be Claude, concomitantly the OR Educator. Shades of my Catholic high school—segregating the sexes! The catch—neither Claude nor I had any previous experience with oncology—other than personal. Additionally, Claude was not pleased about being pulled away from the OR.

When life gives you lemons, make lemonade. I decided to do just that—make lemonade. Claude and I needed to improve our knowledge base. As GYN Nurse-Specialist, I wanted to observe some of the more common GYN operations. That was a piece of cake since the obstetricians with whom I had worked were happy to include me. Claude eased my way with OR personnel. I found the vaginal and abdominal operations interesting. I also witnessed several mastectomies. Observing the positioning of patients and the mechanics involved helped me to explain the resulting post-operative issues to both patients and staff.

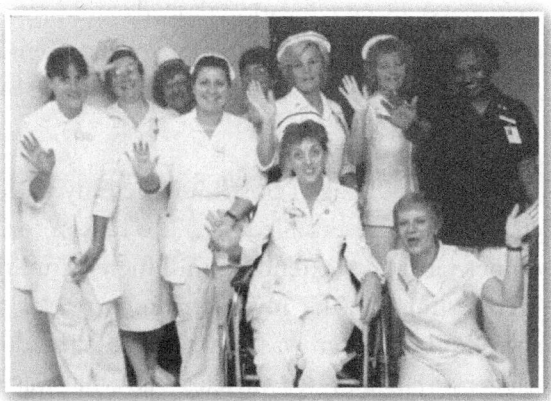

Figure 13 GYN Staff Wave to Retiring Head Nurse, Mrs. Maxwell. *Caps were still worn but now nurses were permitted pants. The Unit Secretary is at right in a navy top.*

I followed-up with pathologists, Doctors Reilly and Davis, observing the process of examining whatever tissue had been removed—the basis of the <u>Path</u>(ology) *Report.* Initially the pathologist dictated *macro* observations while dissecting the specimen (uterus, ovaries, breast tumor) on a butcher block. A microphone suspended above the table was turned on/off with a foot peddle. I learned the difference between a *frozen* and a *permanent* section. A *frozen section* is evaluated at the time of surgery. A sliver of tissue is "freeze dried" and examined under a microscope by a pathologist. It establishes the type of surgery needed while the patient is still under anesthesia. The *permanent section* can take several days to be read because of the number of steps used to prepare it. But it is more accurate.

The histologists, one of whom was fellow St. Paul's grad Mary Ann Damato, were happy to show me how, for *micro,* specimens were imbedded in paraffin. Then microscopic shavings at intervals were taken of the tissue, placed on a slide and put through several stages of stains. Only after days of prep was the slide interpreted by the pathologist. One of my more memorable observations in pathology was dissection of an ovary with "chocolate cysts" caused by endometriosis. The chocolate was old blood. Endometriosis is a condition in which the lining of the uterus (endometrium) grows outside the uterus on abdominal organs and sheds every month with menstruation. It can be extremely painful. Later, when teaching endometriosis, I served the nurses syrupy chocolate candy to help them remember.

The designated GYN floor, 3 SW, was just south of the OB unit. My efforts were concentrated. Each of the educators had been assigned their own units. Mine was all of third floor excluding OB. I collaborated with the Head Nurses (unit managers) about educational needs and provided around-the-clock education and support. As GYN Nurse-Specialist, I enjoyed not only teaching the GYN nurses about many aspects of GYN nursing but also intervening when needed with patients.

When a middle-aged post hysterectomy patient was upset on the day of discharge, the nurses called me. The reason for her hysterectomy had been endometrial cancer extending millimeters into the myometrium—the very thick uterine muscle. The myometrium provides a great barrier to avoid further spread. The woman was upset because the doctor had "told" her that she had cancer *throughout* her muscles—so what was the use? I asked the physician to return to the patient and explain that only the muscle of her uterus had been involved—and that it had been entirely removed. Anxiety prevented her from hearing what the doctor had said. Yes, I did explain, too, but her doctor's pronouncements carried more weight.

A thirty-five-year-old, married woman was post abdominal hysterectomy with bilateral salpingo-oophorectomy: removal of uterus, ovaries and tubes. The operation was for intractable endometriosis. Think chocolate cysts. I was called by the nurses who thought her behavior odd. Nervously the patient explained that the doctor had performed a total hysterectomy. She believed that this meant removal of the vagina, too. Not able to have sex, she was certain that her husband would leave her. I explained that she still had a vagina and, using a plastic model, explained the operation. I notified the physician who would re-enforce my explanation.

A similar belief was held by a twenty-two-year old woman in tears after a hysterectomy for recurrent pelvic inflammatory disease. Pelvic Inflammatory Disease (PID) was usually gonorrhea and difficult to treat in women. Antibiotics would be first line approach—TAH & bilateral S&O would be the last choice. The woman verbalized that sex wouldn't be the same. Her boyfriend's penis couldn't fit into her uterus anymore. I explained anatomy using diagrams, divulging that the penis can never fit into the uterus on anyone. I listened and encouraged her to ask questions.

Though there were probably plenty of patients who took misconceptions about their surgeries or body parts with them to the grave, I did my best by asking open ended questions—*how will this affect your life?*—*What did the doctor say?*—to discover them. I used these situations in my con-ed classes and in-services to make nurses aware of common misconceptions and ways to discover them.

Increasingly aware that women, including nurses, could know very little about their bodies, I originated an eight-week GYN nursing class. It was repeated on a yearly basis. Searching for a GYN nursing text book, I found nothing that fit the bill. Medical textbooks droned on concentrating on cell pathology. I couldn't see the nurses reading multiple journal articles in the library as I had done. So, I settled on a newly popular book—*Our Bodies Ourselves*[3] by the Boston Women's Health Book Collective. It touched on all aspects of women's reproductive health. Lesbianism had a section in the book, but I didn't cover that. As early as 1976, St. Anthony's mission statement declared that care or employment would not be denied because of race, creed or *sexual preference*. Anatomy & physiology, abortion, family planning, menarche, menopause, STD's, fertility and GYN issues were covered in the book and discussed. One of the nuns, a retired RN, registered for the course and purchased the book. Next thing I knew, she had complained to her superior, Sister Gladys, who had complained to the administrator, who complained to Molly. *Complained* is a euphemism. Tempers flared. Never again was I to use this book. Any book used in the future would need to be cleared through Pastoral Care. So much for freedom of speech! But I continued to teach the same subject for years—sans book. My feeling was that it was fine to disapprove of abortion and birth control—but it was nice if you understood what you disapproved. Nurses, as health professionals, had a responsibility to be knowledgeable.

I've described the GYN role first—because it was the most well-defined. There was a GYN unit; there were a small group of gynecologists; there was only one GYN Nurse Specialist (me). For oncology, there was no designated unit; Claude and I were two sexually segregated nurses with no oncology experience. To compound matters, *Administration had never fully informed the physicians of our existence.*

Observing in surgery and pathology had expanded my GYN expertise and initiated networking with departments which impact a cancer patient. I always used them as resources. Pastoral Care, Blood Bank, Dietitians, Oncologists, Pathologists, Rehab Therapists—I consulted them all. They were part of the nursing classes which I offered. But Claude and I needed more.

I discovered that the relatively new (at least to the area) medical specialty of medical oncology was practiced by two physicians at St. Anthony's. One was Michael Lynch a tall, black haired, blue eyed, Kennedyesque Irish Bostonian. His office was behind Bayfront Hospital. The other oncologist who practiced primarily at St. Anthony's, was Julio Ochoa. Dr. Ochoa was a post-Castro Cuban expatriate. Managing to escape, he had left parents and family behind. Educated in Spain, he completed residencies in the US. Dr. Ochoa was not as tall as Dr. Lynch but similarly handsome with black hair and piercing blue eyes. Though his children compared him to "the Fonz," from *Happy Days* on television, I thought he resembled John Travolta, the star of the movie, *Grease*.

The day we met, I bravely entered a nurses' station where Dr. Ochoa charted on one of his patients. I was in full nursing battle regalia (cap/white uniform and stockings). I listened to him pointedly question one of the nurses about a policy to which he had probably contributed. *Oh boy! Self-important*, I thought. When he finished quizzing the nurse, I introduced myself as the new Oncology Nurse Specialist. He might have been unaware that there was going to be one, but he addressed me cordially. I decided to be honest, humble and blunt, "I have a master's degree but have no experience with oncology and would like your help." He suggested that we, Claude and I, meet with him at a certain hour each Thursday morning to make rounds.

The man was awesome. His knowledge, which I absorbed like a sponge, was unending as was his patience. Claude was less enthusiastic but also appreciated Dr. Ochoa's generosity.

Dr. Ochoa taught us the elements of staging a tumor (using the TNM method—T = Tumor, N = Nodes (regional), M=distant Metastases.) and grading it (cells well-differentiated to totally undifferentiated) to determine the proper course of treatment. We became versed in different treatment protocols, not only for each type of cancer but for different stages of the same type of cancer. His words were spoken with a very thick Cuban accent, making the science exotically compelling. Sheep erythrocytes became *cheap* erythrocytes, linen became *leenon*, nausea was *nowsia* and liver became *leeber*. One day, Dr. Ochoa sat at a patient's bedside and declared, "I think we should do a liver scan." The man turned to me dead-serious, "I didn't know I had a leeber. What's a leeber?"

Through Dr. Ochoa, we learned the difference between anecdotal studies (the basis of unproven methods) and legitimate, evidence-based scientific studies. He reviewed basic assessment and treatment of oncologic complications such as congestive heart failure (Lasix and Lanoxin) and hypercalcemia (hydration, Lasix, activity). Here was my *REAL* Med-Surg class!

Always for the patient there was a smattering of hope, "I think we can do something about your . . . pain . . . cough . . . tumor progression . . ." Hope was not necessarily for cure but for the relief of suffering or for enjoyment of something tomorrow. In contrast to Dr. Ochoa, Dr. Lynch was all about acknowledging from the start that there was very little he could do about a diagnosis or that there were limitations to what the patient could expect. Some of his patients lamented that he had been far too pessimistic. On the other hand, Dr. Ochoa's patients sometimes complained that he had not been entirely candid with them about the seriousness of their disease. To make matters interesting, they covered for each other on weekends and holidays.

A fifty-seven-year-old affluent man with two high school-aged children was emaciated and developing pressure sores during his terminal hospital admission. His wife was more interested in playing golf than visiting. She knew he was dying. Dr. Ochoa continued to be pleasant and positive with the patient, making statements like a vague, "I think we can help . . . " To me the patient complained that he just wished Dr. Ochoa would level with him. If he were dying, he wanted to know about it so that he could plan. I was convinced. At my urging, Dr. Ochoa agreed to be honest. No sooner had Dr. Ochoa sat but the patient blurted, "Gee doctor, I hope you've come to tell me that I'll live to see my son graduate next year." Dr. Ochoa did not destroy that hope. I recognized then that it was okay to talk about powerlessness and death with a nurse. But the doctor's confirmation made it reality. Was ambiguity the better approach? I didn't know.

A fifty-two-year-old psychologist with ovarian cancer and lung metastases refused to acknowledge that she was dying. She became angry at Dr. Lynch's "negativity." She commented, "I once knew a woman whose family was so accepting of her impending death that she had no choice but to die."

The surgeon and GP (both "old guard" doctors) of a seventy-year-old Italian gentleman with stomach cancer had informed the family that the man was terminal. He had only three months. The family did not want the man *told* the time limit. He was simply aware that he had an unresectable tumor. When I visited him and his wife, we discussed the situation. He told me that he had fished for years with a friend who had the same condition. He knew that it could be a long time or a short time, that only God knew, and it was in His hands. I was impressed with the man's serenity and very realistic philosophy. Later, I was thanked by his wife for "not telling" her husband that he had three months. According to her, once the doctor had said three months, three months it was going to be. I wondered how his life would be with the whole family shielding him from *The Truth*. That man survived at least another year then I lost touch. Though the surgeon and GP had written him off, advising that seeing an oncologist would be a waste of time, his RN daughter-in-law had insisted that he consult one.

Obviously, each individual and family has its own approach to coping with cancer. Cancer represents multiple different diseases. Not all cancer is terminal. I was privileged to learn from the folks whom I was asked to see. In the beginning, all I needed was a nursing consult. If the nurse asked, it was probably a situation in which she felt conflicted in some way. Visiting the patient lead to teachable moments with the nurse. How could she better approach the patient in this situation? How did the patient interpret her actions or the doctor's actions? What was important to the patient? . . . to the nurse?

It was proven repeatedly that patients can easily misinterpret what is said due to their heightened anxiety. A fifty-seven-year-old woman with an EdD, highly placed in the school system was "opened and closed" when diffuse unresectable ovarian cancer was discovered. She was petrified because her surgeon made such a big issue of keeping her comfortable. It made *him* feel better. But she had deduced that she faced an immediate future of excruciating pain. Once she was exposed to a different perspective, she managed to live—uncomfortable—but pain free until she died at home.

Administration had not paved the way for the Oncology Clinical Nurse-Specialist position with the physicians. Eventually, I became Oncology Nurse-

Specialist for both sexes. Responding to nurses' needs, I was able, not only to lend patient/family/nurse emotional support, but to influence how nursing was conducted. I had no line authority so nurses' goodwill and respect for me were the only means of effecting change or of influencing the care of oncology patients hospital-wide.

Then the bottom dropped out. A fifty-something urologist reminded me of Henry VIII. He had russet hair, a ruddy complexion and a huge belly which proudly preceded him. His demeanor loudly proclaimed: *I am the cock of the walk, the lord of all I survey.* A stinky, fat, lit cigar accompanied him everywhere—in the elevator (illegal); in the nurses' station—everywhere. When he visited his patients, he placed his mouth-moistened cigar on the edge of the nurses' station desk. Like the Saint, he wore his Catholicity as a shield. He used medical oncologists rarely—true of many old guard physicians raised on the principle: if it is unresectable, it is untreatable.

I had seen one of Henry VIII's patients per a nursing request. When he discovered my visit, he blew it into a maelstrom. He wanted absolute control over who saw his patients and lobbied the rest of the medical staff to see it his way. No matter that he had absolutely no practical control over which housekeeper, CNA, LPN, RN or clergy interacted with his patients—he objected to contact with a master's prepared RN.

The brouhaha came to a head when I was summoned to an evening medical staff meeting with the chiefs of all the medical sections and the administrator. Henry VIII was Urology section chief. Joe Cool was GYN section chief. Oncologists were probably represented by Internal Medicine. The Gastroenterology section chief was a kind southern gentleman who pulled a chair out for me at the huge board room table. I sat next to him and faced an inquisition before an unusually silent administrator. The prime inquisitors were Henry VIII and a crabby older surgeon who often confused himself with God. Joe Cool and some of the less pompous others came to my defense. The main contention/fear was that I would "counsel" patients to choose a specific form of therapy, second-guess the doctor's plan or inform them that they had cancer or were about to die. Of course, I denied it all. I was providing emotional support and helping the patient to deal with whatever reality he heard. My consults were always documented in the nurses notes and available for scrutiny—unlike Pastoral Care at that time. One of the participants, partially ameliorated, summarized, "Well you are a very nice girl (I was in my thirties) but who knows who would take your position when you left it?" I was excused.

The result of the proceedings was that the Oncology Nurse-Specialist required a doctor's order to see a patient. The GYN section and the oncologists gave me across-the-board permission to visit any of their patients without a specific order. Though it miffed me that doctors could have that much control (Doctors fill beds, I was reminded), conversely, I was relieved not to see patients whose doctors would throw me to the wolves. There were plenty of patients to see. There was a plethora of projects afoot. Though fuming, I tended to be a glass half full kind of person.

Remember that there was no oncology unit but there was a gynecology unit. Lack of a specialized unit fragmented oncology care. There were no nurses who specialized in just oncology. Many oncology patients were repeaters who returned to the hospital monthly for their chemo and would draw comfort from consistency.

Some of the oncology drugs were themselves carcinogenic with repeated exposure. Special precautions to protect the staff were needed when the drugs were handled. If an IV infiltrated, some chemotherapy agents could be vesicants—destroying the tissue into which they leaked.

Because the drugs were tough on the vascular system, new methods of delivering them through a central line were beginning to be used. First it was the Hickman-Broviac which exuded from the chest like a strand of spaghetti. The under-the-skin part of the tube had a filtering cuff to prevent microorganisms from migrating beyond it; the end terminated in a blood vessel just above the heart. The Hickman-Broviac was followed by ports of various sizes. Ports were totally implanted under the skin—a much better barrier to infection. They could be accessed only with the special needle (a Huber non-coring) which punctured first the patient's skin and then the rubber diaphragm of the port resting just under the skin.

Some protocols for acute myelogenous leukemia (AML) required a month-long or more stay. In the hospital, the patient's immune system, platelets and red blood cells were destroyed in the interest of forming new, healthy cells. The interval between administering the chemo and discharge home could be a lethal one with potentially fatal bleeding or infection. Nurses who encountered AML induction remission chemotherapy needed to be able to plot when to expect what side effects. They needed to synchronize themselves and family members with the blood bank, so vital to the maintenance of life throughout the ordeal. Yet these patients were all over the place. It was as though Administration were saying, *Look, we've got an oncology nurse specialist. Why would we need a special unit?*

I repeatedly, using many different tactics, lobbied for an oncology unit. When an IV chemo agent (thankfully not a vesicant) infiltrated a woman's breast after the Huber needle slipped out of position in her med-port, Administration's answer was to in-service *those* nurses on *that* floor. It flew in the face of logic since the next day the same situation could occur on another floor. If I in-serviced all nurses on all floors, by the time they admitted a similar patient to their unit, they would have forgotten. It merits mention that there already were urology, cardiac, orthopedic, gyn and OB units.

Eventually, permission was obtained to make 3SW the unit for induction remission chemotherapy for AML. But, until I left the position after fourteen years, there was no oncology unit. That was a supreme disappointment. I constantly put out small fires with staff all over the hospital relating to chemotherapy, radiation therapy, and just general cancer misconceptions. Continuing education courses and in-services could never hope to reach all of the nurses who needed them. A few years before my departure, the hospital did develop a tumor registry which provided monthly tumor conferences per the American College of Surgeons' progressive guidelines. The surgeons were a vocal group. Had the oncologists been half as vocal, we might have had a unit. The oncologists, who now numbered four, were low key, don't-make-waves kind of guys. But they were infinitely more likeable than some of the surgeons.

I once read that physicians carry cemeteries in their heads. So do oncology nurses. Friends wondered if being an oncology nurse was depressing. I always answered no. Sobering, maybe, but not depressing. For the first few years as Oncology Nurse-Specialist, I was also involved with young expectant couples via the prepared childbirth classes. To friends, I was known as the *womb-to-tomb nurse*. Witnessing both ends of the continuum maintained my perspective. I joked that I was the *below the belt nurse*. It was important to retain a sense of humor—not at the expense of patients. I had not caused the cancer. No guilt. If I wallowed in maudlin sympathy rather than empathy, I would be unable to don my big girl panties to help the patient. I had the ability to extend myself to be a solid and faithful presence to the patient and family. In my bag of tricks were many interventions which could make the path easier. The interventions covered a broad spectrum of physical, emotional and cognitive approaches.

To stay whole, to stay healthy, I engaged in a wide variety of coping mechanisms.

I might come home in the evening from an abysmal situation and laugh raucously at a *Mork and Mindy* episode on TV. Somehow, Mork's inane "*NanuNanu*" was hilarious. There were multiple opportunities at work to have fun with fellow educators—carving a pumpkin for the pumpkin-carving contest; designing giant Christmas cards for the hospital Christmas card competition. There were dog parties in my back yard. There was tennis. There were crafts. And there was yoga.

I learned to practice hatha yoga and began a wonderful friendship via an experience with a dying patient. Fran was dying of advanced ovarian cancer which had metastasized to her lungs. Her X-ray demonstrated lungs stippled with cancer. Increasingly short of breath and unable to assume any position except head elevated high, pillows under her arms to open her rib cage, she was extremely anxious. One day, her yoga instructor visited and closed the door for an hour. When the door opened, Fran, flat in bed, was more flexible and never again needed to resume that extreme upright posture. The secret was Jeanne Gootson, an incredible yoga instructor who had put Fran through progressive relaxation and guided imagery; then guided her through gentle exercise, focusing on flexibility, followed by more relaxation. She had left Fran with a relaxation tape of her voice and gentle music which Fran used until she died.

Convinced that I had witnessed a miracle and looking to increase my armamentarium, I enrolled in Jeanne's evening yoga class. Eventually, several fellow educators also enrolled. Jeanne was an amazing instructor. She suffered from Multiple Sclerosis (MS). Though better than at her worst, Jeanne still had some visual impairment. From Jeanne I learned even more ways to help patients via slow, calming voice, relaxation, and guided imagery. One evening, after attending yoga class, I returned to the hospital to visit a very upsetting situation. The intelligent, articulate, and well-read woman was in ICU on a ventilator. Unable to talk, she wrote short notes. When I arrived, she wrote, "You look relaxed." She seemed to relax, too, and we had one of our best "conversations." I realized that yoga had put me in a state that had made me more open and accepting—both visibly and internally. Since then, Fran and Jeanne, who became my very good friend, have passed away. Namaste,[4] Fran. Namaste, Jeanne.

Community Activism

Community involvement in our areas of specialization was a must for the educators. Each of us belonged to professional organizations related to our specialty. Several of us joined organizations in the broader community. Since graduate school, I had been a member of NAACOG, the Nurses Association of the American College of OB-GYN. The title reminded me of the little sisters of ATΩ. In principle, I would have much preferred to belong to a purely nursing organization. However, being a step-child of ACOG assured many MD lecturers at programs and conventions. I also attended the huge ICEA convention here at the St. Pete Hilton and enjoyed the plethora of maternity-related topics. Once employed as Oncology Nurse-Specialist, I joined the Oncology Nursing Society (ONS). Later, under their auspices and after testing, I became oncology certified (OCN).

The most significant organization which I joined was the Pinellas County Unit of the American Cancer Society. Initially, I contacted them to see if they had any publications which I could use for my classes. I was amazed to discover that they had many professional (medical) publications as well as ones geared toward the lay community. All were free in whatever quantities I needed. After becoming an ACS "frequent flyer," I was invited to join their Service Committee composed of other health professionals and cancer survivors. *Sure*, said I, welcoming an opportunity to network. Members of the Service Committee were other nurse professionals; physicians, including Dr. Michael Lynch; and cancer survivors representing visitation programs and support groups. ACS had other committees, too—Public Education, Professional Education and Crusade (fundraising). The latter was composed mostly of society women who staged fundraising events or coordinated phone-a-thons or door-to-door solicitation. The ACS was active. More than eighty-percent of their budget was directed to research, education and service. A small paid staff guided us and carried out whatever decisions we made. After a few years, I was elected to the board and eventually became president of the Pinellas County Unit. That was groundbreaking considering that the presidency previously had alternated between MD and a socially prominent Crusade representative. No fundraiser, I was considered "medical." Monetarily, I was not able to donate much but I was generous with service.

Reach to Recovery was a long-standing ACS program lead by Bertha Kopf with her husband, Dave. She raised large sums via her annual fashion show featuring post mastectomy models. The *Reach to Recovery* program volunteers were mastectomy patients trained by Bertha. They visited new hospitalized mastectomy patients—provided that there was a doctor's order. They had a bag of gifts for the patient, but the message was: this has not changed who you are, and you can continue to look good. Bertha's gals were heavily schooled in appearance. She routinely visited surgeons to assure that the referrals kept coming.

Like *Reach to Recovery*, but far less structured were the *Laryngectomy Visitors* and their support group. Laryngectomy is the removal of the voice box (larynx) and vocal cords due to cancer. Some visitors used esophageal speech, swallowing air and "burping" it back—speaking on the vibrating burp. Others used an electrolarynx, a hand-held vibrator, held to the throat while mouthing words. No matter their method, their visit meant the world to people who woke from surgery thinking that they would never speak again. An additional outreach was the *Ostomy Support Group* and *Ostomy Visitors* who helped people adjust to bowel or bladder surgery. Their meetings were held at St. Anthony's and my co-worker Christine, our ET, was their advisor.

Shortly after I became involved with the American Cancer Society, it developed a new program entitled *I Can Cope*, reminding me of the basic childbirth class—for cancer patients. The message was survivorship via knowledge. Some content was psycho-social; some was geared toward medical terminology. Mary Ann Wanuscha, MSW from Bayfront Hospital and I held the first series at St. Anthony's and the second at Bayfront. Later, Bayfront's Pam Rak-Srejma, MSW and I held them episodically.

In the first series, there were just a few participants. I asked our PR department for some publicity. A local newscaster and his retinue of light and camera people arrived at one of the classes and took over. The participants were in a circle. At one point, the interviewer dropped to his knees and, with unbelievable insensitivity, thrust a microphone in a participant's face asking, "How does it feel to have cancer?" Crass! He continued around the circle. One of the folks just slipped out before he could be cross-examined. It made the news. I promised myself—never again. Our purpose was to help—not to exploit. We had just emerged from an era when the word *cancer* was never mentioned. Only in 1974 had First Lady Betty Ford shocked the world by going public about her breast cancer and mastectomy.

Not long after initiating *I Can Cope* (for which I flew around the state to train others), Pam and I realized that *Reach to Recovery* alone did not address enough of the issues faced by women with breast cancer. *Reach to Recovery* focused on maintaining range of motion and appearance. But women with breast cancer faced more: the cancer itself; mastectomy long-term complications; chemo and hormonal therapy; family members' reactions. Pam and I founded the *Breast Cancer Support Group*, creating mild friction with Bertha & Dave Kopf who were highly identified with *Reach to Recovery* and felt that it addressed all needs of the breast cancer patient. Our group met monthly at the ACS office. Sometimes we carried the ball ourselves. Other times there were planned speakers—physicians or prosthetists. Ours was a good group whose members gave and received mutual support. Pam and I worked well together—each picking up on something the other had missed.

The group possessed a unique humor. One evening, a group member shared a dream she had. Her missing breast was crawling its way up I-275 to reunite with her. She nudged her husband awake, insisting that they had to find it. He clapped his hands, "Splat!! A Mack truck hit it. Now go back to sleep." The room roared with laughter. Another woman with bilateral mastectomy bragged that she had two sets of prostheses—one small, the other large—giving her a choice of dressing sexy or demure. Another declared that she kept her gelatinous prosthesis in the refrigerator so that when she woke up on a hot day, it would cool her. Of course, it wasn't all jolly. There were significant and sometimes painful issues discussed, including recurrence. But, overall, it was positive, productive and helpful.

After several years facilitating the *Breast Cancer Support Group*, I had lunch with a surgeon—the first at St. Anthony's to offer immediate reconstruction after mastectomy. He claimed, with this procedure, his patient wouldn't need *Reach to Recovery* or the *Breast Cancer Support Group* because she woke up with a breast. In other words, it had never happened. Politely I disagreed. She had had cancer, she had had her breast and lymph nodes removed (potential for serious lymphedema), she could need chemo or hormonal therapy. Something *had* happened.

Most surgeons who performed mastectomy—all the ones I knew were men—believed that they had saved the woman's life, case closed. They minimized or denied complications resulting from the operation. Yet lymphedema, swelling of the affected arm, could be so severe as to make the arm useless. A woman who failed to obtain a prosthesis of equal weight to her remaining breast could develop spinal complications from the uneven weight distribution. I have known several with scoliotic spines. Some complained of an uncomfortable "wad" of flesh under their arms. Imagine cutting a fabric cone at the base and then sewing the remaining fabric together. It would "bunch." Sometimes the arm and adjacent underarm and mastectomy were numb; sometimes pins and needles. To have the chutzpah to remove a woman's breast it might have been necessary emotionally to minimize the consequences. If a surgeon spoke at the Breast Cancer Support Group, he could receive more feedback than he wanted.

It was not unusual for ACS staff to schedule me for radio or TV interviews related to cancer issues or programs. One morning, I returned to the hospital after having been interviewed on television. Soon, I received a peculiar request. A dying patient upstairs wanted to see the *TV Nurse*. Oh boy!? What could he possibly need? I entered the room with trepidation. The family—wife and adult children—sat or stood all around the bed of an obviously much-loved man. The patient semi-reclined—the strong *pater familias*. He was not worried about dying, he explained, but feared that his family—particularly his wife—could not survive without him. So, he fought letting go. I asked his family how they would manage. While acknowledging that they would miss him terribly, they related how they had prepared for the inevitable. His wife volunteered that she had been learning about their finances and assured her husband that, though his loss would be incomprehensible, she would be okay. He fell back on his pillow in relief, saying, "Okay. That's all I needed to know."

What had I done? Nothing. The "TV Nurse" had been a catalyst. Perceptualism. It wasn't about who I was or what I did—but who I was perceived to be. The Presence. Then the folks solved their own problems—very well, as only they could.

The ACS sponsored various professional education programs about current diagnosis and treatment of the various types of cancer. I attended or presented at many and encouraged hospital nurses to attend, too.

Hospice was an increasingly visible community resource. The same group whose beginnings I had witnessed now functioned. As with family-centered maternity nursing, for hospice, it was a few radicals who got things off the ground. The initial Pinellas hospice, *Elisabeth Kübler Ross Hospice*, was named after the famous physician and author of *On Death and Dying.*[5] After Kübler Ross became interested in out-of-body experiences and channeling the dead, she became too radical even for the founders. The name simply became *Hospice, then Hospice of the Florida Suncoast, then Suncoast Hospice.* It subsisted with donations. Marketing it was like marketing motherhood and apple pie. Who could resist an opportunity to donate? Hospice initially employed one RN and had volunteers. There was no brick and mortar entity. Care was provided in the home. I attended a community forum at which their nurse spoke. Her presentation convinced me that Hospice could be as unbendingly rigid as she accused hospitals of being—only in different ways. According to her, when the patient died at home, his face was never covered with a sheet—even if the family wanted it. There was the "ceremony" which was supposed to bring closure—dumping all the deceased's meds down the toilet (now illegal). I was unimpressed. Later, they employed a few other nurses—one, my former nursing student—on twenty-four-hour call and very stressed.

Two major events occurred which changed the course of hospice history. The first was financial. In 1979, The Health Care Financing Administration initiated demonstration programs in multiple hospices throughout the US to assess their cost effectiveness. The result was Medicare re-imbursement for hospice in 1982 as part of the Tax Equity and Fiscal Responsibility Act (TEFRA). TEFRA's purpose was to reduce cost. Hospice represented a means to encourage lesser use of expensive services by people who were dying and really did not benefit from them (the MRI to see if there is tumor progression; chemo when it is no longer effective). It was about death with dignity. This act was delivered during the Reagan presidency. As a result, Hospice was no longer a charity although donations were still welcome. It was reimbursed like any other legitimate medical service. That financial basis of hospice care was seminal.

Another equally important event for our Pinellas hospice was the appointment of Mary Labyak in 1980 as Program Director and later Administrator/CEO. Mary, an MSW, was a product of the traditional healthcare system and could articulate rational—not radical—goals. She had a talent for bringing like-minded professionals together within the organization and on state and national levels. Eventually, thanks to Mary, and the decision to make hospice reimbursable, Hospice became the largest hospice in the world with in-patient facilities, hospital contracts, nursing home outreach, survivor support and the home care with which it began.

Often my hospital patients were dying. It required a huge amount of attentiveness and guidance to assist some to move from acknowledging the illness; to acknowledging that it was terminal; to understanding that, to qualify for hospice insurance coverage, the doctor was required to claim that the death would be within six months. I explained that the doctor himself realized he was not omniscient but had to make the statement so that the patient could qualify for care. Patients could outlive the six months. Qualifiers like this were necessary because many patients could acknowledge that they were dying—but not so soon. In fact, too many of them waited until their last few days before acknowledging that death was imminent.

Once those stumbling blocks had been surmounted, there could be little time to get them home and into hospice care. Yet repeatedly I made the referrals only to discover, "Well, we're not available to do the intake on weekends. We'll get there in about four days." *Heck, by four days they could be gone. Let's strike while the iron is hot!* Out there in the community, hospice claimed to be the epitome of care when, in fact, it fell far short. Their marketing was better than their service. Hospice spokespersons claimed that hospitals were not doing their part to make referrals. But when referrals were made, the results were not always positive.

I was disgruntled and probably voiced it to my friend Mary Jean Etten who was on their Board. Next thing I knew, Mary Labyak made an appointment to see me. I had read Machiavelli.[6] I understood that it is wise to bring your critics into the fold. That is what she did to me, listening attentively to my complaints followed by an invitation to join one of their committees. I recognized the ploy and marveled at her slickness.

For a few years, I was on one of the Hospice committees composed of nurses and doctors. And then I was on their Board. In the late eighties when they dived head first into a huge fund-raising campaign, Hospice presented a program for the Board making it very clear that each Board member was expected to contribute several hundred dollars to initiate the campaign. That cinched it for me. I could not afford to make a large donation. I donated to St. Anthony's via payroll deduction and ACS where I was an active volunteer. So I resigned. I had been a squeaky wheel. Services offered, and their availability had improved during my tenure, attributable not to me but to the realistic and farsighted monitoring and leadership of Mary Labyak and the continued support and guidance of my friend, Mary Jean, committed to improving end-of-life care. Amazingly, for years afterward, older GP's still approached me declaring that one of their patients needed to go *TO* hospice, not realizing that, at that time, hospice was not a place but a patient/family care delivery system and philosophy. Now Suncoast Hospice has several campuses for in-patient and home care as well as collaborative agreements with hospitals and skilled nursing facilities. They continue to provide a valuable service at the end-of-life. Mary Labyak died under hospice care in 2012.

After three of my patients died leaving bereft widows, I formulated a means of providing continued support to all three—short of running myself ragged. I invited the three widows to have dinner in a POB classroom. I brought fried chicken and Greek salad and dressed the table up a bit. Though I knew each, the women were strangers to each other. As they interacted, the support they shared was obvious. They asked to meet again the following month. For multiple months, we met at each other's homes. There were common themes—*Why did this happen? I don't know how to . . . pay the bills, do repair work, etc.* Of course, it resonated with me, having experienced similar loss. My message to them was positive—you can, you will . . . but it is okay to let yourself feel what you are feeling now.

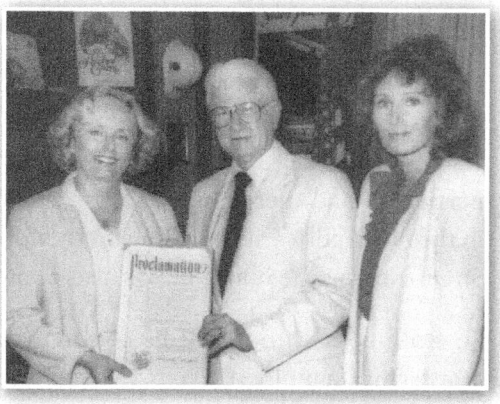

Figure 14 *As a Board Member of Hospice, I was asked to receive the* **St. Petersburg Mayor's Proclamation of Hospice Week**. *The Mayor is Dr. Ed Cole, a pediatrician with whom I had worked in the newborn nursery.*

Based on our interactions, I concluded that the hospital should offer a support group for the newly widowed. I organized a loose outline of what the group might entail—a closed-ended group of five sessions including one guest speaker of their choice. It could be an attorney (D'Arcy Clarie), or a funeral director (Dale Gunter or Terry Brett). Once it was a mechanic (Eugene Ruga). If the participants wanted to continue on their own afterward—fine. Administration's only caveat was that I include Pastoral Care. That made sense. Their monthly memorial service for families of patients who had died the previous month would be a conduit for referrals.

We began one evening in one of the classrooms at a round table of about five women in their sixties or seventies, the Director of Pastoral Care and me. We asked participants to introduce themselves and to share anything about their loss and what they hoped to gain from the discussion.

When it came to the priest's turn, he said that obviously he had not lost a spouse. He remembered that after his father had died, his mother had quickly followed. As the priest explained, "She was in her sixties; the kids had grown and were all out of the house—It was time." Talk about speaking without thinking! For subsequent widow support groups, only the nuns participated (Sister Pat, Sister Gail, Sister Claire)—and they were great! Until I left the Education Department, the groups continued. Many years later, I was pleased to meet the son of a gentleman who attended the support group. His father, now ill, needed continuing care. I was able to share how proud his dad had been of him.

Loaned to Junior College

In the winter term of 1986, the St. Petersburg Junior College Nursing Department needed a nursing instructor for the fourth session clinical group at Clearwater's Morton Plant Hospital. The Clearwater and St. Petersburg Nursing Departments had merged since my previous employment and were now housed in the old Webb's City building on the corner of Park Boulevard and Sixty-Sixth Street North. The building was also home to other health-related professions.

St. Anthony's, mindful of its community obligations, offered my services for that term. I happily obliged. Ten years without an oncology unit was frustrating. I needed respite. But respite was not in the cards. I had never worked at Morton Plant where my clinical group met. Not only did I not know my way around the huge hospital, but I lived a good forty-five minutes away. To make assignments, I left before dawn to arrive before change of shift. Fortunately, the students, on the last leg of their journey, were adept at most aspects of care. We had some good post-conferences. After ten years, some instructors with whom I had worked on the St. Pete campus remained.

One very cold afternoon in January 1986, while I drove from Morton Plant back to the Health Care Building, the car radio blared that the Challenger missile carrying a teacher into orbit had exploded after take-off.

After my brief MPH stint, I served as clinical instructor for the junior college at St. Anthony's where a few nursing students participated in a senior internship. Discovering that a patient on their unit had died, I volunteered several students and myself to clean and wrap the body. I coached them to be respectful since, considering documented near death experiences, we couldn't be certain of the patient's level of awareness or ability to hear. I explained rigor mortis, livor mortis, algor mortis and other peri-mortem changes. We discussed their reactions without the probing, all-hallowed "How do you feel about it?" that I had experienced in college. It was a difficult but good experience for these young (to nursing) students and a better introduction to death than most nurses receive.

Writing on the Wall

Though I continued to work with in-service, con-ed, community projects and counseling, I, too, read the writing on the wall. The character of our department had changed greatly since those early days. Most positions had turned over except for Christine, Joannie and me. Claude finished his master's, worked briefly on our substance abuse rehab unit, and then resigned to work for Comp Care, educating substance abuse units in other hospitals throughout the United States. Edna Clifton became Director of Nurses after Pat Ryan succumbed to lung cancer. Rosemary worked with administration to promote her outreach programs. Our department was not as influential as it had been. *DRGs* had transformed patient care delivery drastically. Several turnovers in the administrative team took penny-pinching to new levels. Middle managers were asked to take early retirement to save the cost of their salaries the size of which reflected their long tenure. They were replaced by new folks who made decisions unaware of their undesired consequences to other departments. The hospital grapevine source, the painters, were eliminated, replaced by contractors. (Later, the folly of this action must have been recognized and the same painters were re-hired.) The well-oiled, organized machine of St. Anthony's hit a very bumpy path.

I had been impressed by St. Anthony's newly formed Home Health Care Department. Bob Greene, MSW, our previous Social Service Director, and I had helped write the application for a state certificate of need to add a home health program. HH offices in the professional office building housed maybe five RN's and a handful of Home Health Aids (HHA's). The home health administrator was interesting—T Ecklund. Just T. T was a tall, tan, ash-blonde in her late thirties who wore dresses and very high heels with no stockings. Scandalous! She was Jewish and spoke with a thick Massachusetts accent. Her graduation from a Catholic school of nursing had prepared her for the politics of a Catholic hospital.

T's Director of Nursing, Jeanne Marie Reeves, was a hot number herself, matching T in the tan and the hair (long and blonde) departments. Her eyelashes were thick and clumpy with mascara. Her figure was Monroe-esque. But she was as real and as down to earth as public health instructor Virgie Pafford had been.

T had a flair for marketing her department. Whenever there was a Catholic holy day or event, she demanded that her staff come in from the field *in skirts* to attend the religious service. She wanted them visible! Internal marketing! She heartily encouraged her staff to attend our con-ed programs. They were undoubtedly the best educated nurses in St. Anthony's! I met them through my oncology and chemotherapy courses and was impressed by their common-sense approach. Unlike hospital-based nurses, they recognized the totality of the patient situation, not just the few days of hospital stay. Because I had followed some of my cancer patients in their homes, as well, I understood their perspective.

It was decision time. I left my position of fourteen years for the brave new world of Home Health Nursing. I had grown immensely during those years, becoming more multifaceted. I had been provider of care, counselor, educator, group leader, community activist, radio/TV veteran, public speaker. I had collaborated with and drawn together diverse disciplines to improve patient care. I had authored a complex self-study book about chemotherapy for nurses. I had creatively developed a monopoly-like game to explain *DRG's*—the very entity responsible for shrinking budgets, making anything less than essential—me—the elephant in the room. The Golden Age of hospital education departments was dust. Some hospitals would become dust very soon.

In home health, there would be hands-on nursing. Good. But there would be areas of Med-Surg nursing of which I had not dreamed since undergraduate school. Not so good. But could anything have been more different from maternity than oncology? I had survived—even flourished. I had a brain. Time to use it for a new adventure.

Endnotes

1. Isabel Briggs Myers et al., *MBTI Handbook: A Guide to the Development and Use of the Myers-Briggs Type Indicator Third Edition* (Sunnyvale, CA: Consulting Psychologists Press, 1998).

2. Sheryl Sandberg, *Lean In: Women, Work and the Will to Lead* (New York: Random House LLC, March 2013).

3. Boston Women's Health Book Collective, *Our Bodies Ourselves* (New York: Simon & Schuster, 1973).

4. Namaste is a Hindu word usually expressed with fingers steepled, palms together and a slight bow. It is a reverential greeting and acknowledgement of the Divine within us. It was how Jeanne began and ended each class.

5. Elisabeth Kübler Ross, *On Death and Dying* (New York: Scribner, 1969).

6. Niccolò Machiavelli, *The Prince* [1532]. *"People should either be caressed or crushed." Multiple world-wide translations.*

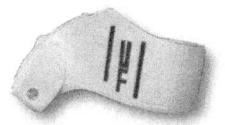

CHAPTER SIX
Out in the Field: 1990-2005

Home Health Nursing

Orientation to Home Health was held in a tiny office. The educator was Veronica Barrimond, a Jamaican RN with a beautiful lilting accent. Her idea of orientation was to sit me down to read procedure books. That was day one. Day two, she took me out for an admission. Never having witnessed one, I assumed that I would observe her. Instead, she had me do the admission while she watched. A more fumbling attempt could not be imagined. The first hurdle was reviewing the multi-page admission agreement with the patient, getting him to sign on the dotted line. It was permission to treat—I couldn't touch him until it was signed. Not very familiar with it myself, it was like *Mirandizing* him. *You have a right to remain silent. Anything you say or do may be used against you in a court of law. You have a right to an attorney . . .* Miranda was way more succinct. As homework that night, I read the agreement and summarized it on a small sheet of paper that I could read to patients until I knew it by heart.

Next came the physical assessment. It had been a long time since I had taken vital signs or performed other parts of the health exam. I had my own stethoscope and sphygmomanometer. Since physical assessment was not taught in my 1965 BSN program, I should have been at a disadvantage. But in the mid-eighties, several Education Department nurses and I had taken a lengthy series of classes about physical assessment. I still had the text. Don't think I didn't bone up! In this first visit, the process was not automatic. I was unable to do it while interacting with patient and family. I was slow. Later, I practiced, practiced, practiced. We were each supplied a glucometer, a hand-held machine for testing blood sugar. It required a finger-stick. I practiced on my own bloody fingers at home until I mastered its use. Eventually, the admission agreement rolled off my tongue as smooth as butter and I was able to perform a complete physical assessment while simultaneously conversing with patient and family. Repetition was my friend since the assessment was done each visit that I made.

When we returned to the office from that first admission, Veronica asked me to document the visit—which I did in narrative form. Remember the English professor who had wanted me to take up writing? I thought my charting would be worthy of his praise. Unfortunately, no one else did and I was required to rewrite it in a specific format. There are few things more humbling than nursing.

Per Medicare guidelines, two instructions were mandated per visit. They were to relate to the illness for which we visited the patient. If we saw her for congestive heart failure but she complained of a breast lump, instruction about the breast lump did not count as an instruction. Believe me, whether it made the chart or not, I would do appropriate health care teaching *in addition to* the two required!

Mona Killough, whose presentation at an orthopedic con-ed program was mentioned earlier, now worked in home health. Veronica partnered me with her so that I could observe routine, non-admission visits. Mona presented me with a home health paradox. "We are required to teach the patient or family— but they don't want to be taught." I found her perspective often correct.

What would we instruct? If the patient had CHF, we instructed him to: avoid sources of sodium, giving examples of what sources were; perform daily weight to identify fluid retention early before it advanced to difficulty breathing; elevate legs and check them for increased swelling; take the diuretic in the morning to avoid night time urinary frequency; if the diuretic also "washed out" potassium, include sources of potassium in the diet, giving examples. For other diseases there were equally as many instructions or more. Diabetes, myocardial infarction (MI), peripheral vascular disease (PVD), joint replacement, diabetic ulcers, pressure ulcers, wounds, seizure disorders—they all had potential instructions. Most patients had more than one disorder. The challenge was to present the instruction in a folksy manner so that it didn't seem like instruction. One patient complained that her regular nurse instructed her as though she were a kindergartner.

At the time, patients could be seen twice daily for months provided there was documentation in the chart to justify the need. Over an extended period, patients could hear the same instructions many times. That was not entirely negative. Their illness, the anxiety they experienced, or the misconceptions which they harbored might not have allowed them to *hear* or *understand* the first few times.

The need for home health was more acute in the atmosphere post *TEFRA* and *DRGs* when patients were discharged from hospitals before they were completely healed or rehabilitated. The types of patients whom we saw ranged from the very wealthy living in glamorous high-rise condos or waterfront "palaces" to the very poor living in roach-ridden shacks or shanties . . . and everything in between. We might go from a home in which we would not dare sit down for fear of tiny roaches running all over us to the spectacular and immaculate home of a captain of industry. Many lived downtown in my district in what I considered high-rise public housing for the elderly, not-so-bright poor. I respected the elderly. But home health convinced me that old age doesn't necessarily confer brilliance. If a person had always ranked low on the IQ meter, that didn't change. If a person historically made poor life choices—smoking, drinking to excess, unprotected sun exposure, irresponsible diet—the rewards which they reaped later in life were not pretty. The ten percent who looked to us for instruction were usually highly educated, highly motivated people, better-off physically and financially, living in better neighborhoods.

I lived in a relatively nice middle-class, working neighborhood. When we arrived at Mona's first visit on my day of observation, it was within a mile of my own home. The patient's house did not look much different from others on either side of it. Inside was a shock. It was the definition of the word "squalor." The terrazzo floor was strewn with dead bodies of huge Florida palmetto bugs—and living cats. The house teamed with cats! The cats had chased and caught countless roaches, leaving body parts to crunch under our feet. The man resembled Truman Capote with the same effeminate voice. He whined that he had to scrape the dead body of one of his cats off the street in front of his house because, "They _will_ go out into the street." As though it were a force of nature about which he could do nothing! Of course, the words *spay* and *neuter* were not in his vocabulary.

We advanced to the equally filthy kitchen where Mona had encased all dressing supplies in plastic bags to thwart the roaches. The man had peripheral vascular disease with open wounds. Our task was to administer a warm whirlpool to his leg for twenty minutes. A motor swished the water in a wastebasket-sized bucket while we performed the assessment. We listened intently to blood pressure and lung sounds over the whirlpool's roar. Afterward, we lifted and dumped the pail, heavy with several gallons of water. We wrapped the wound and cleaned and disinfected the entire whirlpool. Filling, carrying and dumping gallons of water from whirlpools was very common in home health care, making the job physically rigorous. Later, regulations were added for disposal of contaminated waste. We were required to bring contaminated/soiled dressings to the office for proper disposal after being "red bagged" and carried in our car in labeled, impermeable boxes.

This single gentleman, retired military and supposedly homebound, drove to the commissary in Tampa to pick up groceries. He sat for long periods with his legs on the floor rather than elevated as he had been instructed. Outside at her car, Mona announced that we were headed back to her apartment nearby so that she could take a shower before seeing the next patient. She did that every morning of caring for the man. It was sweltering summer in his un-air-conditioned house. Welcome to home health!

After I had my own territory downtown, I was expected to see five to six patients per day. The Admissions nurse would have already admitted them. We were expected to spend close to an hour with each patient. For some, we were their only visitor. They loved to chat. We rotated weekends and holidays to make routine *and* admission visits. Nightly at home, I finished my paperwork and called the next day's patients, providing them with a time frame for the visit. I tried hard to be prompt. Not infrequently in the rainy summer months I slogged through ankle deep water to get to a patient in the field. Outside the office was considered the field. Some days I hummed The Who's *Baba O'Riley*: *Out here in the field, I fight for my meals. I get my back into my living.* [1]

Early in my HHC employment, I arrived at the home of a bilateral lower extremity amputee—my first contact with any amputation—ever. I opened his (pre-arranged) unlocked door greeted by the patient crawling on the floor toward me. He had the physique of a basketball player—long arms and (previously) long legs. Crawling toward me, he looked like a giant spider.

One afternoon, I knocked in vain at a patient's alleyway apartment. In the main house, I found his landlady who unlocked his door. There was the patient—naked, emaciated and white-bearded. He had fallen during the night on his own diarrhea-streaked wood floors. The man lived on a diet of raw eggs. I spent hours cleaning him and his floor while trying to instruct one who did not want to be instructed. He wanted to get back to his raw eggs (possible diarrhea cause) and tricycle treks through St. Pete—regardless of a foot ulcer—and a Medicare requirement to be home-bound to receive care.

I visited a barrel-chested, ruddy-faced, emaciated emphysemic, and former *Ferg's Bar* devotee now homebound and oxygen-dependent. He insisted on chain smoking. The fact that he once had a "blow up" with third degree burns on and inside his nose never phased him. I surprised myself by insisting that, before I entered, he either turn off the oxygen and continue smoking or put out the cigarette and continue the oxygen. He could do as he pleased when I wasn't there against my advice—but he was not going to blow us both up! Standing outside a house like his, preparing to knock, the odor of cigarette smoke hung like a cloud. I left, post visit, reeking of smoke.

An unpleasant, unhappy man in his sixties lived alone in what had once been a nice, two story home, not far from St. Paul's. His wife dead, his children gone, he sat alone. Parts of his feet were amputated episodically because of peripheral vascular disease and diabetes. He just didn't care—continued to smoke (constricts blood vessels), and to be non-compliant about his diabetic diet and blood sugar testing. He was a double-dipper, receiving dressing supplies not only from us via Medicare, but also from the VA for "just in case." He stockpiled them. We visited him twice daily. That he drew money from two branches of the federal government; that it paid for twice daily visits; that he himself did not a thing to improve his situation was a sore point to the nurses who visited him. Ironically, he died of bladder cancer—another disease for which smoking is a risk factor. In a sense, he killed himself. Had that been his intent?

One of my tires went flat while I made a home visit. AAA arrived and resuscitated the tire enough to reach a Goodyear service station. They fixed it, removing the puncturing nail. When I asked, "How much?" they replied, "Forget it. You're out helping people."

I visited a barely literate African-American man in his early sixties who lived on the south side in his phone-less wood frame cottage. It was not my first visit to monitor his hypertension, to instruct him about the disease and his meds and to devise a med system which he could follow. I arrived at the pre-arranged time to find a negligee-clad cachectic woman languorously reclining on his sofa with him at her feet. Think Shug in *The Color Purple*. She fit my preconceived notion of a prostitute—a disease-ridden prostitute. Midway through the visit, there was a loud knock on the door. "Police!" The woman jumped up and ran into the adjacent bedroom—for all I knew, out the window. The patient, Joe

Smith asked, "What'll I do? They're looking for her." *As though I found myself in this situation every day and was an old expert at handling the police! Right.* "Answer the door," I replied authoritatively. He answered the door but didn't open the screen. The police were looking for Janey Jones. He returned, asking me, "What do I do?" "Get her," I said. My great uncle Charles, former Mount Lebanon Chief of Police had advised me: "Don't ever argue with a policeman." I didn't plan to start then.

Joe admitted the police pointing to the bedroom door, then he sat. While I listened to his lung sounds, the thought occurred to me that I could be the first St. Anthony's Home Health Care Nurse killed in the line of duty in a volley of bullets between police and suspect. Amazingly, Janey slinked out when the officer beckoned. He allowed her to smoke but not to change clothes. Carting her off in cuffs, he said, "Thanks, Joe. See ya around." My patient had a more than passing acquaintance with the police! After they left, I asked Joe what Janey had done. "Oh, she beat up her old man when he caught her stealing his things. He already had a restraining order against her." Oh. Then, insightfully, he confided, "I likes who she is, but I don't like what she do."

One of my patients lived in a first-floor apartment with a front window in a dilapidated old boarding hotel near the Mirror Lake Library. It has since been torn down. Alienated from his family, he had a prickly personality. But we got along. With very little money, his idea of a splurge was a Vidalia onion sandwich on white bread with butter. Taking his vital signs, I smelled peanut butter. I mentioned it and he explained that he could not afford dental adhesive for his dentures—so he used peanut butter—smooth, not crunchy!

One night, I was on call, making an evening visit for a patient I had never visited before. The address was a street between Twenty Second Avenue South and Lake Maggiore. The street was very dark—no house number in sight. But, lo, there was a house with a chain-link gate. Beyond the gate, silhouetted, a man stood in the light behind a frosted jalousie door. He was adjusting the TV set in front of him. I stopped my car, got out, opened the gate and was almost to the porch when the man disappeared. I wondered why. Surely, he had seen me. Meanwhile, I read his house number and reckoned that *my* house was just two doors up. When I opened his gate to exit, the man opened his door. I explained that I had been lost but now recognized my destination. "Good", he said. "I would have opened the door sooner, but I didn't have any clothes on." *Whew!! Was I glad that a small detail like that would matter to him!*

Several of my missions involved male genitalia and, each time, I wondered what my very proper father would think. I visited a gentleman in upper-middle class Maximo Moorings. The man, suffering from episodic incontinence, was to be fitted with a Texas (condom) catheter. His wife was away when I arrived, and I was alone with him in his bedroom. He sat on the side of the bed—me kneeling beside him, trying to decide which condom (small, medium or large) would fit. It occurred to me that, in a snapshot, prostitution might not look much different.

Another evening, I was called to insert an indwelling catheter for a male living in a nice upstairs condo on Redington Beach. When I arrived, his wife was just leaving to attend a social function. *What was with these wives? Didn't they know that I would so have appreciated a chaperone?* Remember, I had attended an all-girls high school, worked with women in maternity and had not been permitted to catheterize a man per St. Anthony's policy. Home Health was my first opportunity to insert a male catheter of any kind. But Claude's lessons returned to me. I called Claude for advice on another occasion when ordered to insert a Coudé catheter, firmly curved at the tip to pass around an enlarged prostate.

A "guest appearance" at a gulf-front cottage on Redington Beach was for a sixtyish gentleman whose penile implant had become infected and had been removed. I was to cleanse and pack the open wound between his penis and scrotum—for which the penis had to be held up and out of the way. A stone face was required but there was an inner flinch. I am sure the patient was embarrassed, too.

A woman with respiratory problems was on my list of admissions. On the phone the night before, she asked me to use the unlocked side door. A *Beware of Dog* sign was on the gate. I opened it and opened the unlocked side door. Standing at the entryway to the kitchen, I called out to the woman. Instantly, eight thudding feet preceded a confrontation by two huge, well-muscled Doberman Pinschers standing, ears erect, growling, curling their lips within feet of my face. Swarmed by the Doberman Gang, visions of being the first home health nurse mauled to death by dogs crossed my mind. The bathrobe-clad patient, unfazed, entered the kitchen behind the Dobermans. Dismissively, she motioned me to follow her into the living room, assuring as she turned her back and walked away, "It's okay. Come on." Not moving, I replied, "Yes. But is it okay with THEM?" "Oh, sure it is." Right. Not making eye contact with either of them (confrontation in dog-speak), I followed her and lived to tell the tale.

A bag woman lived in the Magnolia Hotel—often without enough to eat. The Magnolia was a seedy old hotel, kitty-corner from the Princess Martha (the Grande Dame of old hotels—renovated and in good shape). Unfortunately, the Magnolia, demolished a few years later, had seen better days. It was rented by the night or week. I walked up to the third floor via a dark stairwell and passed a common area on the second-floor landing. There, a group of skinny old men with several days beard growth clutched *mysterious* bottle-shaped brown bags while chewing the fat.

To arrive at my patient's room, I walked down a long, narrow, dark hall illuminated by one bare light bulb hanging from the ceiling. The woman was mentally challenged and had, in her words, "escaped" a private assisted living facility (ALF). She had trouble making ends meet—instant social worker referral. She had persistent diarrhea and the cloying odor lingered in the room. All she could do was try to hand-wash her soiled panties. These visits were not ones to which I would look forward. To make life interesting, I occasionally asked one of the two men at the front desk to take me up in the elevator. I felt safer because they had to ride with me to operate it. The old brass cage type elevator, clanking and groaning, reminded me of the one in the movie *Thoroughly Modern Millie*. In the movie, to get the elevator started, Millie sang and tap-danced as it rose to the upper floors. Riding the ancient elevator, it took every bit of gumption I had not to break into song and tap dance. My nursing bag with ten pounds of equipment—no, not a bowling ball—leant gravity to the situation. By then, I had no cap to maintain my dignity.

Another waifish woman lived in one of the crumbling boarding hotels near Mirror Lake. When I mistakenly called her *Mrs.*, she was quick to correct that she had never been married. Prudence, now in her eighties, fully intended to lasso a man before she died. She was a Boston physician's daughter and had lived a country club existence . . . tennis with her brothers, convertible cars. In WWII, one brother had been killed; the other driven to depression, booze and suicide. She had met the love of her life, but he married another. She fled to Italy where she flirted with many but returned to America unwed.

Clad in thrift store clothes, Prudence lived in a cluttered, roach-infested room. From her demeanor, you would think it was the country club. Class-conscious and upper crust, she had a "steady" at the hotel but thought he was too "hypertensive" to make it permanent. She meant *high strung*. For her leg ulcers, we visited her off and on over a period of years. She would fly to Italy seeking romantic dalliances, returning with wounds worse than ever. The front door of the boarding hotel was always locked, so she left a rock to prop open the second story back door. It was reached via a rusty old fire escape. There was a huge sign from the fire department warning to keep the door closed but—"ah piffle" to her.

Prudence thought like a teenage girl. If a male beckoned, previous wound care commitments were forgotten. Then she was nowhere to be found—with not a trace of regret or apology when we caught up with her. Last I heard, she had married her "hypertensive" friend and they were searching for communal digs. Driving around town, I saw her—angular and limping, cloche hat pulled around her face, looking like a bag lady but to-the-manor-born. Perception. Dr. Purkey would have loved it!

Was Prudence homebound? Not really, although we could interpret that qualification for care liberally. Folks needed to get their essentials, make doctors' appointments, etc. They were definitely not prisoners of their own homes. Had Prudence been compliant walking around town? Noooo—despite repeated instructions to elevate the affected leg. That was the reason for episodic admissions and discharge—promises unkept to be homebound and compliant.

Clearly Mona had been on target. We were required to instruct but folks didn't necessarily want to follow instructions. In my mid-forties, I had not entered home health expecting to solve everyone's problems, converting them to the straight and narrow. Being comfortable with ambiguity had been essential for working as Nurse Specialist/Educator. I had been good at it. But home health was ambiguity stretched to the nth degree. It was a true test of the *Serenity Prayer* by Reinhold Niebuhr:

> *God grant me the serenity*
>
> *to accept the things I cannot change;*
>
> *the courage to change the things I can;*
>
> *and the wisdom to know the difference.* [2]

Acceptance, courage and wisdom could be elusive.

More than physical assessment was necessary in home health care. As with oncology nursing, it was essential to know what made the person or family tick (Dr. Purkey's perceptual field). I couldn't just go in there and do wound care, case closed. I assessed the patient's ability to make decisions, and to function safely in his unique home environment. I determined if what he did incorrectly was due to ignorance, lack of resources, life-long quirkiness or outright lost touch with reality. What was his intellectual level? I listened to vocabulary. Did he use million-dollar words, or could he barely put a sentence together? Was he concrete, or could he think abstractly? Could he think hypothetically? Who in his world helped him? Did he need to know WHY, or did he just want to know HOW? Who would cook the meals? How would he get his groceries? Could he get to the bathroom? If not, who would empty the bedside commode? Did he need a home health aid to assist with activities of daily living? Did he need an occupational or physical therapist to strengthen limbs or work on dexterity and balance? Did he need a speech therapist to work on speech, swallowing or cognitive issues? Did he need a social worker to connect to community resources? The goal was to keep the patient out of the hospital and to make him as productive a member of society as he was able.

My subcutaneous size needle, short and very fine, hovered momentarily mid-air, preparing to sink into the soft, pale flesh of my new insulin-dependent diabetic patient. A loud "Ow!!" scared the stuffing out of me, shattering my concentration. If he felt pain *BEFORE* I stuck him, what would he do *WHEN* I stuck him? My thoughts must have been transparent because the otherwise mild mannered ninety-year-old gentleman broke into a smile. "Now we've got the 'ows' out of the way." he grinned, peacefully permitting the injection. A compliment followed, "That didn't hurt a bit." Thus, began the daily ritual— charging ten cents for having his vital signs taken—after all, I was TAKING them—and getting the ow's out of the way for Bill Betts. Bill and his wife, Bertha, married sixty years, lived in a nice, private home ALF. Childless and avid readers, Bill and Bertha were no longer able to care for themselves. He had mild dementia and she had psych issues—probably long-standing. She was indulged by her loving husband. He was DOCTOR Betts, Bertha would be quick to share. PhD. An educator who had met Franklin Roosevelt and worked on one of his projects, Bill had been Dean or President of a mid-western college. Bertha's pride was palpable. I envisioned her the perfect Dean's wife, overseeing social

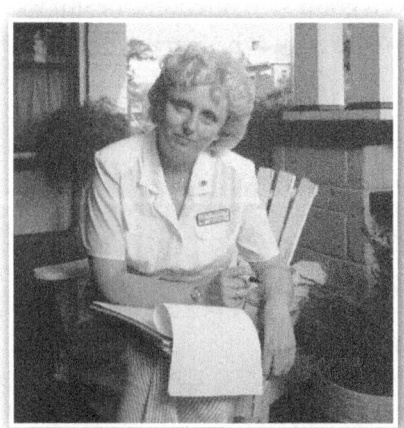

Figure 15 *Photo Shoot Here I am at 7:30 in the morning, sitting on a porch, facing a camera, trying not to squint at the bright lights aimed at me while being told to look empathetic.*

functions for faculty and their spouses. Bill was a kind, quiet and humble man. It shone through his every action. I looked forward to my morning "ow," the ten-cent fee and "that didn't hurt a bit."

T decided that I was to be one of the poster nurses for Home Health. She recruited me to have my picture taken for a promotional calendar highlighting St. Anthony's programs. I was supposed to be on a porch, talking with a patient. I was, indeed, on the porch of an older home owned by two young gay guys who were not patients. Being told to look compassionate, I stared into bright lights and camera—not the eyes of a patient.

On another occasion, several of us from different disciplines posed for large posters advertising Home Health. The "shoot" was in an airplane hangar at Albert Whitted Airport. It had been converted into a studio with seamless white walls and extremely bright lights. In my vignette, I taught an older, bed-bound gentleman, wearing pajamas, how to draw up insulin. The bed was really a low flat table, covered with linen. The "patient" was our supervisor's husband. The headboard against which he "leaned" was held in place by a man squatting behind it. I stood to the patient's left, holding an upside-down vial while the patient pretended to be learning to use a needle to withdraw his insulin. From the position in which I'd been placed, I complained that I couldn't see what my patient was doing. The response was swift. It didn't matter.

Interesting asides to my home health career, these experiences had nothing to do with nursing. I developed an awareness of marketing as a necessary tool to convey a perception. "Things are seldom what they seem; skim milk masquerades as cream." [3] To this day I watch commercials and imagine what's *REALLY* happening. My gullibility was forever tarnished.

After a year packed full of Med-Surg adventures, discovering the extremes of how people lived on Florida's Suncoast, I was happily a home health nurse. I felt very "nursey." We had moved to a separate office on Ninth Street—just blocks from the hospital. Half of the building housed the private duty folks and the other half my Medicare and insurance-reimbursed section. Like the hospital, we were approved by the Joint Commission on the Accreditation of Healthcare Organizations (JCAHO).

A walk-in storage room housed medical supplies: dressings, glucometer supplies, catheters, IV equipment. There was a small conference room for meetings and lunches brought in by representatives of companies seeking to push their products. I usually stopped for lunch in whatever area I was visiting, charting as I ate. The advantage to working predominantly outside the office was the absence of office politics and the ability to breathe clean, fresh air albeit hot and humid in summer.

We were independent. We made our own schedule deciding how often and when to see the patients within our district. On visits, there was a sense of isolation. If I were unsure when assessing my patient, I had no colleague at my elbow to consult. What if I missed something? No doctor arrived to see the patient every day to summarize and make decisions as in the hospital. I felt the responsibility heavily. I was IT. At the end of the day, we each returned from the field to chart and to share experiences in a giant room with a counter around its periphery.

One morning, a nurse was scheduled to see his patient in Jordan Park, one of the oldest public housing developments in St. Petersburg's African American community, founded by Elder Jordan in 1941. The nurse knocked repeatedly at the front door, but the patient did not answer. He had other patients—so he left. Later that day, his patient was found dead in her apartment. The question hovered: *what if?*

Aware of that situation, when I didn't get an answer to my knocks, I circled the house and peered into windows. It was not the safest approach. One day, I knocked on a screened porch door near Crescent Lake. No answer. The screen door was unlocked, so I entered. I knocked on the front door. No answer. The handle was also unlocked. I opened it. I was greeted by a groggy, just-waking young woman pointing a gun in my direction. Fortunately, it clicked that I was her nurse.

Another Saturday afternoon, I was to admit an elderly woman just released from the hospital. There was no answer at her mobile home no matter where I knocked. Doors were locked. It was pre-cell phone. I returned to the office to call the police requesting a safety check. They broke in and found the woman unable to rise from the toilet but otherwise okay.

Since *DRG's*, hospitals were loath to admit patients whose hospital stay might not be reimbursed by Medicare. Sending them home with Home Health was the new option. That was what happened to a gentleman living alone in a private home in Meadowlawn. I don't remember the diagnosis—maybe CHF, maybe PVD. The ER sent him home via taxi with prescriptions. The taxi driver helped him into his house and left him in a chair. The next morning when Jo arrived to admit him to Home Health, she discovered the man still in his chair, incontinent of bowel and bladder. Alone, she was unable to leverage him out of the chair. The prescriptions, of course, remained unfilled. The house was filthy with obvious signs of previous incontinence on matted down thirty-year-old gold shag carpet. Jo arranged for me and another nurse to walk/lift the man into bed which we made with the few unsoiled sheets he possessed. Jo notified the man's lawyer, his only contact. Our private section provided twenty-four-hour home health aids to cook and care for him until he could be placed in a nursing facility the next day. We probably ate the bill.

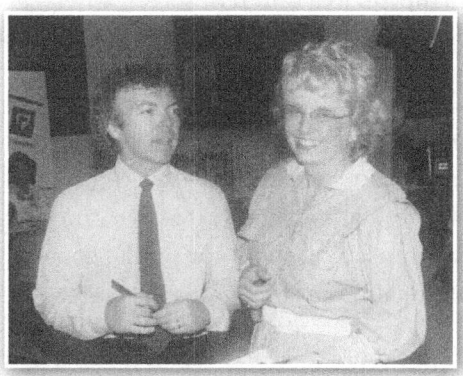

Aside from these glaringly emergent situations, there was the daily need to evaluate each patient, methodically ruling out problems to be reported to the doctor before the next nursing visit or the next

Figure 16 *Dr. Miller, the idea man, and me at Cancer Awareness Day 1987.*

doctor's office visit. Picking up on signs and symptoms of life-threatening situations in my patients was my responsibility alone. Home Health nurses were the equivalent of the 1930s family physician making house calls. The only thing missing was the leaches.

Loaned to the Cancer Center

Back at the hospital which I had left in frustration, change was in the air. A radiation oncology center was being built adjacent to the POB. At last, there would be a dedicated hospital oncology unit. Undoubtedly, Administration had been moved by the prospective financial advantage. Heaven knows I had tried every patient-centered argument!

The medical director of the new center was Dr. Robert Miller, a radiation oncologist whom I knew through the American Cancer Society. He was a very slight man, with permed, blonde hair who talked a mile-a-minute. He reminded me of the *Greatest American Hero*—another television program furnishing counter-balancing laughs in the early eighties. In the series, the protagonist, slight with permed blonde hair, had the ability to fly when he donned his caped suit. Dr. Miller, indeed, flew. His mind travelled at warp speed. He had numerous projects—only one of which was composing music on his computer. He was an Apple enthusiast of WYSIWYG (What You See Is What You Get.) and a devotee of one of their first personal computers, the Macintosh Classic, which arrived on the market in 1990. PC's of the era had three parts: keyboard, heavy monitor, and what I called "brains"—an enormous box. The Classic was brains and monitor all in one compact package. It had fantastic "draw" capabilities and a *Hyper-card* program in which buttons could be created and programmed to morph to a different screen when clicked. It was a primitive, but more versatile version of what is now known as PowerPoint.

Dr. Miller envisioned his Cancer Center to be cutting edge, featuring a computer in its lobby where waiting patients and families could receive further instruction about their type of cancer and interventions for related problems. Aware that I had an extensive knowledge of oncology issues and had a knack for translating them for public consumption, he wanted me to create his educational program.

One problem—I had never used a computer! An *idea man,* Dr. Miller could not conceive of that being insurmountable. *You are only as limited as your own imagination.* He had arranged for the hospital to buy the Classic. All he needed was for the program to be developed while the building was constructed. The Classic was set up in an empty patient room on a closed hospital unit. My Home Health Department backed the idea. T banked on ingratiating Dr. Miller and becoming the recipient of his referrals. I found the challenge scary but titillating.

It took almost a year to create the program. Salary was the same. Dr. Miller approved my initial outline which reflected his general vision. The catalyst/key to *mission accomplished* was summer break at St. Petersburg High School's International Baccalaureate (IB) Program. Remember that toddler who loved to suck his thumb while twisting Joannie's long blonde hair? I had known Jayson since he was two. He was on high school break between junior and senior year. As part of his IB Program, Jayson was required to serve a specific number of volunteer hours. Knowing Jayson, he would have volunteered anyway because he was a totally good kid. He was like his bubbly mother but with an overlay of masculine restraint—the bubbles and excitement visible just under the surface.

Jayson volunteered to help me. Good thing—because as words appeared and disappeared on the screen, I panicked—unaware of the cause or how to retrieve them. Jayson had not worked with a Mac but easily made the transition. Together we sat before that screen for hours, tediously structuring our program while backing it up on a floppy disc, a necessity. Later, I took a Mac evening course at junior college. But Jayson was my mentor. When school resumed for him, I bought my own Classic—I had become so enthralled by it. I worked on the program from home for hours into the night—way more than the hours for which I was paid. My program included layered images in the pathophysiology section that I had drawn freehand with the mouse.

Finally, the Cancer Center opened its doors. The Classic was placed in an alcove in the lobby where few saw or used it. No one was budgeted—nurse-educator would have been nice—to help people to get started with it. In the early nineties, most people did not have a computer at home and would need help. The instigator of the project, Dr. Miller, was too enmeshed with administrative duties to follow through with his creation.

You would think that, having spent so much time developing the program, I would have been disappointed with its virtual abandonment. Twenty-five years in nursing had taught me to expect administrative short sightedness—and my own powerlessness. I counted myself lucky that, at hospital expense, I had acquired skills which would benefit me personally for the rest of my life. In that sense, it had been a well-paid sabbatical. Jayson later graduated from MIT and worked for Intel in Oregon. He designed computer technology, married and became the father of two boys.

Resume Home Health Care

T asked me to become their Educator when I returned from my "sabbatical." I agreed, realizing that teaching nurses was something that I had missed while working in the field. The Educator role was primarily a matter of orienting new nurses and home health aids to home health. Most people who applied for the job had hospital experience but no experience with home health, a relatively new development. While hospital charts documented a patient's positive progress, in home health, we charted his deficits. It was an entirely different perspective—glass half full *vs* half empty. Using the jargon tied to reimbursement was essential. Unlike hospital prospective payment, in home health, reimbursement remained fee-for-service.

To locate supplies, I sent orientees on a scavenger hunt. To orient to the department, I set up museum-like tours with audio-tape recorders and earpieces. The front office clerical staff appreciated their inclusion as a tour destination—introducing them to the new employees. Those creative learning strategies afforded me time to accompany the nurses on their first visits; to set up lunch in-services, monthly HHA in-services; and to maintain the staff's educational records.

Being Educator was multi-facetted—I could teach, role-model with patients, and be creative. My friend Mona had stepped up to CCC (Clinical Care Coordinator), investigating hospital referrals. At the time, both hospital and home health used the Baylor staffing model. Staff worked either Monday through Friday for eight-hour shifts or Saturday and Sunday, plus either Friday or Monday for twelve-hour shifts. The staffing model was advantageous for employees, acknowledging and working with their personal needs while providing consistency for patients.

Within a year of my return, T Ecklund resigned and a new HHC Administrator was hired. In her thirties, she was married and the mother of a middle-school-aged daughter. A one-hundred-and-eighty-degree shift from T, she wore tweedy ill-fitting brown suits. Her demeanor was mannish. Shortly, Jeanne Marie resigned as Director of Nursing. A young, twenty-something new MSN with no home health experience replaced her as DON.

The new administrator and her young DON became the subject of gossip after she bragged to the clerical staff that things would be different (better?) because both she and her DON had master's degrees. Her braggadocio was directed at clerical people with a high school+ education. She tried to pull the same with me, ingratiatingly implying that we master's-prepared people knew what was best *and needed to stick together.* I didn't bite, remembering the BSN who sent the urine specimen through the Lamson Tube System.

Disregarding a commitment to move half of the office to Seminole in two months, one weekend the new Administrator took it upon herself to rearrange everything in the office. Her husband helped. Staff returned Monday to find their space violated. Her surreptitious maneuver was reminiscent of a younger me rearranging supplies in Shands' newborn nursery. At least, I had not done it surreptitiously. A dog peed on something to make it his. Coincidentally, during the Administrator's regime, an Associated Press article was published in the *St. Petersburg Times.* I clipped it.

> *A flum is a flaw in the works, a manager who promotes "needed" change but imposes chaos instead, defending it by explaining that old conformities must be destroyed if the company is to adapt to a chaotic world.*

... flums feed on flux and feed into it as well. Flums flip common sense on its head, embracing all the highly publicized trends and fads and creating disorder and jumbled work processes.

Flums survive because of chaos. They help create it. They hide behind it. They defend their "results" as necessary and temporary, but often the chaos they produce is permanent, entrapping them. [4]

Based on the work of Professor Emeritus Eugene Jennings of Michigan State University, it described our Administrator in a nutshell—constantly changing the physical plant, ways of charting, general procedures. Nothing remained unscathed.

Staff was unhappy. So was I. Her clandestine office upheaval had some drastic effects for me. I scoured the entire office to find my file cabinet of confidential staff records. My tiny but adequate office was no longer mine. I was forced to conduct my business in the large room where nurses noisily finished their charting and discussed the day's events. *Don't pee on me and tell me it's raining.* [5] I resigned the post of Educator. Eager to flee the office, I returned to the field as an Admission Nurse working out of the newly opened Seminole office.

Later, the St. Pete office moved to a building behind Chili's in the Tyrone area. *Increasing visibility* was the stated purpose. The high rent district hidden behind Chili's, was visible only to the employees who worked there. At that time, St. Joseph's Hospital in Tampa and St. Anthony's in St. Petersburg joined forces in a consortium. Middle management jobs and expenses were cut in both facilities. The positions of HH Administrator and DON were up for grabs. Each pair applied. Our "flum" Administrator and her DON were replaced by St. Joseph's Administrator and DON. No one on this side of the bay was aggrieved—until we met their replacements.

Tampa managers believed that their agency could spin circles around ours. These folks had rough edges—a far cry from the T Ecklund era of culture, high heels and dresses. One of their administrative nurses repeatedly passed me in the hall looking straight through me as though, a mere field nurse, I were invisible. Unsmiling, they were more about quantity than quality. The number of patients to be seen per day increased. No more talk of spending quality time with the patient. According to them, they saved us from ourselves. Without them, our agency would have gone under—and it still might. *That* mantra surfaced repeatedly, no matter the administrator.

I have noticed that nurses treat patients only as well as they are treated. It's not intentional—not even conscious. It is bowing under the pall of oppression or walking tall and graciously reaching out under the umbrella of beneficence. Under our newest administration, we were factory workers required to toe the line.

The nurses held in highest esteem were those who could cram the greatest number of visits into their daily schedule. I substituted for one of them on his day off. The patient was an astute eighty-something gentleman, living with his lady friend in a private home in a middle class northeast section. I interrupted him, still limber, digging a ditch in his back yard for a sprinkler connection. He had facial cancer treated with radical surgery. Removing the bandage from his left face, I suppressed my shock. His left eye and the left half of his nose and face were gone, exposing a large cavernous sinus with a moist pink base which vibrated when he spoke. After I performed wound care, packing and dressing it, the gentleman mentioned that mine was the best assessment he had had. His "regular" nurse never listened to his lungs or took the complete vital signs which I had. This was how I learned that the few "rewarded nurses" whose performance met the new administration's quantitative standards—fudged. The more I substituted for this nurse, I heard similar comments. In the field, there was no real oversight and the only review was chart documentation—which could or could not be accurate.

Most of my colleagues continued to function as they should, regardless of flak from above. We were joined by Ariel Grant, a nurse who had been in my orientation group at St. Anthony's in 1968. She was an excellent HH nurse. So was Betty Stewart, another refugee from the hospital before she returned to work in its SNF. Joannie Strayer who had transferred from Education and Joan O'Halloran were both great nurses. Carmen Coleman and Jim Hager (of the flaming orange hair) worked the south side and their patients sang their praise. Other nurses came—and went.

While working in the field, I happened upon a brief article penned by Mother Teresa, a Catholic nun who served the poor of India. I clipped it and still have it. It seemed an appropriate meditation for a home health nurse. Here is an excerpt:

> *We all long for heaven where God is, but we have it in our power*
> *to be in heaven with Him at this very moment. But being happy*
> *with Him now means: loving as He loves, helping as He helps,*
> *serving as He serves, being with Him twenty-four hours,* touch-
> ing Him in His distressing disguise.* [6]

With the advent of the joint venture between the two hospitals, our territory greatly expanded. I could visit extreme south Pinellas Point in the morning and have a late afternoon visit in Trinity just north of the Pinellas County line. Non-nurse schedulers now dictated our day. One Saturday morning I was assigned a fasting blood sugar in Oldsmar. That meant leaving home before seven in the morning, joining the interstate just blocks from the office, and traveling approximately twenty-two miles. Because I had not stopped at the office first, I was denied pay for that (to and from) mileage. Enter the bean counters!

If you hold on long enough, something will change—and it did. In 1997, the bay area's non-profit hospitals, feeling the economic pinch, agreed to form a larger alliance. St. Joseph's, St. Anthony's, Tampa Baptist, Bayfront Medical Center, Morton Plant and Mease became one entity to share services and to minimize operational expenses. The alliance was *BayCare*. We were no longer St. Anthony's or St. Joseph's, but *BayCare* Home Health with a central administrator, Denny Crockett, from the Clearwater (previously Morton Plant) office. Our local administrator remained the same, but we inherited a very youthful DON from Bayfront, Michelle Barlow. A small and cohesive group, Bayfront's home health nurses, joined our new office in St. Anthony's Medical Office Building (MOB). Accustomed to being thorough, they reminded me of our group before the expansion and takeovers. When they voiced their discomfort with the new system, we could only sympathize, pointing to our own three *hostile takeovers.*

Post takeover, a vacancy occurred in a hospital Clinical Care Coordinator (CCC) position. A CCC responded to patient referrals: reading his chart; copying information; determining the equipment he would need; interviewing him; and sometimes getting authorization for care from insurance companies. From there, the information was faxed and phoned to the Intake Coordinator—now Mona. Poor Mona was set up in a large room with people constantly arriving from the field. Phone conversations with referral sources were difficult for her to hear. She scowled and shushed folks. Who could blame her?

The CCC position was cut out for me. Having been an Admissions Nurse for a while, I knew exactly what information the admitting nurse needed and how crucial it was for the CCC to glean as much as possible about the patient, including the necessary DME (durable medical equipment—wheelchair, walker, bedside commode, etc.) and other supplies required. Unlike the hospital, home health equipment was not right around the corner in the supply room. When I was at a patient's home I was virtually stranded and needed to have everything either with me or delivered prior to arriving.

When considering the CCC position, I remembered a weekend situation. I was to admit a patient to administer an evening injection. The weekend CCC, one of administration's shining stars, had faxed the admission paperwork to the office. The patient was discharged from Northside Hospital that afternoon. I assumed that the CCC had visited. It was winter and already dark. I arrived at what *should* have been the address on the south side only to discover an empty lot on a dead end in a known high crime area. I scrounged through the paperwork in my dark car, illuminated only by the tiny over-dash beam of light. The CCC had copied the address incorrectly on her referral. The home was really just above Lake Maggiore. When I arrived and knocked, I was greeted at the door by a very nice, *African American* gentleman. The referral said he was *white*. Perhaps the CCC had been listening to his accent on the PHONE. He was from the north and lacked any trace of southern accent. Don't get me wrong. That he was African American was not an issue. He could have been purple for all I cared. The point was that the CCC had not done due diligence, not visited the hospital, not provided reliable information. Was there something more crucial to patient care that she had failed to mention? Later, the CCC resigned to become DON of the Pinellas jail infirmary. I kid you not!

I took the CCC position at St. Anthony's alternating with CCC's Patty and Woody. The way St. Anthony's discharge planning was structured, anyone with an order for home health was referred to us. We were required to give the patient a choice of agencies—but our agency name was at the top of the list and we could push the concept of continuity of care because of the hospital affiliation. It kept us busy. Patty was a quiet worker, preferring to work her own units, venturing out on personal errands when her referrals left her time for a break. Woody was another story. From New Hampshire, she was the original hippy, animal lover, and green advocate. Like a triathlete, she carried her water bottle with her onto the units. I thought it a silly affectation but soon revised my opinion. Most days we *were* running a marathon.

Eventually, I was sent to Bayfront to fill in for the CCC's there—Jeanne and Eileen—both delightful people. I networked with a large group of medical professionals—CCC's from other agencies; nurses who worked for insurance companies and authorized treatment for their patients; doctors whom I had not known; and Bayfront's nursing staff.

At the start of the *BayCare* alliance, St. Anthony's entire OB unit had moved to Bayfront. The move made sense. St. Anthony's unit was usually in-the-red due to high tech, expensive equipment; increasing liability premiums (A baby and his family had twenty-one years to sue.); staffing adequate for emergencies even when there were few patients.

The *St. Petersburg Times* discovered that Bayfront, allied with two Catholic hospitals, had agreed to stop performing second trimester abortions. *First* trimester abortions occurred in doctors' offices or family planning clinics. The *Times* drummed up public sentiment against the consortium. Bayfront, a private non-profit, leased the city-owned land on which it sat for a nominal fee. City council questioned Bayfront's new affiliation and its potential interference with a woman's right to an abortion on public property. After the brouhaha exploded, Bayfront withdrew from *BayCare*. Bayfront retained the former St. Anthony's maternity staff. St. Anthony's was left without an OB unit while we retained Bayfront's home health staff.

Working at Bayfront, I discovered, if not a miracle, then a blast from the past. I struck up a conversation with a nurse who had worked with Michelle Barlow, our DON. Chuckling, she said, "Yes, I knew Michelle when her last name was Tousignant." Tousignant? That was an uncommon name. I had met a Tousignant years before.

It was in the late seventies at St. Anthony's. Mr. Tousignant was a scrawny taciturn New Englander with a fuzzy black mustache. He reminded me of my husband's Uncle Norm (pronounced *Nom* in Maine). The gentleman, thin and weak, was in and out of the hospital. His family was large—eight children— mostly raised in New England. As death approached, I was present intermittently during all shifts to assure a hospice-like experience. It was important for the entire family to be with him, setting their own limits on visitation. His wife scowled perpetually. His children were grief-stricken. Given the possibility that he could still hear, I encouraged them to review their lives together in his comatose presence, reviewing scrapbooks, saying their peace to him. The youngest, a sixteen-year-old daughter was present at times—acting like a fidgety sixteen-year-old.

Now more than twenty years later, returning to our office, I asked Michelle if that gentleman had been her dad. He was. Though neither of us remembered the other in appearance, we remembered the situation and hugged. Michelle, then sixteen, now was mother of her own sixteen-year-old daughter.

In 1997, the *Balanced Budget Act (BBA)* mandated the development of a prospective payment system for home health care. Just like *DRG's* in the hospital, the point was to eliminate fee for service payment, and replace it with payment for categories of care. In home health, not just the disease but the functional status were factors. As always, the only means of justifying a certain level of care was excellent documentation by all members of the health care team. The requirement only came into effect in 2000, but our agency participated in a pilot program before that. By then, nurses' charting was completed on a Palm Pilot, a hand-held computer worked with a stylus. It was downloaded over-night. Returning from an admission, nurses were required to review the *OASIS* (*Outcome and Assessment Information Set*) information to determine the best re-imbursement with the lowest number of visits possible—but not too low or the reimbursement would be less!

The Utilization Review Coordinator reviewed the assessment with the nurse and finished the financial paperwork. Saundra Houston, former Head Nurse of St. Anthony's GYN unit, had been a Home Health Patient Care Coordinator (PCC), supervising staff in several districts. She was moved from that position and joined two other Utilization Review Coordinators. That title was a euphemism for *Payment Assurance Coordinators*. Saundra was a tall, well built, former military woman in her fifties. Her manner sarcastic, Saundra's conferences with nurses were not always pleasant. I discovered two graffiti's which reflected her attitude perfectly:

> *Let me drop everything and work on your problem.*
>
> *I can only please one person a day. This is not your day.*

While I worked between St. Anthony's and Bayfront as a CCC, good fortune arrived in the form of Sandy Calvert. Sandy replaced the St. Joe's Administrator. Sandy was a tall, heavy-set red head—beautifully quaffed, beautifully outfitted and beautifully made up every day. She was as real as your next-door neighbor—hailing from the south, communicating in a pleasant, courteous and easily understood manner. A white Oprah. In us she inherited a handful of discontents. Her mantra was that we put the *fun* in dys*fun*ctional. She was a benevolent leader, marshalling our disparate forces while answering to a centralized home health administration with its own agenda, buzz words, and pet ideas. She and Michelle worked well together and were supportive of staff. I should have realized that it wouldn't last. Another Sandy aphorism: *No good deed goes unpunished.*

During Sandy's administration, each of the CCC and Intake nurses were required to reapply for their jobs at least twice at the direction of Central Administration. The rationale was downsizing—like a litter of puppies being culled.

We were each individually interviewed. For me, the interview was an interesting exercise—like taking a math quiz when it wasn't attached to a grade. I was not so far removed from being a field nurse and I cared not which of the positions I was awarded.

Intake in Margaritaville

As it turned out, I was brought in from the hospital to overlap Mona's hours in Intake. By this time, she had moved to a large, more sequestered, two-desk office adjacent to the conference room. We dubbed the office *Margaritaville* because our legal names were both Margaret. Every Cinco de Mayo, we put the *Margaritaville* sign on our door. Staff returning from the field in the afternoon were treated to virgin Margaritas, chips and salsa while Jimmy Buffet tunes permeated the office. One year we even had a piñata. It was our shot at breaking the tension in what had become a very intense business.

Intake was the hub of a communication network. All day we received referrals from doctor's offices, hospitals and nursing homes. We took the information and then called it in to the CCC's in the field to visit the referring institution. The territory we covered was Pinellas County south of Ulmerton Road. We punted referrals north of Ulmerton to the Clearwater HH branch. When the CCC faxed the completed referral and backup material, we entered the information into the computer, assigning ICD-9 codes. It took time to learn and we frequently received "feedback" from the UR Coordinators.

Handling a phone referral from a doctor's office took the patience of a saint. Pulling out essential information was like pulling chewing gum from the bottom of a shoe. The CCC's did not visit physician offices for referrals. So, the nurse who visited the home first would only know what we were able to glean.

After making copies, we delivered the admission packets to the PCC's who accepted them as though we had delivered the newest strain of smallpox. It was their task to pull staff like a rabbit out of a hat to make the visit. The minute we knew that the admission would require a same-day visit, we alerted the PCC— way before the paperwork arrived. We also ordered DME, injectables or IV's. For managed care cases, central administration housed a managed care section which we alerted to obtain authorization for visits. We recognized many people just by the sound of their voice on the phone and developed phone relationships with them to grease the wheels. "English" Wendy at Northside and Nini in Managed Care were just a few.

We started the day later and stayed longer than most of the staff due to the timing of referrals. We often received PT/INR bloodwork results which had been drawn earlier. PT/INR's monitored the effectiveness of Coumadin. Too high—the patient could bleed to death. Too low, he could develop blood clots, pulmonary embolus or stroke. Sometimes the levels were way out of whack and we searched high and low to find the doctor after his office hours for an order to modify the Coumadin dose. When we left at night it was dark. Only Sandy remained.

Mona and I worked together well even though our styles were different. I tried to be neat and methodical—though it didn't come naturally. I kept a legal pad next to the phone, recording the gist of the call and anything I needed to do relating to it. Mona had been doing intake for so long that she just left little sticky memos to herself all over her desk. The number of referrals we handled per day was high—usually into the teens. I measured my day by how many pages on my legal pad had been used.

When Mona had abdominal surgery it became a nightmare. She was out of work for a while with repeated operations, an open wound, and long-term antibiotic therapy. Jeanne Glousser—Mona's exact opposite—took her place. A slim New Hampshire Yankee, Jeanne was a perfectionist. Oddly enough, we also worked well together and enjoyed each other's company. When Mona bravely returned to work, she was still on IV antibiotic therapy. Whoever worked with her hooked her up and ran it.

In 2004, Florida experienced a very bad year for hurricanes—the worst for any one state in a hundred years. Charley, Frances and Jeanne crisscrossed Florida. During the Hurricane Watch, nurses reminded patients of their evacuation zones, informing them that staff would not visit during the Hurricane Warning. Patients requiring daily care were counseled to return to the hospital if the care could not be provided by a family member. To prepare the office, we unplugged computers and covered them with plastic—our salvation because the roof leaked. Sandy communicated with staff via voice mail throughout the hurricanes.

Not long after the hurricanes, there was another administrative upheaval. Michelle resigned to work as administrator of another home health agency. She was replaced by a BayCare Clearwater branch nurse. Soon, Sandy was let go and resurrected as Administrator of another unrelated agency. Her replacement, also from the Clearwater office, was a short, plump, wimpy extension of

Denny's arm. Denny Crockett, BayCare HHC Administrator, was an empire builder. He *obviously* had read Machiavelli. He placed his own people in key positions. Mona and I should have taken note.

Under Denny, we had been required to reapply for our positions several times. This time the announcement was made that one position would be eliminated in Intake. Mona and I, both part-time, had filled the slot of "one-plus" Intake Coordinator. Jeanne was the other. That our daily volume could be handled by just one Intake Coordinator defied logic.

We each had the opportunity to think about it. If we let it, the situation could pit us against each other. I hated that. Mona was older, heavier and had recently been seriously ill. Intake Coordinator was a perfect position for her and she had seniority. I realized that I might have a few more options to work elsewhere. I would not be manipulated into stabbing Mona in the back. The decision was made. I would take the moral high ground. I would not apply.

Meanwhile, Mona had done her own thinking. A few months short of retirement age, she had decided to retire and encouraged me to apply. Assured that she was serious, I proceeded with the interview. At the onset, the administrator informed me that the Intake job had already been filled. *Before all were interviewed? What a façade!* But, I could have the position of HHA Supervisor. *Really?* That position was titular only. Much as I enjoyed the aids, it would be very poor use of my accumulated knowledge and skills. I was sixty and my age would be somewhat of a liability in the job market. But it also represented a rich nursing background—more than necessary for Home Health Aid Supervisor. The decision was made before I left the interview. No. I would not accept that role. My letter of resignation followed. After Mona and I resigned, we were replaced by TWO of Denny's Clearwater RNs. Phony? You bet.

Over forty years, my optimism and love of patient care had eroded to full blown cynicism. Extrinsic factors like legislators who had never looked a patient in the eye perverted patient care into a reimbursement-focused operation. Intrinsic factors of empire-building and carnivorous politicking pushed staff to see more patients; patients to see fewer staff; and the agency to be more profitable. In the 1987 movie *Wallstreet*, the character Gordon Gecko had exclaimed, "Greed is good." That mantra had found a home in home health.

> *The optimist underestimates how difficult it is to achieve real*
> *change, believing that anything is possible and it's possible now.*
> *Only by confronting head-on the reality that all progress is go-*

ing to be obstructed by vested interests and corrupted by human venality can we create realistic programmes that actually have a chance of success. [7]

An optimist, I had learned the hard way that my naïve belief that we existed to serve the patient was not everyone's truth. By eschewing management from the start of my career, I had forfeited the power to make positive change or to take things in another direction. I had witnessed middle managers treated like disposable tooth picks in the scramble for power. Disillusioned, I needed a break. It was Halloween and I decided not to seek gainful employment until after the Christmas holidays.

Pet Therapy

There was plenty to do at home. One of my great stress relievers since 1981, had been my Samoyed dogs. Samoyeds were amazing. Big, white, soft, yet powerful sled dogs, they had been reindeer herders in the Russian Arctic. In 1993, my first Samoyed show-dog, Angel, opened a huge world of possibilities for us both. We showed in conformation, dabbled in obedience and tracking. We took a tricks class and participated in herding trials. We traveled around the state, participating in dog events, making new friends. I was a founding member of the Samoyed Fanciers of Central Florida and its first newsletter editor. But probably one of the best things we did together was to participate in *Project PUP* (Pets Uplifting People).

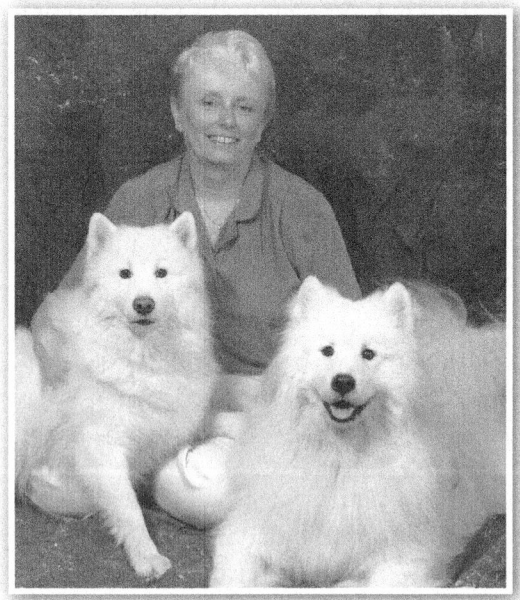

Figure 17 *Pet Therapy Team*. Project PUP volunteers: Angel on left and Noah on right. They were wonderful representatives of their breed, greeting each patient with love, warmth and a Samoyed smile.

Through *Project Pup*, Angel and I were the first therapy dog team to volunteer at St. Anthony's. Our assigned unit was the Skilled Nursing Facility (SNF). We slipped into a pattern of presenting a "show" in the day room (dog jumping through hoops and over sticks, walking through my legs as I walked, etc.) and then visiting patients who could not leave their rooms. Both staff and patients were therapy recipients. Soon, Angel was joined by Noah. After a few years, they were joined by Gracie. Many miracles were observed during their ten-year tenure. Dogs have a wonderfully calming, pleasant effect on most people.

To an aphasic patient, Angel voiced her soft "woo" repeatedly until the woman, smiling, burst out forcefully, "Speech therapist!" There was a man whom Noah encouraged to use his incentive spirometer by following the ball going up and down while the man breathed into it. A woman who had not spoken suddenly babbled about her German Shepherd. Occasionally, in home health, I admitted patients who remembered the dogs fondly. I volunteered invisibly behind my dogs—observing a skilled nursing facility's care with a nurse's eye—perspective which I would soon use.

During my mini-vacation, I recognized that home health care had afforded me the opportunity to grow as a nurse. The Med-Surg nursing which I had dismissed in school had become my bread and butter. Visiting people from one end of the social spectrum to the other had been fascinating. I had become more accepting of diversity and more flexible as a person. A consolation: if unable to find a new position, I could easily become a taxi driver. I knew the streets of St. Petersburg like the back of my hand!

Paralleling the hospital, the economic constraints of the prospective payment system had forced administrative change during my home health tenure. The focus had become "getting by with less." As a young nurse, I would never have guessed the dominant roles that internal politics and economics play behind the scenes in nursing care.

Endnotes

1. Peter Townsend, Baba O'Riley. Recorded by The Who, (Nashville: Universal Music Publishing Group, 1971).

2. Elisabeth Sifton, "The Serenity Prayer," *Faith and Politics in Times of Peace and War* (New York: W.W. Norton & Company, 2005).

3. W.S. Gilbert and Arthur Sullivan, "Things Are Seldom What They Seem" *HMS Pinafore* [1878].

4. John Cuniff, "What is a Flum? A Manager Who Brings About Chaos," *St. Petersburg Times* (April 30, 1993).

5. Judge Judy Sheindlin, *Don't Pee on Me and Tell Me It's Raining* (New York: Harper Perennial, 1997).

6. Mother Teresa, *A Gift for God* (New York: Harper Collins Publishing, 2003).

7. Julian Baggini, "In Praise of Cynicism," Originally in *The Guardian*. Published in *St. Petersburg Times* (July 20, 2003).

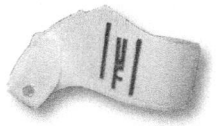

CHAPTER SEVEN
From Womb to Tomb: 2006-2012

Job Hunting at Sixty

In January of 2006, I noticed an ad in the Sunday classified section for a Nurse Liaison (CCC equivalent) at Menorah Manor, a SNF within a mile of my home. I remembered that Almeda Martin, my director at St. Petersburg Junior College, had lived there after a stroke. My friend Mary Jean Etten, an expert gerontologist who had served on the governor's task force to review state-wide nursing home care, had engineered Almeda's admission. Menorah Manor was respected in the community.

My experience with SNFs was limited. I had visited several of them following-up on cancer patients. My grandmother and mentally handicapped uncle had been in one. Generally, my impression was negative—air permeated with the smell of urine; disoriented people walking around aimlessly. The few DONs I had met were dysfunctional and/or alcoholic. A friend had been in an austere SNF privately owned by an attorney. His huge motor boat parked behind the facility telegraphed his fiscal priorities. When my friend was no longer able to private-pay and qualified for Medicaid, she had been forced to find another nursing home.

I decided to give Menorah Manor a whirl. I was well-qualified for their admission nurse position. Director of Nursing, Anabelle Locsin, was the first of seemingly endless interviews. Eyeing her name tag, I was amazed that she had her doctorate. No old out-of-touch alcoholic there. She conducted a good interview, asking appropriate questions. Her last question almost lost me the position. "What do you like about gerontology?" "I don't like gerontology," I blurted, conjuring images of Lois Knowles feeding bananas to her menagerie of geriatric performers. The words spoken, Anabelle's jaw dropped. Struck by how ridiculous it sounded, I covered, "I like people, no matter the age." Anabelle guided me back to the front office to Leta Medina, the Director of Admissions and we had a brief, pleasant interaction.

The next interview was with Marshall Seiden, the CEO. With him was Judy Ludin, the Foundation Director. I had worked with Judy when she was on staff at the American Cancer Society. Marshall asked some pointed questions while Judy observed. He gruffly pounced on the fact that I had never worked in a SNF and was not familiar with their prospective payment system. Feeling a little plucky, I shot back that, in both hospital and home health, I had been aware of the prospective payment system. A quick study, I was certain that I could learn the SNF equivalent. Guiding me to my next interview, Marshall mumbled something about us having been born in the same year. Foolishly I had placed my date of birth on the résumé. I quipped "Guess we'll both need to look for an ALF soon." His face reflected instant surprise. Marshall was not accustomed to employees or potential employees being so blunt.

My next interview was with a young man whom I took to be an administrative assistant. I later learned that he was Administrator, a married father of two pre-teen boys. He asked a few questions about my résumé then asked what I did for fun. I mentioned being involved in the dog sport with my Samoyeds as well as my research into their origins in this country. "Oh, you should talk to Leta," he said, "She shows her dogs, too." Finding Leta in the hall chatting, I waited until she was free and struck up an animated conversation with her about our dogs. She had Goldens. We walked and talked to the front entrance. I left the building tabulating how many folks had interviewed me—five counting Judy. You'd think I was running for president! But Marshall had made a strong point that, if I were hired, I would be the face of Menorah Manor to the medical community. They had to be very careful about whom they hired.

Within the week, I was called by the Director of Human Resources, Gail Fullam, and offered the position at a salary greater than my previous one. Returning to finalize the deal, I was interviewed by Gail, a cordial and attractive woman of Portuguese descent with a Rhode Island accent. She asked one very incisive question. "Having worked so long at St. Anthony's/BayCare, would you be tempted to return out of loyalty should they make you a better offer?" In a matter of seconds, I recognized what a very good question that was. I had been a very loyal employee. Things had changed. *Times* had changed. I looked forward to turning over a new leaf. After a few minutes of reflection, I looked up at her and said simply and honestly, "No." Nothing negative about my former employer just . . . no.

An Elder Healthcare System

Orientation to Menorah Manor proved quite an undertaking. I discovered that MM was not just a SNF, but a comprehensive health care system focused on the elderly. Anabelle arranged for me to spend a short time with each of the three RN Resident Care Coordinators (RCC's). To market Menorah Manor to healthcare facilities, I needed to discover all that Menorah Manor had to offer. It was the only Jewish nursing home on the west coast of Florida. While its first responsibility was meeting the skilled nursing needs of Jewish elderly, it had expanded its outreach to elders in general. Judy and Leta had worked closely with Jewish organizations (Maimonides Society, Hadassah, JCC), synagogues and temples (collectively: shuls). "Community" was code for "*Jewish* community." There were plaques all over the walls honoring donors. Menorah Manor was a faith-based, not-for-profit organization. Having worked for a Catholic non-profit for more than thirty years, I felt at home.

There were a few differences. No Christian holidays were celebrated here—only Jewish ones. All food was kosher. Kosher foods conform to Jewish dietary laws (Kashrut). Biblically-based, they govern how animals are slaughtered and the parts of their bodies which can be consumed. Dairy and meat cannot be served together. A rabbi oversees the kitchen. Unlabeled, potentially non-kosher food could not be brought in from outside, except for the employee dining room. A large chapel with an Ark housed the Torah but the room could be divided into three sections for resident activities.

Upstairs, three floors housed specialized units. There was a small unit for short-term rehab patients; two units for long-term alert patients who could socialize; and two units for palliative, end-of-life, bed-bound patients. A third unit housed early dementia patients who were mobile, could socialize and could find their way around the building freely without risk of wandering outside. There were alarms in elevators and at doors to the outside which sounded when at risk patients tried to pass. A specific procedure for "elopement" assured a rapid response.

Second floor housed dementia patients. Dementia is a collective term for diseases like Alzheimer's, vascular dementia, Lewy body dementia and others. To exit that floor, a code was required for the elevator to open. Second floor included two separate areas—early dementia was the smaller unit. Residents on this unit interacted, played games, worked at crafts and enjoyed a large secure patio with a garden maintained by volunteers. The other two dementia units housed people who were mobile but walked aimlessly, spoke or acted repetitively and purposelessly. It would be entirely possible for someone with dementia to be admitted on the early dementia unit; to be transferred to a secure unit when becoming a wander risk; then, with progression of the disease, to be transferred to the more advanced unit. When virtually bed-bound, they could be cared for on the palliative unit. Placing patients appropriately throughout the building was the key to Menorah's success. Alert and oriented patients were not frightened or appalled by people with advanced dementia. Dementia patients avoided being rudely treated by alert patients who did not understand them. The delineation allowed staff to work with the kind of patients with whom they were comfortable—a good deal for everyone.

Patient rooms were unique. Except for a few private rooms scattered around the units, most were semi-private, built so that each patient had his privacy and each patient had a window. A three-quarter-wall divided roommates preventing them from seeing each other. Only the bathroom was shared. Visiting many nursing homes as Nurse-Liaison, I never encountered a SNF set up so well.

The composition of patients according to payer source was more than seventy percent Medicaid. The rest were Medicare, private insurance or private pay. Medicaid did not fully cover the cost of providing care. If Menorah had been a for-profit, obviously the care would have had to be scaled back—in quantity and/or quality. Thanks to donations from the Jewish Community (and from some of us employees), the care and services available were outstanding in relation to other area nursing homes. In quite a few nursing homes, when one became a Medicaid patient, he was either discharged or placed in a three or four bed "ward"—clearly for lower income, in a more austere area of the building. Not so with Menorah Manor. Unless a patient chose to share her payer source, no other patient knew. Everyone was treated the same.

A podiatrist, a wound care physician, an audiologist, a dentist, psychologists—all operated in either the Menorah clinic or at bedside. A two-page list of staff physicians was useful for patients to choose the doctor who would follow them there. There was an X-ray room, but x-rays could also be completed at bedside.

Bayfront was contracted to perform lab work.

The cook, Bill, prepared outstanding meals. Arriving for work, I caught whiffs of home cooking. On Friday nights, I quietly hummed the tune to *Bei Mir Bist Du Shein*, a Yiddish song: "To me you are beautiful." It was popularized by the Andrews Sisters and enthusiastically sung by the post Yiddish Lotto crowd of residents. Later, on Friday evenings, gussied-up residents and family members lined up, some in wheelchairs, for the Shabbat dinner (like Sunday dinner) which signaled the beginning of the Sabbath. For Shabbat, the chapel was transformed into a restaurant with white tablecloths, wine glasses, and brisket. Brief prayers were said and a candle lit. Families were urged to accompany their loved ones for this special dinner. People of all faiths were welcome. A religious service followed on Saturday morning.

No one wants to be in a nursing home. But if circumstances dictated that being in a nursing home was inevitable, Menorah Manor was the place to be. A myriad of opportunities existed for the enjoyment of patients and families—a well-stocked library; board games and puzzles; television; at least twice daily activities; a hair salon; a gift shop with treats as well as essentials like stamps and cards. The MM bus took groups out to lunch or for shopping episodically.

Menorah Manor reached into the community with its specialized expertise, as a mitzvah but also for marketing. There were two directions for outreach:

The *Adult Day Center* was a Monday through Friday operation. Elders—usually with very early dementia—could be dropped off or picked up by MM to spend the day while their families worked or engaged in a little R&R. Meals were provided on tablecloths with good china to encourage polite and mannerly behavior. There was a room for naps. They watched TV or engaged in games designed to improve memory in the living room. The dining room converted to a craft room for seasonal creations to which they pointed with pride. Julie Forsythe, LPN and manager, administered medications and plotted their progress. The group took Menorah's bus for field trips. Occasionally there was a cookout beside their back door overlooking Bear Creek. When some of these folks eventually required in-patient care, the transition was easier because Menorah had become like home.

The other outreach was the *Geriatric Assessment Program* which met weekly in the library. Around a large table, Dr. David Levine, MD; psychologist Dr. John Carnes; and Jeanette Brownstein, MSW—all gerontologists—interviewed the patient and family member(s). The people assessed lived in the community, alone or with spouse or adult children. Usually, there had been a change in behavior, a new tremor or gait disturbance. The patient's primary physician had either overlooked it, or ascribed it to normal aging, or had been unsuccessful treating it. Families were self-referred—no need for a doctor's referral. The physician and psychologist billed Medicare or insurance, but there was no fee for Jeanette's time. Apart from the actual assessments, her time included record keeping and availability for long-term follow-up and counseling. Her role included counseling and referral to community resources. When completed, the patient's primary physician was sent a copy of their findings and recommendations.

I attended one of the assessments and was awestruck by the dynamics. The woman had been referred by the Neighborly Community Center. Small and scrawny with stringy, greasy hair and questionable hygiene, she entered the room clinging to her over-sized son. While we waited for the session to begin, I asked her what she wanted to happen here. She hoped that they would find a reason why she was so unsteady on her feet. Dismissive of her concern, her son chided that if she just held on to him, she could walk fine.

For an hour, all three professionals interacted with patient and son, assessing emotional, cognitive, functional, and physical status. Dr. Levine drew blood and wrote a prescription for a brain scan. The history revealed that mother and son had stayed with out-of-town relatives over the Christmas holidays. Prior to the visit, she had been drinking excessively. During the visit without alcohol, she had had a seizure—possibly alcohol withdrawal. Since then, her gait had been "off." Her son believed that her judgment was off, too. She lived with him. But he worked away from home during the day. There were long stretches of alone time.

Two weeks later, mother and son returned to discuss the evaluation results. Cognitively, her judgment *was* a bit off. Though there were no signs of Alzheimer's, perhaps there was some vascular dementia, making it inadvisable for her to spend long periods alone. The scan revealed a previously undiagnosed cerebellar CVA (stroke)—likely the cause of her impaired gait. One of her meds could have compounded the gait problems. An alternate med was suggested. She would benefit from physical therapy. Everything was discussed in an hour long round table with the three professionals. A copy of the team's conclusions and recommendations was sent to the family doctor.

Mother and son were introduced to the MM Adult Day Care Center where the patient could receive physical therapy as an outpatient. Weeks later, I watched the same lady walking in the hall with a walker and a therapist. While in the Day Center she used our beauty shop and had a nice clean do. With regular, balanced meals and fluids, she had filled out. No longer scrawny and greasy-haired, she was coming into her own.

A well-kept secret, Menorah offered physical, speech or occupational therapy on an outpatient basis. One need not have been an inpatient. Rehab team members were extremely talented, enthusiastic and creative. Motivation was their forté. Overflowing with specialized equipment, the gym looked out over Bear Creek.

Adjacent to MM's main building was the one-story ALF, *Toby Weinman Assisted Living Residence (TWALR)*. In a U shape, TWALR's open end with a patio faced Bear Creek where alligators and exotic birds could be observed in their natural habitat. Residents grew herbs and tomatoes in waist-level boxes set up by volunteers. The ALF could accommodate twenty to twenty-five people and kept kosher. Rooms featured showers with a low lip and built in stool. Bathroom lights blinked on with entry. There were inconspicuous hand bars along the halls. A variety of room types and sizes met multiple needs for married couples or individuals. The dining area was spacious and there was a small library.

Jewish Hospice Program worked conjunctively with the Hospice of the Florida Suncoast, providing rabbinical and volunteer support to Jewish patients in their homes or at MM. Sometimes, when a patient was dying in the SNF, one of the ALF residents volunteered to sit with him.

Appreciating a Rich Jewish Heritage

My old friend from my Final Transition classes, Rabbi Luski, was the rabbi for Congregation B'nai Israel next door. But we had our own rabbi in Pastoral Care. Rabbi *Gabriel* Ben-Or did, in fact, resemble an angel with curly blonde hair.

When Rabbi Ben Or left Menorah, he was replaced by a dynamic woman, Rabbi Leah Herz. With bubbly disposition and sandy, curly hair, she resembled Shirley Temple. No taller than that tap-dancing tyke, Rabbi Leah, a mature woman with a grown son, ministered to staff and patients alike. She could resoundingly blow a shofar taller than she. The shofar, a ram's horn, is blown in shul during Rosh Hashanah and Yom Kippur.

Purim, the holiday based on the Book of Esther, was always a big event. Esther was married to a Persian king who was unaware that she was Jewish. Haman, an evil court advisor, plotted to destroy the Jewish people. Esther's cousin, Mordecai, discovered the plot and informed Esther. Revealing that she was Jewish was dangerous but, to save her people, Esther bravely informed her husband. The Jewish people were saved, and Haman was hanged. It is a great feminist tale of triumph illustrating that we need to be brave enough to do the right thing (á la Sister Beatrice).

The feast was cause for celebration at Menorah. Each year a pageant depicting the story was performed. In different years, the roles of Esther, King, Haman and Mordecai were played by staff, patients or tiny kindergarteners from the Jewish Day School. The funniest was a pint-sized, costumed Esther who turned to her husband and coyly improvised, "King, honey, I gotta tell you something." Essential to Purim celebration were hamantaschen, triangular fruit-filled cookies. Another essential was making cacophonous noises to drown out the word "Haman" whenever it was uttered—to signify that he will be forever damned for his heinous plot.

Purim signaled the marketing portion of my "Liaison" work. Most agencies like ours provided treats to physicians at Christmas and Easter. We were different and capitalized on it. Whatever we gifted them had to be kosher. For Purim, we provided hamantaschen; for Rosh Hashanah, apples and honey; and for Passover, chocolate matzo. I was the deliverer to doctor's offices, praying that my chocolate wouldn't melt, or my apples wouldn't rot in the hot car while I dragged them all over the county. Usually I designed the card accompanying the gift. I liked using a little creativity in the job and was grateful to be encouraged to do it.

A lapsed Catholic in a Jewish facility, I felt very at home. I believed the Shema in Deuteronomy 6:4: *Hear, O Israel: The Lord our God, the Lord is one.* Those words are placed in a mezuzah, a small cylindrical or rectangular case affixed to the doorframes of Jewish homes—including Menorah Manor's front door. What Catholics would call "actual grace," Jews would call a "mitzvah"—a good deed. I witnessed many mitzvah, large and small, while working there. Menorah Manor's raison d'être was to provide a warm, hamish (homelike), Jewish environment. *Anyone* would feel at home among these caring people. A lapsed Catholic in a Jewish SNF? Ish Kabibble? (What's to worry?)

Consummate Professionals

I discovered that I would report to both the Director of Nursing, Anabelle, *and* to the Director of Admissions and Marketing, Leta. Both would complete my evaluation. *No one can serve two masters.* (Mathew 6:24) Like Solomon's baby, would I be torn in half? (Kings 3:25) I preferred to answer to nursing. Soon, I revised my opinion. It worked just fine. After I devised a new assessment tool and wrote the procedure for it, Anabelle and I realized that we were fairly in sync. She had bigger fish to fry, assuring safe nursing practice on the units. She was always copied in on the results of my assessments and would ask questions if she had them. Episodically, when concerned about an unusual patient situation, I asked Anabelle's opinion and discovered that we agreed. Anabelle and I were each satisfied with her benign neglect.

Leta was the heart of Admissions. She had global responsibilities, about which I don't believe even Administration had a clue. Leta constantly greased the wheels to make everyone happy. She remained connected to SNF patients and ALF residents—dealing with their problems—legitimate or picky (roommate kept light on after 8 p.m.; staff wouldn't let her keep money in her room, the brisket wasn't cooked right).

One son who was hen-pecked by his mom (our patient) brought her a baseball cap which read: חי **MAINTENANCE**. The symbol is Hebrew for "Chi" or "Life." It is pronounced like a coughing "Hi" and is ubiquitous in Jewish circles. His mother was one of many who could wear that cap. Always cordial, always calm, Leta deflected lunacy allowing team members do our work.

We set up luncheons with hospital case managers to introduce me as their new liaison. For the lunches, I created and presented a PowerPoint about Menorah Manor. The lunches were delicious and artfully prepared by Bill the chef who accompanied us to set up tablecloths, centerpieces, and meal. We always made verbal note of the kosher food and tried to debunk misconceptions—one being that you had to be Jewish to be admitted to Menorah Manor. I developed and distributed a one-page grid of all the services offered by Menorah Manor with contact names and numbers to be used as a resource for the case managers.

Moves were a big part of Leta's life. She coordinated all moves within the SNF and ALF; making sure that the room didn't need "touch-ups" like flooring, paint or plaster; communicating moves to other departments; arranging with Housekeeping to perform the actual move. If someone had a communicable disease (C-difficile, Shingles, MRSA, ESBL), and needed isolation or cohorting (placing with a same-disease roommate), call Leta. Plumbing was backed up. Call Leta to notify maintenance. A visiting family member was hypoglycemic. Call Leta to arrange for lunch at the gift shop. Is it any wonder she had frequent migraines? Leta was one of the most genuinely generous and giving people I have known.

A few months into my employment, Julie Hally was hired to fill the admission coordinator position. In her late twenties and recently wed, Julie was a beautiful young woman—slim and tiny with a permanent tan, long shiny black hair and a quick smile. Born in Columbia but raised in the U.S., Julie was energetic, idealistic and sincerely loved gerontology which she had studied at USF. A people-person, she made instant connections with new arrivals and their families. She was the designated team member to get the admission paperwork signed. The number of papers far exceeded what I had handled in home health. Julie entered the information about the new patient into the computer, made and distributed multiple copies for various departments, and warmly greeted the new patient on his arrival.

Julie reminded me of my former student, Christine, who, as an enterostomal therapist, was now a wound care consultant at Menorah. Over the next few years, Julie had two pregnancies. Each time, her belly was almost bigger than she was. Particularly in her first pregnancy, I enjoyed following along, sharing her journey and providing information if needed, getting a taste of my original specialty. My office was a cubicle outside Leta and Julie's offices. I spent the bulk of time out of the office, visiting homes, other SNFs and hospitals in Pasco, Pinellas, Hillsborough, Manatee and Sarasota counties.

One of the most enjoyable people at Menorah was Gwen Kaldenberg, MSW, Director of the Bressler Dementia Unit. Gwen was my size and height with strawberry blonde hair and a quirky disposition. She was unfailingly positive and generous with her time when, episodically, I asked her to accompany me to assess a dementia patient. The dementia unit was Gwen's baby. She was careful and protective of her existing patients and deserved a say on any newcomer's admission and placement based upon the extent of dementia. She felt a keen responsibility to assure that current residents on her unit were not harmed or agitated by a new patient.

If the patient had advanced dementia and only an early dementia room was available, we could not admit him. Probably that perpetuated hospital case managers' perceptions that it was difficult to place patients at Menorah Manor.

When they called, they asked only, "Do you have a bed? "or "Do you have a male/female bed?" They were woefully unaware of just how many types of beds we had and persisted in asking the same questions despite multiple explanations. Placing the right patient in the right bed was responsible for our positive community reputation. We rarely had empty beds on dementia and, when we did, they were filled quickly. Those who were there were well cared for and constantly stimulated by two dedicated activities therapists.

Gwen was a riot. We chatted up a storm on our travels. We developed our own shorthand communication—just a look or staccato phrase in the patient's presence. One of my acts of bravery was to invade the body space of prospective patients to test the likelihood of aggression—always ready to take a quick step away. To sweeten the deal, when we traveled a distance, we rewarded ourselves with lunch at *Sweet Tomatoes.*

It was impossible to escape the Prospective Payment System (PPS), even in a nursing home. Since 1998, SNFs had been mandated to use a prospective payment system for Medicare. Like home health, it relied not solely on medical diagnosis but included functional and cognitive status. It factored in what had happened to the patient in the hospital in the weeks prior to admission to the SNF. The SNF version of PPS relied on the Minimum Data Set (*MDS*), a lengthy multipage assessment performed within a few days of admission. It was like home health's OASIS. The MDS was repeated episodically to monitor change. Based on the *MDS*, patients were placed in categories called *RUGs* (*Resource Utilization Group—similar to hospital DRG's*) which determined reimbursement for that patient. Of course, the emphasis was on getting a higher paying *RUG*.

Fortunately, Menorah did not rely solely on floor nurse assessments for the *MDS.* There were three *MDS Coordinators*—two LPN's and an RN Director, Joan McCabe. These three created patient care plans and held patient care conferences with both patient and family to assess progress toward goals. Joan later became Risk Manager. Joan was an affable tall blonde Ohioan. I enjoyed her use of colloquialisms common to the Ohio/Pennsylvania area like "younz and youse."

In the beginning, Joan came down hard on me. Concerned with MDS, she constantly pointed out what *other* information I had failed to secure that might improve the *RUG* but would be of no earthly use to the actual care. Heeding her advice, I restructured my assessment sheet twice to reflect her concerns. I also attended an all-day seminar in Tampa about MDS. It was more than I wanted to know. Eventually, Joan helped me get my act together and we worked cohesively.

We both attended the very early morning daily Nursing meeting with the DON, ADON, and RCC's. In the meetings, patient care and progress throughout the house was reviewed daily. Often Joan and I had similar thoughts—expressed differently. Sometimes I was the recipient of dirty looks for having the audacity to admit a difficult patient or a patient with needs which were difficult to meet. Generally, I took it with a grain of salt and used my time to speak as a means of making the new patients' needs as clear as possible. The meetings provided feedback about how my admissions fared.

A very self-effacing man at MM was a VIP in my book. His name was Ray Teasdale. Shortly after I arrived at Menorah Manor, Ray was appointed Activities Director. He had worked in activities on the dementia unit for years. Tall, his head shaved, he resembled Daddy Warbucks. In a rare moment of personal transparency, he explained that as a child he had suffered teasing and bullying. He never wanted to make anyone feel the way that he had felt. He treated each patient and every staff person with dignity and respect. Each person was treasured for their specialness. Ray and his staff engineered multiple activities throughout the day both in the SNF and ALF.

Observing Ray's activities, I recognized that patients could fare better at Menorah Manor than they had in their homes. Families found that difficult to understand, having desperately tried to keep their loved one at home. They felt guilt, relief, or—more often—a combination. At home, usually the most stimulation had been the TV. Patients coming from home could be poorly nourished because of their lack of energy or cognitive inability to make meals. Here, the meals provided were wholesome and attractive. The activities almost never stopped. Music filled the halls on most days. Al, in the Activities department, played a mean piano as did some patients' family members. There were current events discussions, Monday morning cooking by the women residents, painting, balloon volleyball, bowling, Thai Chi, lectures, visiting singers, and programs with children from the Jewish Day School. An Elvis impersonator had the women swooning. All thanks to Ray and his department.

The atmosphere reminded me of an old Andy Rooney/Judy Garland movie where someone says, "Let's put on a show," and everyone contributes. At an annual extravaganza with different themes, staff put their hearts and souls into providing variety shows—magic, dancing singing and stand-up comedy (Dr. Levine & Son). I was a can-can dancer with administration women and a singer for nursing's version of the *So Long* song from the *Sound of Music*. DON, Anabelle, performed a "fire dance" from her native Philippines—dancing in native garb with a bowl of real fire on her head. The Staff Kazoo Band performed episodically, wearing parrot head visors as we played.

Ray enlisted my dog "expertise." For several years, at Westminster time, I masterminded a real dog show with real judges—one of whom had judged at Westminster. Another was our evening receptionist, Arlene. We laid down a rubber track for the dogs, roped off the ring and put on a "benched" show, placing the dogs on display while patients filed by them to enter and exit. There were ribbons and a trophy for Best in Show. Win photos were by Judy and Marshall. The Administrator was the ring steward. I was the announcer. We had a bogus need for cleanup when I surreptitiously liberated plain water from a syringe. Heidi, Medical Records Director, answered the call of "Clean up to Ring 3." Folks loved it. We made the paper. We made good impressions on those who were gracious enough to bring their dogs. But, best of all, in sharing a little dog show flavor, we made our residents' day.

Patients and Their Families

Life was very good there. Of the one hundred and eighty beds, we were able to keep all but five to ten occupied while being a bit picky about who was admitted and where they were placed. My actual patient contact was minimal—just the pre-admission interview. But I was privileged to interact with some of the long-term patients on a regular basis as our paths intersected around the facility.

A one-hundred-year-old woman, well-coifed, rode her electric scooter, purse hanging from her arm. She rolled out onto the first-floor patio garden to pick hibiscus for her room. Her hearing was bad, but she peered up at bystanders, smiling, raised a clenched victory fist, and declared in a throaty voice through clenched teeth, "Yeah!"

An elderly man with his walker made his way over from the ALF every morning, interrupting the admissions "stand up" meeting to wish us all a good morning. Sometimes he brought candy, other times, he brought flowers. Whenever I toured prospective ALF residents or their families, he graciously invited them to tour his apartment, pointing out a large portrait of his beloved wife of many years.

One pleasant lady, mildly confused, shuffled around the building. To her it was a social club, replete with activities. In a grass skirt she performed the hula beside similarly clad employees during one extravaganza.

Deb had mild dementia and swore that she had once been five-foot-four. Now she was closer to four-foot-eight. She loved Julie, calling out to her in an adenoidal New York voice, "Jew-ly." Whenever I toured folks on her early dementia unit, Deb always asked if I wanted to show them her "apartment," a semi-private room.

A very dignified, well-dressed woman whom I always addressed as "Mrs." on the dementia unit enjoyed reading the paper and completing word puzzles on her "front porch." The front porch was the hallway outside her room. The puzzles she only *imagined* solving. She had dementia, but she knew when it was Friday, wishing me a "Shabbat Shalom." Her daughter kept her immaculately dressed, providing outfits and coordinating costume jewelry explaining that her mom had always been a sharp dresser. The aids dutifully adhered to the program, dressing her just so.

An emaciated Catholic woman with an orange beehive would only move to a more appropriate unit if she could see the Catholic cathedral from her window.

A wheelchair-bound, roly-poly man from Morocco via Paris promised to speak French with me if I would teach him a few Russian words.

We had our own tragic love story. Hans had been a young Jewish Pole who joined the Russian army for survival during World War II. Postwar, he moved to Canada where he married and had children. When he was widowed, he moved to the east coast of Florida, where he met and fell in love with Fanny. A subsequent stroke robbed her of the ability to speak (aphasia). When she was admitted to Menorah Manor, Hans relocated to Benjamin Tower next door. Daily, he walked over to help her with meals and to support her in any way that he could. He made certain that her hair was done, her nails polished, and that she was not alone. Her look of devotion toward him mirrored his. When Hans became ill, he was moved back to Canada by his daughter never again to see his beloved Fanny.

My limited patient contact was satisfying. But as Liaison, the more I was out marketing or assessing prospective patients, the better.

Technology: A Blessing and a Curse

Electronic Medical Records (EMR) were mandated by the federal government in 2009. The target date was 2014. Penalties would be assessed in 2015 for non-complying institutions. Information Technology (IT) had come a long way from the birth of personal computers and my Mac Classic. It was now an era of technical sophistication. One example: the smart phone—a hand-held computer capable of exchanging information—both text and photo—virtually around the world!

Charting was no longer to be hand written but *entered* on computer. In one respect, it was a boon for nurses. Some physicians' handwriting was impossible to decipher without the potential for misinterpretation. Care could be safer and more accurate with *EMR*. With connectivity, the physician could access lab work or x-rays for his hospitalized patient without having to be physically present in the hospital or SNF twenty-four/seven. Time could be shaved off his day by not having to walk to radiology to access an x-ray. Referrals could be made, and information transferred to other health facilities or home health agencies considering admitting the patient.

Menorah Manor was no slouch, becoming one of the first local SNF's to initiate EMR. A bonus—statistics were kept about key elements of patient care. Anabelle and comrades poured over the statistics constantly, picking up loose ends. Sometimes I wondered if their attention was focused more on statistical reports than on actual patient care and face-time with the caregivers. But who could blame them? When the AHCA (Florida's Agency for Health Care Administration) team arrived for yearly surveys, armed with the power to award their precious stars or to shut us down, their evaluation was based on these easily available statistical computer runs. That I was cynical should be no surprise. From home health, I had learned that *If it was not charted, it was not done* should be: *If it was charted, it was not necessarily done.* Once again, man-made constructs, even computerized ones, can fall short. It is possible to look far better (or far worse) on paper or computer than in reality.

HIPAA, the <u>H</u>ealth <u>I</u>nsurance <u>P</u>ortability and <u>A</u>ccountability <u>A</u>ct, had been another federal mandate back in 1996. Summarized in one word—it would be PRIVACY. The patient has a right to privacy. HIPAA anteceded and eventually led to the *EMR* mandate. *EMR* made sense. Now, case managers in the hospitals could send history, physical, med sheets, and other appropriate information to the SNF with the referral via a web-based network. *Curaspan* or *ECIN* were the two networks used by local hospitals. But hospitals required the SNF to pay to participate.

Access to patient information within a hospital during a visit was a prickly issue. For years, all that was required to enter a hospital and have access to patient charts was signing-in. In some hospitals, I would just walk in the front door and sign in. In others, the sheet was in Materials Management, Case Management or the Emergency Department. Parking could be very far away. The job required extensive walking. I eschewed high heels and walked fast.

Hospitals are responsible to *JCAHO* (the Joint Commission on the Accreditation of Healthcare Organizations) for maintaining *HIPPA* standards and for demonstrating accountability for control of people who enter their buildings. Hospitals also have high risk of liability for any injury to patient, visitor or staff. Several of the *for*-profit hospitals concluded that it was best to shift the responsibility for monitoring visiting professionals to an independent on-line credentialing, company. There were several. *REPTRAX* and *Vendor Clear* were two with which we dealt. The HCA hospitals (Largo Medical Center, Edward White, Northside and St. Petersburg General) chose one. IASIS (Palms of Pasadena) chose the other. Only liaisons vetted and approved by the on-line companies were permitted access to charts. The existence of these intermediary credentialing agencies was a good deal financially—for the credentialers. I wish I had thought of it. Hospitals paid the on-line intermediary to maintain the records. SNFs paid them to approve one or more of their nurses at greater than two hundred dollars a year per liaison. It was not a good deal from my perspective as Liaison.

Each company considered me a vendor. A nurse, not a vendor, I visualized Dali's *Chest of Drawers* sculpture. My chest would open like a vending machine and a can of Pepsi would emerge!

For credentialing, the company requirements included: yearly chest x-ray and yearly flu vaccine—more than my own employer mandated. Radiation has a cumulative effect. They wanted proof of all vaccines since childhood. They demanded scanned copies of license to practice, college diploma, employment history for the past year, physician's statement that I was in good health, a copy of Menorah Manor liability insurance, and my photograph. In addition, there were five on-line multiple-choice tests with a 100% pass requirement. Some tests were easy. A difficult one concerned electrical safety in the Operating Room. Apparently, everyone was in one class of vendors, including industrial reps demonstrating OR equipment. Please! I would never see the patient until he was well out of there.

Once credentialed, when I signed in at a hospital, I entered my code and received a sticky name badge with my photo, name and time of entry. After the visit, I was required to sign out on the computer. This process of credentialing with a constant stream of individual hospital policies to sign off on throughout the year was never-ending. Each year required an update and a new fee. These so-called "advances" mostly succeeded in complicating access to patients and their information.

Expansion during the Recession

The time frame was the first decade of the Twenty-First Century. On September 11, 2001, terrorists had hijacked four airplanes, ramming two into New York's Twin Towers and one into the Pentagon. A group of resourceful citizens had derailed the hijackers' plans for the fourth plane and crashed it into a Pennsylvania field. The death toll was astounding. Within two years, the US was immersed in a bloody and prolonged war against the Taliban and al-Qaeda in Afghanistan and Iraq. The war's objective was finding al-Qaeda's founder, 9-11 mastermind, Osama bin Laden. An intelligence claim that, Iraq, under President Saddam Hussein, had amassed weapons of mass destruction was later disproved. Nevertheless, Hussein and his regime toppled. Hussein was executed in 2003 and US troops discovered and killed Osama bin Laden in 2011.

Domestically, President George Bush was in his first term of office on 9-11. The home-front reaction was jingoistic. War stretched on interminably. The cost—in resources, in human life and limb, and monetarily—was staggering. Not just the US experienced the strain. Oil (much of which came from the Middle East) and food prices rose. Risky lending practices in the US led to loan defaults. Unemployment soared. Homes were foreclosed. The homeless became increasingly visible. By 2008, we were in full *Recession* which, some argued, was the worst since *The Great Depression* of the 1930s. Its effects were felt well into 2013. Barack Obama, riding on the campaign slogan of *Hope*, was elected President in 2008. Coping with financial crises, his administration was hog-tied by an extremely divisive Congress. One of the factions, the Tea Party, was the most vocal. Of note, Congress passed the *Affordable Care Act* in 2010, which opponents dubbed *Obamacare*. Its purpose was to provide comprehensive health reform, increasing the quality, affordability and the percentage of insured citizens. Though its opponents were many, the ACA was upheld by the US Supreme Court (National Federation of Independent Business v. Sebelius, June 2012) By 2016, it had twenty million participants.

Into that precarious and financially perilous atmosphere, Menorah Manor's Board and executives made the decision to step forth with expansion. I assume the idea had been brewing for some time. My first inkling was when Marshall asked if I thought I could bring in enough rehab patients to fill a forty-bed unit. *Remember, short-term rehab patients offered the best reimbursement.* We had a boat-load of long-term Medicaid patients whose payments fell far short of the cost to provide care. Completely understanding why Marshall would want forty rehab patients—*I wanted to win the lottery*—I replied truthfully that I had trouble filling twenty beds with rehab patients. If I did not provide the answer he sought, I should have realized that there were others, including pricey consultants who would.

The concept included a large spa-like rehab area where patients never so much as glanced at a long-term patient. Elegant separate dining facilities and a whirlpool would complete their experience. According to the plan, on admission, rehab patients would not enter via the front door but through a side door directly to their own private elevator up to their renovated accommodations. That sounds good albeit elitist. But how do you teach random ambulance drivers to know the difference between long-term (front door) and short-term (side door) patients? The gym would be redesigned with separate areas for short-term and long-term patients. Food on the plush unit would be different from the rest of the house and would be served restaurant-style with a chef cooking to order. Staff groused about the demeaning effect that the proposed caste system would have for aware patients on other units.

To begin the renovation of 4N and 4NE, one of those twenty bed units was emptied out, the patients transferred elsewhere in the facility. Grumbles and groans followed. Logistically, during renovations, a minimum of *twenty empty beds would not garner revenue.* Already, we were in the hole! When one wing was finished, patients from the other wing were transferred to the renovated unit to empty out the next wing for renovation. The whole deal took at least six months—*six months of at least twenty empty beds*—while we scrambled to place the long-term patients somewhere other than the new unit.

Simultaneously, Menorah Manor's Board secured loans to begin construction of *Inn on the Pond*, an ALF to rise at the former site of the Jewish Community Center in Clearwater. Early in the depths of the recession, loans were next to impossible to secure. This ALF would be much larger than *TWALR* and would include a memory support (dementia) unit. Leta campaigned to secure financial commitments from prospective Jewish residents before the first shovel broke earth.

Consider the atmosphere. Home owners overextended with high-risk loans were being foreclosed and left on the street—sometimes literally. Here we were creating two new ventures simultaneously while cutting one source of income by more than ten percent for as long as those twenty beds remained empty. A leap of faith? The Comptroller was nervous. I understood why. Digging in their spurs, she and Administration pressured Admissions to fill every last possible bed that remained, failing to grasp the extrinsic factors beyond our control. We took to the road extolling our virtues to case managers and doctors' offices.

Cost-cutting had been noticeable for some time. Wonder-Chef, Bill, was gone, replaced by a series of less talented people. Food for employees was targeted. When I had been hired, meals were served free as an employee benefit. During or prior to construction, a nominal fee was set. Then the fee was raised. Finally, lunch was no longer provided. Staff was responsible for their own meals except during Passover when leavened bread was not permitted in the building. There were no raises during those years.

Out of Touch

Just before construction began, Leta's husband was offered a job in Seattle where their married son lived, and another married son would soon follow. It was Leta's dream to have her family together and to enjoy her future grandchildren. While happy for her, I would miss her dearly.

Following Leta's decision, there was a spate of disastrous Admissions Directors. Apparently, the only requirement was being Jewish. Sixty-something, a grade school remedial reading instructor had no experience in health care. She was lovely but nervous. Her memory extended no more than five minutes. I thought she might be a Geriatric Assessment Program (GAP) candidate. Seriously. Nervous, red welts flamed on her arms and neck. After numerous complaints, late one afternoon, Marshall closed her door. The next morning, we learned the new Director was history.

Lori, Julie's other half, not short on self-confidence, applied for the job. Lori was opinionated and a little pushy. She jumped to conclusions. But she was energetic and enthusiastic. Lori knew Menorah Manor. She had experience in a physician's office and needed no tutoring on medical lingo. She lacked Leta's calm maturity and measured words, but she must have impressed Marshall because we heard her scream of delight when told the Director position was hers.

Lori inherited the task of master-minding the huge exodus of twenty people out of the unit being renovated. It sounds easy but wasn't. What little security long-term residents had was easily threatened. Lori accomplished it positively, optimistically and cheerfully, literally joining Housekeeping to move beds while lavishing them with praise. Martha, Director of Housekeeping, loved her for that. Lori was able to sweet-talk patients and their families into cooperating with the moves. She monitored the welfare of the residents just as Leta had. Lori also arranged moves at TWALR; organized work to be done on the rooms between residents; and marketed to fill beds when TWALR residents dwindled. Though episodically she made cringe-worthy assumptions, Lori stepped up to the plate. Commuting from her home in Tampa daily, she was unfamiliar with key marketing opportunities in St. Petersburg. I drove her to the Neighborly Senior Services locations, high rise apartments for the elderly, and the local Jewish Community Center (JCC). She discovered neighborhood newsletters and took out ads. Lori, in my estimation, did a great job—an unbelievably positive alternative to the remedial reading appointee.

Apparently, Marshall didn't agree. One afternoon, the Administrator informed me and the newest Admissions Coordinator, Jen, that Marshall was terminating Lori as we spoke. The very difficult moves and relocations were complete. The rehab unit was up and running due, not in small part, to Lori.

With the rehab section completed, we were free (*urged*) to "fill" the twenty-plus empty beds, it was easier said than done. Remember the economy. People were not rushing to hospitals in droves to have elective surgery like hip or knee replacement. When they were hospitalized, their situations were more complicated because they had postponed treatment or sat on symptoms. When an extremely ill person was admitted to Menorah Manor, it wasn't always clear if they would be long or short-term. The goal was a huge volume of short-term rehab patients but none long-term. Rehab patients' actual turn-around time on our unit was swift—staying only a week or so, leaving an empty bed to be filled—again. Hospital case managers had grown accustomed to MM turning down patients during the renovation and were slow to refer. Now we marketed to them constantly. Every Thursday, I delivered platters of kosher bagels to different hospital case managers . . . all while attending to the referrals we received. The pressure was on.

Another Admissions Director was hired. Qualification: she was "big in Hadassah." She had worked for a college foundation. We honestly hoped she would fit the bill—despite her inauspicious lack of any experience related to healthcare. Undoubtedly, she had connections and could be valuable marketing to the community. But referrals? Comprehending medical records or explanations of them?

She evoked memories of Tallulah Bankhead—sixtyish; long, chestnut hair obscuring one eye; deep, raspy cigarette voice; the odor of cigarettes swirling around her. I winced at the first impression she would make on families.

The long hair in desperate need of a headband and the smoking were not the biggest issues. At every turn, the woman resisted learning the ever-essential admissions computer program. She called out from her office, "*What room did we give Mrs. X? I'm too lazy to look on the board.*" The board was in her own office. She had an annoying habit of sniffing—more as a statement than a physiologic need. She thought nothing of invading our space; sitting at our desks; using our phones and computers as we stood by—displaced.

Daily admissions Stand-Up Meetings—the office was too small to sit—became a nightmare. They had been fifteen-minute multidisciplinary meetings to review potential patients and to discuss placement in the facility. Now the meeting was an hour-long misery and gab session. Multidisciplinary eyes rolled. Professionals had better things to do. Julie or Jen eventually took control of the meetings—someone had to.

The new Director wanted to direct the route I took from one referral visit to another. Why did I visit this patient before that one? I had been visiting referrals for six years. As far back as 1990, even my home health supervisor had not questioned my routes. Situations are variable. There were good reasons for my choices.

To every department member complaint, the Administrator responded that we needed to teach her. She did not want to learn. Now I reported solely to the Admissions Director. Now, per the Administrator, I was to teach the woman with the higher salary who would evaluate *me*. *Was that yellow rain?* The situation continued for months, crippling the department. It was our problem because we complained.

Having reached retirement age, that was what I did. I didn't feel the need to clarify. Admissions staff and the Administrator knew what had precipitated it. I gave a month's notice. A week after my last day, the Admissions Director was let go.

Reflection

Administrative debacles had been the lightning rod. But it was time.

Years before, I had believed that working in the nursery would prepare me to care for my own babies. *Life is what happens while you're busy making other plans.* I arrived at sixty-six never having birthed those babies. I had made peace with that. At Menorah Manor, the womb-to-tomb nurse was confronted with what escapes no one. Old age is a process which could scare the begeesus out of anyone—if they let it. I might not have endured an out-of-control labor, but the labor toward my Maker was guaranteed.

Daily for six years, I had read "histories" of people referred to us. The pleasant ones were the quick rehabs after elective surgery. But reading histories of how some had come to need a nursing home for their final days—which could morph into years—was cumulatively wearing. People with dementia had had careers, hobbies, amazing intellects and community involvement. They had been doctors, state legislators, social workers and nurses. Yet, gradually, they lost all that they had been—like flour powdered through a sieve. Others had suffered sudden strokes or heart attacks, leaving them with altered states of consciousness or incapacitation. Dialysis, feeding tubes, ostomies—all on a march to the tomb. Loss of money, possessions, home, family, pets. One minute walking around, the next forever dependent on the care of a few good nurses. Which one of their stories would be mine? Insouciant youngsters (me years ago) and some of my death-denying contemporaries could avoid a comparison which I could not.

The glories of our blood and state

Are shadows, not substantial things;

There is no armor against Fate;

Death lays his icy hands on kings . . .[1]

Endnotes

1. James Shirley (1596-1666), "Death the Leveler," *Immortal Poems of the English Language* (New York: Washington Square Press, 1965), 104.

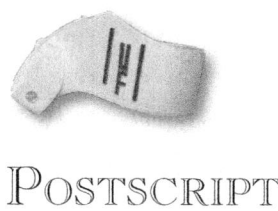

POSTSCRIPT

Writing this memoir has been an amazing trip down the rabbit hole. It is surprising how much that gelatinous grey ball retains after so many years—the sights, the sound of certain voices, the feelings. It has been a *re*-living—with perspective from the comfortable distance of age. Patients, nurses and other health professionals have touched my life. Each contact we have impacts another for the better—or worse. As for my nursing, I hope that my impact has been positive. Certainly, I am the better for having known so many positively wonderful people.

I have always considered the profession a calling and myself a professional. Dean Smith's observation that most of the professional "becoming" occurs after graduation proved true. Interpersonally, I grew into the ability to be therapeutic with individuals, groups and fellow professionals. I impacted individuals' lives on a very basic level. I used my creativity to educate both patient and nurse. I lacked personal ambition to "rise" in the profession, preferring to remain in the trenches rather than become manager or theoretician. I understood the "big picture," but was often powerless to impact formal structures within the health care system.

An usher in the theater of other folks' lives, I cared for women and their families bringing babies into the world. I helped people handle grave illness and loss. I reached out to survivors of loss. I cared for patients in many settings—my favorite their home—where the unvarnished, unabridged person lived. I soothed and comforted. The little girl who craved a cap and white stockings would never have guessed the broad range of professional possibilities that nursing would afford or the number of metamorphoses.

Flying below the radar, making changes from within was my modus operandi. I was a product of my sex, my place in time, and the mid-century Catholic culture in which I came of age. I was no different from my maternity care study, Dorene—also a product of her sex, her culture and society's limitations. My way was not to *lean in*[1] but to *reach around* unobtrusively. My successes were many on a 1:1 level. One day at a time, one minute at a time, I made a difference to patients. As an educator and a role model, I made a difference. A mover and a shaker? No. To effect institutional change, sometimes I might have been speaking a foreign language. The beauty of it is, like it or not, change came anyway. Time does not stand still.

Years ago, up to my eyeballs in oncology, I was asked about "burnout." We recognize how Post Traumatic Stress Disorder (PTSD) affects the military and first responders. They have seen things no one should see and possibly done what they were raised not to do. On a subtler level, nurses experience that, too. They see what the average person does not see and deal with appalling situations over which they feel powerless. It is called *Compassion Fatigue or Secondary Traumatic Stress (STS)*. Flight from the nursing battlefield is not always a realistic or financially feasible option. For nurses, there is no honorable discharge, no purple heart.

I have witnessed long-term, good nurses *close off*—like a flower closing its petals. They retreat, placing institutional structure above individual patient needs; minimizing patient contact; adopting passive-aggressive behavior; charting rote; doing bare minimum. At the beginning, I judged them. Now, I understand and know that at times I have done the same. I never identified patient contact as the stressor. Administrative politics and injudicious leadership were *my* nemeses.

When I had enough, I moved on—within nursing. If I experienced anger, it was directed toward management or systems. I balked when the patient was the last consideration. I balked when management paid top dollar to extrinsic consultants, underestimating the wisdom of front-line employees within their walls who made their system work.

I knew when my time had come. *There is a time for everything and a season for every activity under heaven . . .* (Ecclesiastes 3:1).

At my "retirement" party, a respected nurse-colleague hugged me and whispered in my ear, "You are a good nurse."

That was all I had ever wanted to be.

Endnote

1. Sheryl Sandberg, *Lean In: Women, Work and the Will to Lead* (New York: Random House LLC, March 2013).

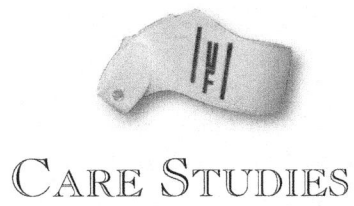

CARE STUDIES

I choose "care" study rather than "case" study. The individuals documented are presented, not as butterflies pinned under a microscope, but unique, strong and courageous women making the best of their challenges.

Dorene's story is the first, written when I was a fledgling maternity nursing student. Dorene introduced me to a culture beyond my ken. I was nineteen. She was twenty-two and pregnant with her eighth baby.

The remaining care studies concern people who have died in my care. When I was challenged by their times of crisis, journaling defused my feelings and clarified my thinking. A nursing educator, I applied their lessons, the most important: discover a patient's unique reality to nurse him.

These are my cemeteries. More appropriately—my memorials.

Care Study: Dorene
Summer 1966

This care study was written as a nineteen-year-old undergraduate student but edited here for brevity. Its intent, other than to document Dorene's story, was to show Miss Hilliard what I knew about maternity.

I met my care study purely by accident. I had just entered one of the clinic rooms to observe a med student examine a mother. The med student sat at the desk charting while the woman with a massive abdomen lay flat on her back. He enthusiastically exclaimed that she should be happy: she was expecting twins! The woman, in her ninth month, whimpered softly. I asked how many children she already had. Four. I responded, "It really must have been a surprise to find out about the twins today." She enthusiastically replied, "Yes, ma'am. I thought I was through having twins." The med student explained that Dorene had delivered twins the previous August, a little more than nine months before.

She was a very dark skinned, African American with broad facial features and no makeup. Her short, black, curly hair was a little disheveled; her pretty, colorful shift wrinkled; white plastic sandals on her feet. While the doctor examined her abdomen, I noticed a silver-colored ring on the ring finger of her left hand. It was not a wedding ring but a dinner ring with the stone turned inward toward her palm.

Finished, the med student left to find Dr. Turner. I helped Dorene to sit up to relieve her discomfort and tried to focus on her feelings about the babies. Her replies were simply, "Yes'm" or "No'm."

Dr. Turner—very white, very tall with very orange hair—was very intimidating to his country clientele. He mumbled a few words about adhering to her diet so that her "blood would not go up." She should return next week. After he left, I helped Dorene off the exam table. We smiled at each other. Outside, Miss Hilliard told me that this could be my care study.

I had mixed feelings. I didn't know how or where to begin. Here was a single woman with four children living and two dead. I wondered about the ring. Did she want us to think it was a wedding ring? What had caused the deaths of her two children? The only clues I could find were in the prenatal record.

I discovered that Dorene, twenty-two years old, lived with her mother on the northeast side of Gainesville. There were five pregnancies prior to her present one, her last was the delivery of twins the previous August. Her first pregnancy— at fifteen—had ended with the delivery of a stillborn male child at thirty-eight weeks (out of forty) gestation. This and the four following pregnancies were delivered at Shands. During her last delivery, Dorene had been pre-eclamptic and had been administered intravenous magnesium sulfate ($MgSO_4$) therapy.

With this pregnancy, Dorene's first clinic visit was on May 9, in her thirty-sixth week of gestation. Her Pap smear and VDRL (syphilis test) were negative. She weighed one hundred and sixty-seven pounds compared to her normal one hundred and fifty-eight pounds. A trace of albumin was present in her urine. Her blood pressure was 140/80. Suspected of multiple pregnancy, her x-ray confirmed twins, both in vertex (head first) position.

On her first visit to clinic, Dorene had been instructed to lose weight, take iron three times a day for "low blood." Doctors were simplistic in their instructions. They assumed the patient incapable of understanding anemia (low blood) and high blood pressure (high blood). It just caused more confusion. I met Dorene on her second visit and "adopted" her as my care study.

Only in my second week of obstetrical nursing, I felt overwhelmed. It was difficult to separate the important from the unimportant; the nursing responsibility from the medical responsibility; to categorize the physical needs and to differentiate and prioritize her more obvious needs:

> 1) Lose weight. *This was the thinking then, but, considering that she had only gained ten pounds for a twin pregnancy, it would be different today. The real issue was water weight.*

> 2) Adhere to a low salt diet and understand that it related to her blood pressure.

> 3) Practice exercises to relieve backache and pelvic pain.

> 4) Know the signs of pre-eclampsia.

> 5) Receive emotional support. Dorene needed acceptance of her feelings rather than the imposition of feelings upon her.

6) Advance beyond the "Yes'm, No'm" stage into one of verbal communication of her feelings—physical and emotional. I needed to know more about her home situation, preparations under way for the new arrivals, and Dorene and her family's reaction to the new arrivals.

Unfortunately, Dorene's next clinic visit was scheduled for the day I was in pediatrics class. After class, I read her chart and discovered that her blood pressure had dropped to 130/80. She had not been taking her iron pills because she could not afford them. I wondered about her income.

On her next clinic visit, Dorene was dressed in a nicely pressed baby blue maternity outfit. Her hair was combed; she wore no makeup and looked very pretty, indeed. I told her so and she grinned sheepishly. While we waited for the doctor to arrive, I introduced myself as Miss Choffat and began to talk with her about her pregnancy. She acknowledged being upset when told she was expecting twins—afraid of what her mother would say. Now she was resigned. Her major discomfort was back-ache. I explained and demonstrated pelvic rocking to her. She seemed pleased and anxious to try it. Dorene added that she had tried to squat just the other day, but her abdomen was so heavy that her mother had to pull her up.

A medical student entered, examined Dorene, then left to find a resident. I helped her to sit up and talked with her about preparations for the babies. She told me that she had or was planning to get all that was needed for the expected twins. She said that she and her mother lived in a three-room wooden building behind her grandmother's larger house. I was unable to grasp where she, her mother and four children slept, only that she and her mother slept in the same room and that they had two beds. She had a refrigerator, but her gas stove was not working so they were using a wood stove. When I asked about a bathroom, Dorene replied that they had a bathroom with a tub and that her mother was planning to install a shower. A good idea, I responded. After the babies were born and even now, it is best not to sit in a pool of water which could travel up the birth canal and transmit an infection.

Dr. McClean arrived with med student in tow and grilled Dorene *and* me. I don't know which of us fared worse! Examining Dorene, he sternly asked me: the complications of twinning; the length of gestation; and the incidence of twinning in the population. Discovering that I did not know the answers to the first and last questions, he angrily retorted, "This is your care study and you don't know? I should think you would be curious enough to find out, don't you Dorene? If I were your teacher, I'd flunk you right now!" Between caustic comments, he threatened Dorene with a thirty-dollar blood transfusion if she did not take her iron tablets and with convulsions if she did not adhere to her diet. Her blood pressure had risen to 140/95 and there was a trace of edema. Dorene complained of dizziness. Dr. McClean admitted her to the hospital for "observation and management of pre-eclampsia."

Dorene looked as though the props had been kicked out from under her, sobbing that she had been afraid of this. She worried how her children would get along without her since her mother was a patient on the fourth floor and her grandmother was the only one available to look after the children.

I didn't know whether to cry or be angry with Dr. McClean. He made me feel so small, stupid and worthless to maternity nursing. But he had no right to barge in, belittle me in front of my patient, ignore her as a person when he talked to me, and then threaten her. I feared that he might have ruined my relationship with Dorene. After this encounter, what reason would she have to trust or have confidence in me? Later I discovered that Dr. McClean's tirade had accomplished just the opposite.

Selfishly, I was glad that Dorene had been admitted. Here was my chance to do some prenatal and diet teaching. For Dorene, it was a traumatic and unhappy experience. She would need a lot of support.

Then I discovered that Dorene was on Tox Precautions and was receiving Phenobarbital. Toxemia Precautions were for patients whose symptoms were so extreme that they were in danger of seizures. I was not permitted to teach her—or even sit and talk with her for more than ten minutes at a time. However, I would be able to give her morning care the following day.

I was discouraged. If unable to teach her, what could I do? Morning care must be kept to a minimum and Dorene should be disturbed as little as possible. How could we build a relationship under those circumstances? The medical goal could be stated very simply, *Get that blood pressure down!* To achieve it, Dorene had been placed in a room with the blinds drawn; no visitors permitted; nursing care kept to a minimum. She was on bed rest with bathroom privileges. She was placed on a half gram sodium diet. Her meds were Hydrodiuril, Phenobarbital and Seconal. All measures were to drive the diastolic pressure downward.

Nursing goals were not so easily stated. The first step was to execute the orders and enforce the limits set by the doctors. Additionally, I wanted to provide comfort and support for the patient and to allay the anxiety caused by her hospital admission. The goals seemed contradictory. How could a nurse expect to allay anxiety and loneliness while keeping patient contact to a bare minimum? Physical comfort could not be achieved with a lick and a promise. Though I would follow the doctor's orders and I would not carry on any formal teaching, I would not rush through morning care but would take enough time to make Dorene physically comfortable to enable her to communicate her needs to me if she felt like it.

The following day proved my approach correct. When we arrived on the floor, Dorene had been crying most of the morning. She had experienced a few irregular contractions and had a white vaginal discharge. That concerned me since I knew that twin pregnancies rarely go to term. I recognized that Dorene might be in early labor. Entering the dark room, we found her crying silently. Miss Hilliard told her that "Peggy" would be taking care of her this morning and that she might feel better after a bath. Dorene whimpered "Yes Ma'am."

As I began the bed bath, Dorene's spirits lifted. We talked about pregnancy— even laughing about how, when she lay on her back, her abdomen rolled to one side or the other. I did some indirect, conversational teaching, asking her if she had read any books about pregnancy and babies. Yes. And she had a book at home which mentioned twins. She wished that she could show it to me. Surmising that Dorene wanted to help me learn more about twins so that I would be prepared for future Dr. McClean inquisitions, I felt better about the fiasco of the previous day. It seemed to have drawn us closer. We were "partners in crime." The climax of the morning came when Dorene burst out, "Peggy, I got to pee!" This was the icing on the cake. It was the first time Dorene had called me by name. I had introduced myself to her as *Miss Choffat*, uncomfortable with *Miss*, and aware that it was a mouthful for anyone to handle. Miss Hilliard had slipped, calling me *Peggy*. Dorene had picked it up! My role as nurse-friend had begun.

One goal had been realized—establishing a trusting relationship with Dorene. I had also learned a little more. Neither Dorene's mother nor her grandmother worked. Dorene worked at a private home for twenty dollars a week until she became pregnant. She also received Aid to Dependent Children (ADC) which, I found, contributed a maximum of eighty dollars a month no matter how many children were dependent. Obviously Dorene was not wealthy. She could need assistance with her budget to meet the needs of her present family, the new arrivals and herself. When she was discharged, I hoped to discuss diet and finances with her at her next clinic visit.

The next clinic visit never came. Dorene missed it and made another appointment for June. At that visit, she was again admitted for pre-eclampsia with a blood pressure of 140/110. Surprisingly, she was not put on Tox Precautions but was given only tranquilizers rather than the usual $MgSO_4$ or phenobarbital. I visited her as soon as possible. She was unhappy about her admission but relieved to have a roommate this time. That night, I returned to the hospital to visit Dorene briefly and then read her past charts which had been sent to the floor from medical records.

Her record was thick as a telephone book, beginning with her first pregnancy in 1959—a stillbirth at thirty-eight weeks. Two weeks prior to delivery, the father of the child had beaten Dorene's abdomen. After the stillbirth, Dorene had several nightmares; expressed guilt concerning the infant's death; and anger toward his father. Subsequently, she was referred to Psychiatric Out Patient Clinic (OPC) where she was interviewed once. Based on that interview, the psychiatrist charted that she had worked out the emotions which had flared immediately post-partum. He considered her intelligence dull normal and her insight nil.

Apparently, the other pregnancies had progressed more smoothly. Each child had a different father. The last pregnancy was complicated by pre-eclampsia. With no prenatal care, the twin pregnancy was not detected until delivery. Both twins were placed in the premature nursery. A period of adjustment to the idea of twins had been necessary for Dorene.

That night while I reviewed her charts and formulated a plan, Hurricane Alma hugged the Florida west coast sending driving rains to Gainesville. I had discovered that, on a low salt, low calorie diet, Dorene had virtually starved herself at home. She ate only one unappetizing meal a day with drinks of Coke® to ease her hunger. Obviously, she needed to be taught better nutrition including specific foods to avoid and why.

When Dr. Mullee examined her, I had noticed that she was terrified of the examination. She needed to be told what is going to be done and why. She needed support during any procedure. I updated the nursing care plan, deciding that the next morning I would fill out a prenatal history and do some labor teaching using the birth atlas.

The next morning Dorene was depressed and non-communicative. I sat at her bedside and began to take a prenatal history in an informal, conversational manner. When I introduced home preparations for the baby, Dorene began to cry. She was not at all prepared for the babies, having neither diapers nor bottles. She did not have a place for them to sleep. She was concerned about her mother, recuperating from her recent illness while caring for Dorene's children. She expressed shame at not being married and at having so many children saying, "They gave me this ring, but it doesn't do any good. I'm still not married." Dorene also expressed shame that she had no housecoat or other personal effects in the hospital with her. By "not having things like other people in the hospital" she was stripped of her last speck of pride.

I did my best to comfort Dorene, but it was difficult. I worried that I had "over-stimulated" her and adversely affected her blood pressure. When Dorene was calmer, I asked if she would like to see how labor progressed. She was interested. Using the birth atlas, I described labor, the relationship of the baby's head to the urinary and GI tract and the sensations which this caused. I explained simply about the cervical "doughnut" and its dilation and effacement. I explained the transitional phase and how, when the contractions become harder and closer together, the sooner it was going to be over. Dorene pointed to the pictures and asked about the water breaking. I explained that this could happen any time but sometimes it did not happen until just before delivery. When I left, Dorene was pensive.

But I was in a tizzy. To put it mildly, I had bitten off more than I could chew. Dorene was in her thirty-ninth week yet she had not prepared for the twins. Obviously, she needed a public health nurse and, perhaps, financial assistance. My first reaction was to go to the team leader who listened to my story before ranting about unwed multigravidas like Dorene. Since that was a blind end, I checked with the Maternal infant Care (MIC) nurse, Mrs. Thorpe, who promised to write a public health referral and to talk with Dorene about methods of contraception. She would be happy to coordinate nursing care for this patient.

The next day, while giving Dorene morning care, I reviewed what it meant to be on a low salt diet. I compared edema to the way a salt shaker attracts moisture and I mentioned the ordinary foods which contain "hidden" salt. Although the information was received well, Dorene was still depressed. I felt that little was accomplished. I attached a note to Dorene's prenatal sheet to instruct the reader to call me in case of labor. Her expected date of confinement (EDC) was just a week away!

It was early that Friday evening. Betty and I had just settled down in the library to study before heading up the hill to the dorms. At seven thirty, the phone rang. I was wanted in labor and delivery. Betty and I rushed up, donned our gowns and entered the labor room. There we found Dorene, thrashing around in her bed, moaning. A glucose IV running in her left arm and a blood pressure cuff around her right arm—neither deterred her thrashing.

When we entered, she stopped thrashing long enough to grin sheepishly and say, "Hey, Peggy. You gonna be with me 'til the babies come?" I assured her that I would be. We began a four-and-a-half-hour vigil of vital signs and reassurance. Dorene's contractions were irregular and of poor quality, five to six minutes apart. I administered a soap suds enema and a prep with the assistance of Mrs. Wilson. I told Dorene what I was going to do, asking her if she remembered our talking about it. She said that she did but, in case she did not, I refreshed her memory. After the enema and prep, the main task facing us was that of reassurance and support of an obviously frightened patient.

Considering the poor quality of her contractions, the pain which she experienced must have been more emotional than physical. All pain is real enough to the patient. Betty and I did all we knew to relieve Dorene's pain. I rubbed her back with each contraction, instructed her in deep breathing, wiped her face with a cool washcloth and let her suck some of the water from it. When she complained of being hot, Betty fanned her. I held her hand. None of our ministrations were very effective. Dorene continued to moan, groan and thrash while her contractions remained of poor quality.

Our weekend curfew was one a.m. We had to leave at midnight. The labor nurse offered to drive us up the hill to the dorm. Dorene's eyes became as big as saucers, "You're going to leave me, aren't you? Don't leave me, Peggy. Don't leave me!" The thought that I would leave seemed to terrify her. I became increasingly aware of Dorene's dependence on me and shuddered at the responsibility. Dorene continued to plead, "Don't let me hurt anymore, Peggy," or just called my name repeatedly. I was glad that Betty was there, too. Betty supplemented my performance. Reassurance and vital signs were all I could manage. Betty timed contractions and recorded the vital signs which I dictated.

As the night wore on, Dorene's labor continued unproductively. Dr. McCurdy or Dr. Mullee would appear, examine her and pronounce that she was "not doing anything." At that, she became upset, recognizing that, despite her contractions, nothing was happening. I explained that her doughnut was getting thinner even though the hole was not much bigger. She was eighty percent effaced but only three centimeters dilated.

At eleven thirty, I left the room for the first time to write some nursing notes. Dorene became extremely agitated, crying loudly, "Betty, tell Peggy to come back. Peggy don't leave me!" I explained that I would be back soon but to little avail. When I returned, Dorene was still crying but now clutched Betty's hand. Truthfully, I was relieved. I was uncomfortable with such intense dependence.

At midnight, we were forced to leave. Despite all explanations, Dorene panicked, crying loudly, screaming at Betty not to let me go. When she realized that Betty was also leaving, she was really in a dither. I hated to leave Dorene. Simultaneously I was relieved. We were exhausted, completely drained. Since Dorene was only three centimeters dilated, it was unlikely that she would deliver until morning. Meanwhile, to help her sleep, Dr. McCurdy ordered 200mg of Seconal.

At one point, a nurse had sternly "laid down the law" concerning Dorene's fussiness. Dorene had been quiet for a while. Should I have been firm? I tried firmness but could not manage it. In perspective, what were our goals with this patient— to keep her quiet or to make her as comfortable as possible? From her chart, Dorene's pattern in her previous labors had been the same. Perhaps this is what her ethnic background told her to do. Perhaps this is the way she thought that labor should be—travail. If so, as nurses, we needed to allow her to labor in her own way, supporting and comforting her by our presence and reassurance.

The next morning, we returned to the hospital at eight with trepidation. To our surprise, Dorene was still undelivered, sleeping peacefully. We did not disturb her but used the time to talk with the nurse about how the night had passed.

Dorene had remained agitated after we left and had continued to call either for her mother or for me. She became nauseated and vomited. She was given Seconal 200mg., Nembutal 200mg., Paraldehyde 15cc. rectally and Morphine 15mg. Finally, she had dozed off. Contractions, effacement and dilation remained the same. The nurse had tried every method of calming Dorene from being very motherly and soothing to being firm. Neither approach was successful.

When Dorene awakened, we resumed our vigil of vital signs and reassurance. She was sleepy, waking only with contractions of increasing intensity. While awake, she was contrite about the way she had behaved the previous evening. Dorene claimed that she was "trying to be good." Since she was more relaxed, I was able to do a better job of getting her to breathe deeply. It all went smoothly from this point on, contractions were forty-five seconds in duration and they were coming closer together. Betty and I resumed comfort measures which we had employed the previous evening.

At nine thirty-four, while Dr. Turner performed a digital examination, the membranes ruptured and Twin A's head which, until this time, had been floating, became engaged in the pelvis. Dorene looked up at him, smiled and teased, "Now look what you did!" Dr. Turner directed that we had better get her back to the delivery room. Realizing the meaning of his words, she looked frightened with eyes again as big as saucers. Betty and I reassured her that we would stay with her during delivery and that soon her labor would be over.

Once in the delivery room, things proceeded quickly. Dorene crawled over to the delivery table on all fours. Betty and I were on either side: Betty taking blood pressure and pulse while I took fetal heart tones. We both held her hands and tried to encourage her as much as possible. At nine fifty-seven, soon after Dr. Turner was seated on his stool, Twin A, a girl, was spontaneously delivered in vertex position with just about one hard push from Dorene. I told her that it was a little girl. She sighed, smiled and began to bet the doctors that the next one would be a boy. The membranes of Twin B ruptured, and amniotic fluid gushed violently due to polyhydramnios (excessive amniotic fluid). Dr. Turner asked Betty to take Dorene's blood pressure. Cardiac failure was possible due to the rapid decrease of intra-abdominal pressure.

Finally, at ten twelve, Twin B, a boy, was spontaneously delivered but failed to breathe or cry. Dr. Sanders, the pediatrician standing by, initiated respirations after intubation.

Shortly after the birth of Twin B, two fused placentas were delivered. Dorene seemed happy and relieved but took little interest in the new arrivals. Although there was a 1° perineal tear, Dr. Turner did not repair it. Dorene was quickly whisked to the recovery room after syntocinon was added to her IV and after morphine sulfate was administered IM.

In the recovery room, Dorene was groggy from the morphine. The twins were brought to her before they were taken to the premature nursery. She made no move to hold them. Now our primary responsibility was observation. Being a grand-multigravida, Dorene needed constant massaging of her fundus and close observation of the height of the fundus and the amount of lochia. Blood pressure was her most important vital sign. If it rose, it could indicate eclampsia. If it fell, it could indicate hemorrhage. Between vital signs, Betty and

I cleaned Dorene's buttocks and perineal area, gave peri-care and placed sanitary pads between her legs. Dorene talked and slept intermittently. She was still apologetic for the previous night's behavior. She mentioned that she wanted to be a nurse like Betty and me and that she wished she had finished school.

At noon, we moved Dorene from the recovery room to third floor where she was placed on Tox Precautions. On transfer, her blood pressure was 140/86, pulse was 84 and temperature was 37° C. Her fundus was firm at U+3. Lochia was rubra and heavy. Before leaving, I asked how she would like to feed her babies. Our previous discussions had concerned the nutritional and financial benefits of breast feeding as well as the satisfaction. She had turned up her nose and said that it would feel funny although she had agreed to think about it. Asked again, she involuntarily turned up her nose, grinned and said, "I'll do whatever you want me to, Peggy." I told her that I wanted her to do what would be most comfortable for her. She repeated her feeling that breast feeding would feel funny. I said, "You would rather bottle feed?" She would. I left Dorene to the sleep which she needed.

Both patient and I had just shared an earth-shattering experience. I needed time to grasp it. Before labor, I viewed Dorene as a twenty-two-year-old woman of low intelligence, a multip and the mother of four children. But during her labor I realized that she was a fifteen-year-old girl who had begun to have babies before she herself had had a chance to grow up. Highly dependent upon her mother and her mother's opinion of her actions, she relied upon her mother to make decisions concerning her (Dorene's) children. In her family, she was more sister than mother to her own children. Her family represented a mother-daughter axis.

Considering that, it was easy to understand her lack of maternal behavior in delivery and recovery. She had not enjoyed her pregnancy, nor had she looked forward to having another baby. Instead, she had denied her pregnancy until her ninth month when she finally appeared at clinic. During labor, she had been panic-stricken, desiring only to be put to sleep and to "get it all over with." Considering that Dorene is close to being a child herself, how could she be expected to show much interest in her newborns? It was *she* to whom the traumatic experience had occurred. She needed time to gradually shift attention from herself to her two small babies.

We could have placed one child in each arm in the delivery or recovery rooms. It was obvious that she was not ready for that. I could have told her that I wanted her to breast feed. But I did not want to force my ideas of what mothering should be upon her. The fact that Dorene would do whatever I wanted indicated her need for approval. I wanted to help her value her own choices.

Preparations had not been made for the babies' arrival. Diapers, bottles and a crib were needed. I checked with the housekeeping department to see if diapers could be given or sold at a discount to patients. I was told they could not.

I continued to visit Dorene for the next two days. On Tuesday I gave her morning care. She did her own peri-care. She had attended Mrs. Thorpe's classes and said that she enjoyed them. Twin B was transferred to the newborn nursery, so I had the opportunity to bring him out to be fed for the first time by his mother. Instead of holding him in her arms, Dorene held him out and away from her body, using only the palms of her hands to touch him. She burped him the same way. I explained the necessity of always keeping the air out of the nipple and of holding the nipple so that it would not block the baby's airway. She was receptive but found it difficult to accomplish while holding the baby at arm's length.

I undressed her boy, to demonstrate that everything was normal. She held him in her lap while we examined the Life Magazine pictures of a newborn and compared her baby's reflexes with the ones illustrated. I wanted to promote bonding with her baby and to understand the reasons behind her baby's actions.

Dorene mentioned that she hardly knew her other little baby. I walked her to the premature nursery where she gowned and scrubbed and sat in the rocking chair holding her baby girl. Dorene seemed nervous once inside the nursery—possibly because she was the only mother in there and she felt out of place. After she had been given her baby, Dorene held it in her arms, closer than she had held the little boy. After looking it over for a while, she shifted her attention to the very premature McClure baby in an Isolette with whom she was fascinated. I explained that this was what a child looked like inside its mother when she was six months pregnant. Dorene was astonished and I assured her that her babies had looked the same.

That afternoon, I met Mrs. Maxey, Dorene's former public health nurse. Mrs. Maxey is an African American woman well-acquainted with her patients and their needs. She had followed Dorene since 1959, with her first pregnancy. Then, as now, Dorene had repressed and denied her pregnancy until she could no longer ignore the obvious. Over the years, Dorene repeated the same mistakes. In September of 1965, after the last set of twins arrived, a discouraged Mrs. Maxey closed out her case. A month later, one of the twins died, presumably of dehydration. Mrs. Maxey believed that, had she not closed Dorene out, she could have prevented the twin's death. She has resolved to continue to follow Dorene.

When Mrs. Maxey first learned of the most recent pregnancy, she had displayed a motherly anger welcomed by Dorene's mother and grandmother who were both critical of Dorene's repeated pregnancies. Dorene told Mrs. Maxey that it was the birth control pills that she had been taking that made her pregnant.

Mrs. Maxey planned to call Dorene's mother to identify what preparations had been or could be made for the babies. She said that she would be happy to take me on a home visit sometime in the future.

That evening, Dorene and I had a long talk. She told me that she had arranged to have a hysterectomy performed in three months. I asked her if she had ever taken birth control pills. She said that she had but forgot to take one and that was why she had become pregnant.

She usually knew that she was pregnant only when her mother told her. We discussed her first pregnancy and the shame and anger which her mother had expressed. She told me that in the fifth month of her second pregnancy she had taken quinine, a folk-method of inducing abortion, but to no avail.

We talked about her life as a child, raised by her grandmother while her mother was deserted, remarried and deserted again. Allen, the father of the two sets of twins, was particularly fond of the first set of twins and had supported them until one twin died. Allen, the surviving twin, bore his name. With this last pregnancy, Allen Senior had refused to support or marry Dorene. Her mother warned her to have nothing to do with the twenty-one-year-old construction worker. Dorene was confused and torn between her mother and the father of her children.

The next day, Dorene was discharged with her baby. Nurse Maxey had come through with supplies! At the time of discharge, I had the opportunity to talk with Dorene's mother but only briefly. She was very much the authority figure. Thin and nervous, she was proud of her new grand children despite her distress at the financial burden they imposed.

Dorene had been curious about her labor and delivery experience, primarily from the viewpoint of, "How did I act? What did I do?" These questions both Betty and I had attempted to answer in a manner which was least embarrassing for her. We confirmed her memory of the previous Friday night but assured her that we had understood how she had felt. We also allowed her to tell us what she remembered about delivery and were surprised that she remembered betting with the doctors about the sex of the second twin. She was amused when we told her about her comment to Dr. Turner when her membranes had ruptured. I believe that she left the hospital with good memories of her labor experience and some closure.

Almost two weeks after the birth of her twins, I called Dorene at home to ask how she was doing. She seemed surprised and happy to hear from me and said that she would welcome a home visit. Twin A had been discharged the previous day and the twins were doing just fine. Mrs. Maxey had already visited to monitor the babies' weight and Dorene's blood pressure. Dorene's mother and grandmother left her at home with her thirteen-year-old sister and six children to attend the funeral of an uncle in Del Ray. They would return on Sunday. Dorene had been left with the responsibility of six children whom I could hear in the background. Dorene excitedly announced that she had decided to name her twins Nancy and Jack.

As we approached the house the next day, Miss Hilliard was pessimistic about what to expect. According to her, our primary responsibility would be merely keeping the new babies alive. I was startled. I had not realized the prognosis was so bleak. When we arrived, I was prepared for the worst.

Dorene lived in a three room, gray shingled shack behind the larger concrete house of her grandmother. The home was composed of a living room, a bedroom and a kitchen. In the living room was a couch, a television set and nine months old Allen sitting in his walker, screaming. The cluttered kitchen had a stove and a refrigerator. There was no bathroom and no toilet. In the bedroom, Dorene sat on a double bed feeding her twins. She seemed to be doing a fine job of temporarily keeping house and home together despite a few problems. One was sibling rivalry caused by the new arrivals—evident from the older children's—especially Allen's—persistent need for attention. Dorene had observed it but did not make the connection.

A related problem was prioritizing her time. She was so rushed with all her children that she apparently had not planned her time so that the formula would be at least room temperature before feeding it to the twins.

Other than that, things seemed to be going well. The babies were obviously thriving. Dorene's lochia had almost disappeared and her breasts were no longer engorged. She had no further physical problems since her discharge from the hospital.

I was proud of Dorene and her progress post-partum. Unable to sit with her to talk as we had in the hospital, I realized the *home* Dorene was not the *hospital* Dorene. The nature of our relationship had changed. No more clinging dependency. She no longer endowed me with super-human powers. She would no longer confide in me as freely as in the past. Still I was a nurse-friend.

Days later, Mrs. Maxey and I made another home visit. We found Dorene and Allen Senior in the bedroom feeding both twins. Dorene introduced us. Allen and I shook hands. He was a tall, handsome and polite young man. Dorene explained that the doctor had ordered her mother to take a vacation from her hectic household because of its effect on her hypertension. Allen was there to help Dorene manage the household, resolving Dorene's conflict between obeying her mother and being with him.

Dorene was now permanently hypertensive. The twins were gaining weight and seemed to be doing beautifully. Mrs. Maxey reminded Dorene that she was not to have intercourse before her six weeks post-partum checkup. Dorene promised she would not. When Mrs. Maxey asked Dorene about her upcoming hysterectomy, Dorene deflected the question. Was she not too young to have it done? Mrs. Maxey shrugged but later told me that she intended to follow through until Dorene had the operation.

I was mildly disappointed with the visit because I had very little opportunity to talk with Dorene at all. Mrs. Maxey did most of the talking. When she was through, she asked me if I had anything to say to Dorene. With such a big audience, I found it difficult to do more than praise Dorene for the job she was doing.

I realize it is not ethical to *force* a woman to be sterilized. Whether or not it is our place to *convince* her is dubious. Our role is to teach the facts and to allay (unfounded) fears. Then, at least, an informed decision can be made. Dorene needs that hysterectomy both physically and financially. She has proven unreliable about using other methods of contraception. For her health and for her finances, she cannot afford to have another child. Yet her feelings about having her "womb" removed must be recognized and dealt with in an understanding way.

Dorene's life continues but the trimester ends. Just as I begin to understand her needs, I must leave her with so many of them unmet.

This care study has been a four-month history of a patient-nurse relationship. It has been the history of the patient. But this care study is only a beginning.

Care Study: Mrs. M
Late 1976

It occurred early in my first year in oncology. As with every patient who followed, Mrs. M educated me far more than I ever helped her. She was prickly. Not easy at all. She held my feet to the fire.

Dr. Ochoa requested my help with a patient who was remote, aloof and unwilling to accept her diagnosis. Mrs. M was a sixty-two-year old married woman with endometrioid carcinoma of the ovaries, diagnosed and surgically removed several months before. But the cancer had metastasized, spilling its ascitic fluid throughout her abdomen. Now she had a pleural effusion—its fluid displacing her lung. Though Dr. N was her primary care physician, Dr. Ochoa was the oncologist to administer a chemotherapy regimen plus Megace, a hormonal therapy. Her thoracic cavity was drained (thoracentesis), and nitrogen mustard, a chemical relative of nerve gas, was instilled to prevent repeated effusions by scarring her pleura.

I first met Mrs. M on rounds with Dr. Ochoa. She moved very little, held her head stiffly, spoke minimally. The slightest movement brought a rush of nausea. Nausea was predictable from the chemo. Her eyes held not the typical pleading look of misery but one of disdainful scrutiny.

I returned after rounds, sat beside her bed and introduced myself as one who talks with people who are on chemotherapy—avoiding mentioning the word *cancer*. I was unsure of her comfort level with it. She had no questions and spoke little. The silence was uncomfortable. She looked as though she felt very sick and I said so, commiserating that it was miserable to always feel like throwing up.

Angrily she burst: "Yes, I come in to get one thing fixed and end up with five others." She had been admitted for shortness of breath, had her lung drained, chemotherapy begun and now she always felt nauseated.

I asked how it had all started—meaning whatever she chose for it to mean. She replied that it had begun with her surgery in June when "they had not been able to remove it all." "The tumor is causing this fluid?" I asked, feeling on thin ice. "The *cancer*," she said, impatient with my euphemism.

That was our first encounter. Several others followed, marked by long silences punctuated by sporadic bursts of anger about her medical treatment. "Everything Dr. Ochoa gives me makes me sick." On occasions when asked if she would like a drink, a bath, or anything for her comfort, she countered with, "I don't care what you do."

Days later, I was aware that Mrs. M was not responding to her chemotherapy. Her nausea persisted way past the time it should have stopped if it were caused by chemotherapy. This time when I entered, Mrs. M sat propped up in the bed. Something was different. There was no stony stare. When asked how things were, she answered, "Not so good." I sensed that something was up and sat on the bed near her legs. I waited. Through pursed purple lips she cried, "I don't think I'm ever going to get out of here." I touched her leg. "I know. It's hard." More tears. "I want so much to see my grandchild but it's not due until May. I want to go up north and be with my daughter. I've spoiled my family's vacation." Pauses. Tears. Dabs with tissues. "I'm not usually like this." "I know. This is very difficult for you." "I haven't finished my Christmas shopping yet; but I'll never make it . . . It always means so much to me to see Dr. N. He always knows what to do . . . "

And so, it went. Not much said by me. A lot of crying. A wet washcloth to cool her face. A heavy feeling leaving the room.

Time passed. Symptoms increased: More abdominal pressure from growing abdominal masses. More vomiting, probably from bowel obstruction, a hallmark of ovarian cancer. Upper backache, a cough and hiccups from her compressed diaphragm. Sometimes Mrs. M interpreted the symptoms as progression of cancer—sometimes not, repeating, "I came in with one thing and ended up with five others," as though medical care were to blame for continued symptoms.

Nursing staff continued her daily care. The priest and I continued to see her. At times, she had us puzzled—talking about voting in the election, going up north—as though she felt she would live forever.

Her responses were understandable given who she had always been. Mrs. M had been a secretary where she was well known for plastering the workplace walls with anti-Nixon Watergate articles. During the House Judiciary Committee Watergate hearings, she had stayed awake into the wee hours, glued to the testimony. She was a dyed-in-the-wool Democrat and a confirmed Nixon-Ford opponent.

Mrs. M was well-read and very politically-oriented. Retiring less than a year before, she finally had time to take some junior college courses and piano classes.

A woman who valued control, Mrs. M had informed no one outside the family about her hospital admission. She kept a record of everything that happened to her in the hospital in a diary at her bedside—enough to make nursing and medical staff paranoid. "She writes down everything I do," complained one nurse. She had already chosen Christmas presents for the family and had methodically stashed away money for them over the previous year.

Gradually, I identified Mrs. M.'s priorities: seeing her daughter, if not grandchild; submitting an absentee ballot for Jimmy Carter to assure the future for her children and grandchildren; most of all, being in control.

As death drew near, the physicians said as much to _Mr._ M. I urged him to send for their daughter—while Mrs. M was still aware. Arrangements were made for her to cast her vote for president via absentee ballot.

As for control, nursing staff and I made every attempt to see to it that Mrs. M's care was according to her specifications. Her bath basin to her left for possible emesis; fracture pan (bed pan) under the basin; tissue in hand with tissue box to her right. The call bell was entwined in the left side rail, no ice in her water and a straw in her water pitcher. The clock, her glasses and diary were on the over-bed table to the right. A washcloth was placed over the sink drain to prevent an irritating drip that defied the plumber's ministrations. She knew the name and action of each drug that she took and tried to predict its effect. Even in getting her up to the "potty chair," or raised in bed, the sameness of the procedures reassured her. Nurses understood her need for control and adhered to the program.

Mrs. M's controlling nature distanced her from people when she needed them most. She circumvented that effect in other ways. She never turned down a backrub though it did very little to alleviate her back pain. The physical closeness afforded by the rub was the therapeutic part. Transferring her from the bed to the "potty chair," I always asked her to put her arms around my waist as I put my arms around her and rocked backward to lift and pivot her toward the chair. As she sat on the edge of the bed until her dizziness passed, she rested her head on my chest while I, arms around her, rubbed her back. It was at these times that she would say, "I don't think that I'll ever get out of here." Usually, I said nothing—just rubbed. I knew she was right.

One day, Mrs. M asked right out of the blue, "Peggy, what are life support systems?" Surprised, I responded, "Things that keep your body going like that IV of yours." "But what else?" "Oxygen, ventilators . . . " "I mean the things they pull the plug on." "Ventilators keep you breathing." "I don't want any of those." After she discussed it with her husband and doctor she was made a *no code*.

When her daughter arrived, Mrs. M asked me to teach her all the things that we did for her. I worried what her daughter's reaction would be. I needn't have. At thirty-one, her personality was much like her mother's—matter of fact, caring, willing to do anything she was shown how—including doing her mom's Christmas shopping with that very specific list.

Her coughing increased with the pressure on her diaphragm. Mrs. M constantly coughed, hiccupped and burped. One morning after one of her worst nights, I found her rolled bolt upright in bed, confronting her two physicians who sat on either side. "How much longer is this going to go on? Is it ever going to get any better?" she demanded. "Well, I think we can help your cough by giving you codeine," said Dr. Ochoa. "But will it cure it?" "It will not cure it, but it will help you feel better." "Then I might just as well cut my throat or jump off the Skyway." I registered her anger and hopelessness. What she said was true—codeine tended to confuse her, the last thing she wanted. But no-one had better options.

After her doctors' retreat, I stood by Mrs. M as she sat on the side of the bed, preparing to transfer to the bedside commode. She asked, "Do you think I was too strong when I spoke with the doctors?" Truthfully, I *had* felt very sorry for them. She had pushed them to the wall, confronting them squarely with their own powerlessness. I replied in what I hoped would be a smooth, warm voice, "You were only telling them how angry and frustrated you feel." "Yes," she said leaning her head against my chest. "And sometimes you have to make a lot of noise before they'll listen to you." As she rested in this position, my arms around her, stroking her back, she whispered quietly, "I'm never going to get out of here. I'll never be better."

Time passed. Mrs. M's emesis was predictable at least every twelve hours. She had diarrhea. Abdominal pressure caused urinary frequency. So weak that it was difficult to get on and off even the fracture pan, she requested a catheter. She had begun to use nasal oxygen. Each new tube represented further surrender of control and independence. She complained that the light splint used to stabilize the IV felt heavy. An NG (Naso-Gastric) tube was inserted and connected to suction to decompress her stomach and intestine. Lung sounds were diminished. She probably contracted pneumonia. With fevers, she was extremely diaphoretic. I wondered where all the perspiration came from. She was no longer drinking.

Mrs. M continued to maintain control. Her daughter made the dictated daily entries in her diary. Mrs. M directed nurses to put her TED hose on at certain times. A creature of habit, she found comfort in sameness—no matter the fact that phlebitis was a minor concern and that she would never resume her diary again.

Mrs. M spun in and out of reality—but the unreality was predictable to those who knew her. She was sure that UN Ambassador Daniel Moynihan had visited her room. In a panic she had her nurse phone her husband, only to ask him to call the FBI.

That morning, she was very agitated. Weak as she was, she reached up to me and pleaded, "Peggy, don't leave me today." I took her hand, sat down and asked, "Are you scared?" "Yes." "Of what?" "I don't know. I just don't want to be alone." I had a sinking feeling because that day, *of all days*, I was tied up giving in-services every hour. But I sat there quietly until she calmed, then I called Pastoral Care for a priest to spell me until her family could be summoned.

Later, during a brief visit with Mrs. M and her daughter, Mrs. M confided that she had died the night before at one thirty a.m. She had felt herself come out of her body but had pulled herself back and had survived. That episode had accounted for her earlier state of panic and desire not to be alone.

For the next two days, Mrs. M became increasingly unresponsive. Tracheal suction was used as the fluid rose in her chest and bubbled over with each breath. She did not act but reacted to what was done to her. I sat with her, touched her hand or arm, and wiped her forehead with the cool cloth which she had always liked. I watched and listened and prayed that each breath would be her last— that, suddenly, her heart would stop. But she held on. I wondered why.

Was death a gradual process of concluding that there is no other way? Was it an incremental process of letting go culminating in relinquishing that final link with humanity symbolized by my hand touching hers?

I visited Mrs. M in the afternoon when I checked on her before I left for home. I planned to return that evening to teach childbirth class and would check on her then. She was carefully positioned on her side, stertorously mouth breathing, apparently oblivious to her surroundings.

Reading the paper by the window sat her husband. Previously, I had sensed that she had been the strong one in their relationship. I had seen his face flush and his lips purse to keep tight control. The threat of her loss had been almost too much for him to bear.

Watching him with his newspaper by the window, there was a change. He talked about his wife and what was happening to her—not using her name or the pronouns *she* or *her* but the collective pronoun *they*. Not *us* or *me* or *my* but *they* (as in those people who are dying). In a flash, I recognized what had happened during her unending suffering. He had gradually relinquished; he already defined himself as separate from her. A survivor, he was not dying with his wife. Though he loved her as she had been, he accepted that she would never be that again. The only conceivable end to her suffering was death.

That evening, after teaching prepared childbirth class, I returned to the floor, noticed the housekeeper's bucket outside her door and I knew immediately that Mrs. M had finally relinquished all.

Care Study: Fran
August to September 1978

It will happen again . . . but I hope not for a while. Not until I have time to digest and assimilate it. Three of my patients have died within the past two weeks. I followed two for two years but neither made the impact of one brave woman whom I've known for just two months.

From the moment I met Fran, I knew that she was dying. Early one morning, Dr. Lynch visited my office minutes before I arrived. He left a note asking me to see one of his patients. She was a fifty-two-year-old divorced psychotherapist with Stage IV ovarian carcinoma. The woman had been intellectual and controlled during the year following her initial diagnosis. For *this* admission for paracentesis, she had come unglued. Worse—Dr. Lynch projected a downhill course with worsening cachexia (weight loss and muscle atrophy), weakness, and probably bowel obstruction.

I knew the picture well, recalling previous patients with ovarian cancer. One had been the extremely vital sixty-two-year-old secretary, Mrs. M. Another had been the twenty-eight-year-old mother of a two-year-old, who had travelled to MD Anderson Hospital in Houston for its promise of advanced treatment. She had died at St. Anthony's, babbling with brain metastases. There had been the dark, complicated woman with three inches of post chemo black hair who looked for all the world like a concentration camp refugee except for her enormous belly packed tight with ascites . . . She had died with a permanent scowl on her face—a victim.

Dwelling on those experiences was pointless. I didn't—except for seeing their faces flash before me. I set my jaw for an experience which did not bode well. The enticement, of course, was the personal invitation extended by the good (and handsome) Dr. Lynch at such an early hour. Obviously, the situation troubled him. I knew from experience that anything I would do would be appreciated. No miracles expected.

The fact that the patient was a psychotherapist intimidated me—especially since the reason for the referral was not that she needed an explanation of treatment or comfort measures but that she was upset. No, it was clear in the message, and later in the progress notes, that the patient understood the status of her disease and her treatment. She was upset AND a psychotherapist. While most of my professional preparation and experience had been emotionally oriented, faced with approaching a psychotherapist about her unenviable situation, I felt a rank amateur. None of those convenient gimmicks—reflection, re-phrasing, or summarizing would work. I envisioned her spotting the logic behind my every move. Her nurses' comments didn't help. They felt that the patient tried to "psych out" everyone who entered her room. With great trepidation, I swallowed hard, knocked and entered room 581.

From the area of the bed emanated a terse greeting. I entered and extended my hand to a tiny woman, tanned—I wondered if by Adriamycin® or sun or both. Addressing her by her full name, I introduced myself as Peggy Newton mentioning that Dr. Lynch had asked me to see her. Accepting my hand and leaning forward, with a commanding manner and tone reminiscent of a stage actress, she replied "Yes. I told him that I wanted to see you. He asked me if I would." Control. Very important. I asked to sit down. Eye contact very important. Slow, deliberate movements. No fidgeting.

"He's probably told you that I work with people who have cancer. I understand that you've been having a difficult time here lately . . . "

A series of revelations followed, the essence of which was that Fran did not want to die. When her primary ovarian cancer was discovered, it had already metastasized to her lungs. She had traveled to Texas to a retreat run by an MD and his psychotherapist wife.[1] There she was taught that there is a precancerous personality. We make ourselves sick. Cancer can be conquered through meditation, guided imagery and other techniques. Obviously, the method had failed. She felt cheated and angry but mostly afraid.

Fran opined, "A friend of mine had cancer and died right around the time I was diagnosed. The way her family treated her, it seemed that, even if she wanted to change her mind about dying, she wouldn't have been able to." Magical thinking like this had isolated Fran from friends and family to whom her decline was obvious. She wanted no part of people who were sending out what she considered *strong invitations* to die. Remaining neutral and dealing with minute-to-minute concerns was my only recourse to be of help to her.

Some Fran-isms:

> *When Dr. Lynch told me he wouldn't abandon me, I told him that, if he wasn't easier to get by phone, then I'd abandon him.*

I need to hear Dr. Lynch say, "Hang in there."

I have this intruder script that says I should never have been born, wasn't meant to be, and should not be here now.

You like my hair? I rather like it, too. (About an inch long growing back post-chemo)

I need my over-40 glasses.

I'm more worried about my debts than the cancer. It is a terrific invitation to die to get rid of the bills.

I want someone to hold me.

Everyone is special. I learn something from everyone (discounting my praise).

A lot of people laugh at this, but I really believe that people are good.

I asked Dr. Lynch if there was anything else he could do. When he said "no," I said, "Of course not." Because, if there were, I knew he'd be doing it.

Maybe this has brought me and my family closer together (one brother). But I shouldn't have to die for that.

On X-ray, Fran's lungs were stippled with cancer. Increasingly, she was extremely short of breath, unable to be in any position but jack-knife—the head of the bed elevated as high as possible with pillows under her arms. She was anxious. One day, her yoga instructor visited, closing the door for an hour. When the door opened, Fran, flat in bed, was more flexible and never again needed to resume that extreme upright posture. The secret was Jeanne Gootson, her incredible yoga instructor, who had put Fran through progressive relaxation and guided imagery—then talked her through gentle exercise, focusing on flexibility, followed by more relaxation. She left her with a relaxation tape of her voice and soft music which Fran used until she died.

I knew Fran for forty-nine days. Every one of those days I left her room thinking, *she's dying.* Somehow, we became friends. Not that she was a saint. She issued imperial commands. "I want this NOW." When I or the other nurses entered that room, we were consumed—uprooted as though by a tornado, jostled in the wind, flung against walls, but always placed gently down on our feet. Leaving her, I felt exhausted, used—yet exhilarated as though I had been an instrument used correctly.

One of the nurses said that, no matter how bad the night had been, after being with Fran, she felt better. Fran was quick to praise: "You make such a difference to my life."

About St. Anthony's, she would declare tearfully, "Everyone here has been so nurturing and supportive. They each deserve a lot of warm fuzzies."

Fran died in her own home at peace with her fate, her brother at her side.

On a later evening, Sister Kathy, who had also worked with Fran, some of the nursing staff and several of Fran's friends including yoga teacher, Jeanne, and her husband, congregated for a brief memorial service in the hospital chapel. For the music, we played a currently popular song which mirrored so much about our collective relationships with Fran.

You Needed Me
I cried a tear, you wiped it dry.
I was confused, you cleared my mind.
I sold my soul, you bought it back for me
And held me up and gave me dignity.
Somehow you needed me.
You gave me strength to stand alone again
To face the world out on my own again.
You put me high upon a pedestal –
So high that I could almost see Eternity. You needed me. [2]

Endnotes
_____

1. O Carl Simonton and Stephanie Mathews-Simonton, *Getting Well Again* (Los Angeles: Tarcher, 1978).

2. Randy Goodrum, *You Needed Me*, sung by Anne Murray, (Los Angeles: Capitol Records, 1978).

Care Study: Mary Jane
1980 to 1985

Mary Jane was a woman in her mid-forties who lived in a mobile home park on the outskirts of the city with her husband who worked as a dispatcher. When she was diagnosed with AML (Acute Myelogenous Leukemia), she was the first person to take advantage of the fact that leukemia patients were admitted to 3 South only. She was admitted in 1980 for induction-remission chemotherapy. The process was bumpy. Fated to die within three months without chemotherapy, she lived an additional five years before returning to die when her leukemia recurred. During those five years, I visited her in her mobile home and kept up with her by phone. On her last admission, I spent hours with her. This is an edited letter I wrote to her doctor after her death.

I think you know that you and I share the same philosophy about the emotions of our patients. We both believe in a strong dose of hope—focusing on what they *can* do and *can* control rather on what they cannot. We are both interested in restoring their control in all the little ways that they are likely to lose it—basics like getting their food or medicine when they want it, when or how they believe it would help. We are both well aware of the symbolism intrinsic in our gestures and actions. I admire you when I see you dealing with what could be interpreted as a very demanding patient. You understand that their behavior only mirrors their helplessness and terror.

We both know that no one can say how long another will live. The dying person must live until he dies. Living and the quality of that life might be the only things within his control.

Many of our patients have hope of a life beyond this one. Even those who are not overtly religious, like Mary Jane, talk about their hopes and beliefs and are consoled by them. I usually ask patients about this—and, in ten years, oddly enough, the only one who feared the hereafter was a priest!

To others, hope is having some control over life and its quality: doing things that are important; tying up loose ends; feeling the love of those who are close; not suffering; not being alone. In this sense, Mary Jane had hope.

According to the literature, dying patients fear abandonment most. The words that you so avoid, "I can't do anything more for you," epitomize the medical abandonment which I see commonly in some other patient-doctor relationships. But "truth" can be told without abandonment or loss of hope.

I suspect you worry about destroying hope (of medical miracles) partly because you wonder, with empty hands, what can you bring to the patient? The answer is simple. It is your attitude of: *we can get through this together.* It's not anything that you don't already do or believe. You don't abandon your patients. You do everything medically possible to alleviate their suffering. You don't give up on their comfort even when you've given up on their ability to survive.

Sometimes I worry that I unwittingly add to your perception that everyone expects you to have the ultimate answer. That puts an unfair and unnecessary burden on you. Of course, I look to your medical expertise because I respect it. But I don't expect you to be a miracle worker and hope you don't expect it of yourself. When I share a patient's emotional/social concerns, I don't expect you to fix it—only to be aware of the context—just as you make me aware of the medical context. You can't accept the total responsibility and burden of all that goes on with patients. We are a team—physician nurses, lab, dietary, pharmacy—and we support each other.

It has been a joy to work with you all these years. Not only are you an excellent physician but a caring, loving physician. You once told me not to get involved—thank God you don't take your own advice.

I hope you know that Mary Jane's affection for you far outweighed her desperate need for a miracle. She felt your love and support throughout and knew that, more than making these past five years medically possible, you have made them bearable.

Peggy

Care Study: Sofia
1988 to 1989

From the 1959 Cuban Revolution through 1961, a wave of close to a million Cuban exiles arrived in the US seeking asylum. Fidel Castro, leader of the Revolution, nationalized institutions and cracked down on perceived enemies. A number of exiles later returned to re-claim Cuba under US sponsorship and were defeated at the Bay of Pigs Invasion in April 1961. In October 1962, the US (Kennedy) and Russia (Khrushchev) were on the brink of nuclear war during the Cuban Missile Crisis before Russia backed down.

Sofia represented my encounter with the Spanish speaking world of Cuban expatriates. Unlike Miami, where there are entire sections of predominantly Spanish-speaking people, St. Petersburg was home to just a few, including oncologist Dr. Julio Ochoa. In Miami, grade school and high school Spanish classes were a necessity. Here, true to my French heritage, I had studied high school French and Latin. Now, facing a woman with an incredibly thick Cuban accent who was most comfortable in her own language, I doubted my ability to help. I felt like a dull-witted American gringo ...

When Dr. Ochoa first asked me to see Sofia in November, I could only understand a few words of what she said and despaired of her ever understanding me under the mask. She was in protective isolation because of low white blood counts after chemotherapy. WBC's fight infection. I encouraged Dr. Ochoa to speak to her in Spanish, though I was present, so that she could understand him better. He indignantly replied that she understood English perfectly. His quick retort cued me that he cared very much about Sofia. Out of respect *for him*, I would try to work with her, doubtful that anything would come of it. My presence, though token, might at least help Dr. Ochoa.

Daily I concentrated intently on deciphering what certain sounds meant. *Ee . . . k? M's* were *ng's!* I was frustrated watching the way her tongue made words—or didn't make them the way I was used to hearing them. I could easily understand Dr. Ochoa's speech patterns but compared to Sofia, he spoke the King's English. Sofia was very polite but also very private, sharing only that she didn't want her family to worry or to realize how very sick she was. I doubt she knew what to make of me. She probably responded only because she saw me as an extension of Dr. Ochoa.

Right before Christmas, it was clear that her platelets, the blood component involved in clotting, were not rising as expected. Dr. Ochoa intuitively spoke to her entirely in Spanish as she sat in the chair. I watched from a hassock, looking from one to the other as indecipherable words were spoken. I absorbed a deep sadness from both. Sofia's face transformed to stone, her color gray. After Dr. Ochoa left, I touched Sophia, noting that I could feel the unhappiness of those words. I asked her to translate. She briefly recounted *what I had intuitively known that he had said.* Tears welled in her eyes. "I have faith in Our Lord. He will not let anything happen to me while I have people who need me." I encouraged her to let the tears come, that she had been through so much and that sometimes, crying is a release. But the stone face returned: "Help me back to bed." Though obviously overwhelmed with feeling, she could not release it . . . at least in my presence.

On the day of discharge, she left candy for me and the nurses at Christmas. I called her a few times at home—but then didn't, thinking that she could call me if needed. Subtle changes of which I was not consciously aware had occurred in our relationship. Incredibly, I had begun to understand her English.

On her next and subsequent admissions, Sofia was concerned about her mother and sister, trying to place them in a nursing home. When that was resolved, thanks in a large measure to Dr. Ochoa, she was more open. Sofia was still guarded about her feelings and her prognosis—returning to the stone face. But she began to relax, smile, tease, and express herself in English with the same gusto and inflection which I'd heard in Spanish. Feeling more comfortable with me, she exposed more of herself, her peculiarities, her prejudices, her opinions and, most important, her life.

Sofia had been raised in Cuba where she attended a private girl's convent school. With marriage, she had become mistress of a household of six servants. She worked on their small farm, tending chickens, even performing minor surgery on them. She recounted the births of her four boys, two in Cuba and two here. The Castro Revolution changed everything. Alone, she smuggled money out of Cuba to Miami, returning on a dangerous flight back to Cuba and her family. Her entire family escaped to Miami just in time for her third son's birth. Finally, they migrated to Chicago, a place of potential opportunity.

After Cuba, Chicago was cold and dark, their apartment small. The former

Senora with servants worked hard. She was discouraged. Many of her Cuban friends continued to pine for life as it had been. But she said, "No. I will not look backward. I will look forward." Once she had taken her sick child to see the pediatrician. Noticing her tears, he admonished her saying, "Your tears won't help. You will only distract my attention from the boy." Those life experiences formed the determinedly positive Sofia whom I was beginning to know.

Sofia's father remained in Cuba thinking that he could protect their property and wait-out the Castro regime. Impossible. Finally, he bribed an official, flew to Mexico and took a *salvavidas* (floatation device) across the Rio Grande becoming a *wetback*. Wetback was a slur used to describe illegal Mexican immigrants who entered the US by crossing the Rio Grande. It was Sofia's word, not mine. I had never heard the term before.

Sofia and her father had shared a close relationship and similar perspective. On his deathbed, he said, "I feel better." Sofia strove to emulate her dad's positive and uncomplaining ways and to encourage her fatalistic mother to follow suit.

They worked hard in Chicago. Her husband, the former factory owner, worked in a pizza parlor. Sofia was a seamstress in a large wedding gown factory. She had no idea of how to run the large sewing machine but asked to be allowed to try. Eventually, they charged her with training other employees how to create a gown as quickly as she did.

A Spanish nanny had followed the family to this country. Since the nanny was nervous, not well-educated, and spoke no English, Sofia worked outside the home while Maria remained home with the children.

With time, Sofia learned to operate some rudimentary commercial computers and used her skill in two Chicago hospitals. Her husband, twenty-one years older than she, became mentally handicapped, making Sofia the primary decision maker.

During several hospitalizations over the next six months, Sofia shared other aspects of her life. She studiously avoided "heavy" topics and graciously commented that she enjoyed our interesting conversations. So did I, but I wondered how I could possibly consider this nursing. And then I realized (justified?) that she was achieving emotional closure on her life by reviewing it with a supportive, non-judgmental listener. Sofia would not ask for help and needed the control that she was accustomed to having as head of her household. She rarely had visitors, cards or any evidence of supportive others because, as I later learned, she simply didn't tell people that she was sick or told them not to come. It wasn't that she didn't *need*; it was that she didn't *ask*. When home, she insisted that I call *her* because she didn't want to bother me when I was busy.

On one call, her usually perky hello sounded somber. She had been given bad news at the doctor's office and realized that she must plan and pay for her funeral. She had just completed that task. I could tell that she was tearful, but, as usual, I just could not persuade her to elaborate on her feelings. As usual, before hanging up, she said, "Thank you so much for calling."

On her final admission, Sofia's face was ashen, her eyes haunted. She could say little but reached for my hand. She allowed me to give her the bedpan but, after the brutally painful "hot, burning" diarrhea which sounded like a garden hose emission, she stubbornly set her jaw and refused to let me remove the pan. I was a "higher class" nurse. I protested but, if another nurse had not arrived, she would still be sitting on that pan. Fortunately, later I was able to convince her that I do bedpans.

The next day, she communicated that her life was increasingly limited. "I used to like to cook. Now, I cannot do. I cannot get off the toilet seat any more—it is too low." Each was said as though these were not temporary but permanent changes.

"You've had a very hard time and are worn out," I acknowledged. "Ah, yes." "Do you remember when you told me that, when you go, you want it to be easy?" "Ah yes," eyes tearful but downcast. "You have heard them call a *Code Blue* here, haven't you?" "Yes." "Do you know what that means?" "It is when someone has a heart attack." "Yes. It's when their heart stops or they stop breathing. We push on their chest and sometimes put a tube in their mouth to make them breathe. Sometimes, doing something like that can make it harder—especially if the person is going to die no matter what. We have some papers that you could sign saying that you don't want that done . . . " "Ay no," somewhat impatiently. "I trust you and Dr. Ochoa to do what is best for me."

"Sofia, I've known you a long time now." "Si." "And you know that I care very much how you are feeling." A modified acknowledgement. "Then share with me what's going on inside you. I can see that your mind is going a mile-a-minute and that you have a lot of feelings inside . . . " Silence. "Please help me to help you." Stone face. Silence and one tear tumbling over her cheek. She made the sign of the cross. "He loves you." "I know He does."

The next day, thankfully, she felt better. I continued to press her that, physically and emotionally, she needed someone with her. Did she have any friends or relatives? Serendipitously, at that moment, an older cousin from Clearwater called. Sofia had previously told her not to come—but, today she said *come* or maybe Isobel said *I'm coming*. It was all Spanish to me!

Her cousin was there for two days and the change in Sofia was remarkable. The stony withdrawal disappeared. Her smile and animated laughter returned. She talked about going home. She arranged with her best and life-long girlfriend to come down from Chicago for two months until "the end." She was certainly realistic and had progressed a long way from the isolation and withdrawal which had always said non-verbally to me, "At the heart of it, I'm not worth anybody's trouble."

Just when things seem better, they get worse. On Friday morning, visiting early, I found Sofia's room full of bright fluorescent over-bed light, drapes drawn closed—the reverse of how she liked it. A student nurse, instructor and staff nurse fussed over her with vital signs. She was clammy and gray, eyes closed, moaning, turning from side to side.

"Sofia?" Eyes open. "Ay, Peggy, not good, not good, pain." She pointed to her epigastric area. Her vital signs were stable. In a quick but quiet succession of movements, I turned off the lights, opened the drapes and sat down next to her, attempting to change the enervating environment. The students withdrew.

I phoned Maria for her. While she was on the phone, an LPN appeared to administer oral Flagyl. Sofia, panicking, motioned her away with the expression of a drowning woman. I told her to continue her phone conversation and asked the LPN to leave the Flagyl which I would administer and chart. Then the students returned with the milk Sofia had requested. The room, since my arrival, had been a three-ring circus. Sofia's escalating anxiety was palpable. I sat with her, talked with her soothingly and did fingertip massage, effleurage, of the epigastric area. The light massage calmed her as she described the previous night. She apparently had had multiple needs which had been met slowly or not at all. She was unaware that there had been *three deaths within twenty-four hours* on that unit. She had not been able to get the staff to understand her. Now her tongue was so swollen that, even had she spoken the King's English, she would have been difficult to understand.

"You must have felt so helpless." "Ay yes." "And it's a shame because it is not your fault . . . " "Ay yes." She remembered a former Chicago boss who had made it difficult for her because of her accent. She had asked him how many languages he spoke. He had answered *one*. Then she had replied, "Well I speak one and a half—Spanish and half English." He had never troubled her again. Sofia's anxiety slowly faded as we both chuckled.

Though she felt bad physically, I could see the anxiety dissipate. With calm, quiet effleurage the epigastric pain disappeared. The nanny would arrive within an hour.

Before I left for home, I visited Sofia. She looked fair but relaxed. She said, "You know I think this morning it was nerves." I was sure of it and promised to return for the night shift since no one from the family was able to stay overnight.

I arrived at ten p.m. The night began slowly but quickly escalated into short two hour or less intervals of sleep punctuated by explosive diarrhea and panic. Fortunately, she accepted that I could do bedpans. Dr. Ochoa ordered a PCA (Patient Controlled Analgesia) pump with morphine which is also constipating. Sofia was very hesitant to use it. The entire night passed as though in transitional labor. She was awake at dawn. I opened the curtain for her to see it. Previously, it would have been pleasurable for her. Now, her panic continued.

She called home and told the whole family to come. Panic. Time passed punctuated with "ay, ay, ay," and then silent, prayerful lips. Her adult son called. She closed her eyes. The family was on its way. In addition to tachycardia, she complained of tingling in her hands and feet and a rash on both arms. She was not hyperventilating, breathing normally. Her vital signs were relatively stable. I tried very hard to remain calming and soothing, silently questioning if I had done anything to contribute to the panic.

Sofia grabbed my hand and began to talk about her sons in Spanish, animatedly and tearfully, flowing into English. Here she was, finally opening-up, crying, making eye contact and I hadn't understood the opening paragraph! When she paused, quietly, firmly and with eye contact I said, "Sofia, the first part of what you said was in Spanish and I didn't understand." Still crying she went on to quickly explain in English. Between her pressure of speech, her accent, and her swollen tongue, all I could understand was that she had something made for each of the boys and, possibly, some money, too. She felt an urgency to talk with them about it.

"You love them very much." "Yes, I do. I am not afraid to die because I know that I will be with Our Lord but . . . my family . . . I had hoped that I would be the last one in my family to go because I knew they all would need my help, but I will be the first instead . . . "

"You had been with your dad when he died." The nurse in me was trying to tidy up by working into death fears. "Ah yes, my father . . . I was very special to him." "You had a special relationship with your father . . . you took after him." "Yes." And then she went on to describe quickly what I gathered to be how he had favored her in his estate, But I wasn't sure.

"I know that your mother and sister were a concern . . . " "Ah yes. But now I know that they will be taken care of—but my husband . . . Did you know that I made all the funeral arrangements for my mother, my sister and me? It is all paid for. I knew it had to be done." "That must have been very hard to do—heartbreaking to do." Crying, "Ah yes. I told them everything, like I don't want any flowers."

"Do you remember Saint Theresa, the Little Flower?" I asked. "No, I don't want any flowers," sternly as though I had contradicted her. "No. Do you remember Saint Theresa, the nun they called the Little Flower?" "Si." "Remember how she is supposed to shower down blessings from heaven like flowers?" Nod. "That is how I see you one day—sending flowers down from heaven for your family—just as you have given them to your family and others throughout your life." Her face was totally red and covered with tears. Behind glasses and mask, mine was, too. I reached up to get some tissues and said, "I think we both need this." She had been vaguely looking at me while she had shared her feelings. Now she watched me, first appraisingly and then meltingly. She said, squeezing my hand and pulling it to her, "Peggy, I love you so much." "Sofia, I love you, too." "And I love Dr. Ochoa, too." She didn't fool with the little tissue but took a whole towel to dry the tears. I wiped her face with a cool, damp cloth. "I wish I could go to sleep and not wake up. Where is Dr. Ochoa, where is my family? Ay, ay, ay."

Word came that Dr. Ochoa had been reached and he had ordered an injection of morphine to calm her. I agreed that medication would help her anxiety and said so. Sofia, who was having a very difficult time talking, signaled to me *No*. I guessed, "You want to stay alert until you can talk with your children and Dr. Ochoa—and then maybe . . . " A nod. "Do you have to use the bedpan now?" A nod and a twinkle, "You witch!" I took that to mean *you are a mind reader*.

After twelve hours with Sofia and without sleep for more than twenty-four hours, I was not in top form when Dr. Ochoa arrived. When he asked Sofia how she was, she pointed to me. I tried to succinctly summarize. Dr. Ochoa was very comforting, matter-of-fact and kind. He reassured Sofia that he would look out for her family. Sofia grabbed his hand, thanked him for all that he had done and said that she loved him. I was touched by his assurance that he was still her doctor and would still take care of her. If ever there had been a sense on her part of letting him (us) down or a fear of separation when she was no longer actively trying to get well, that had certainly been assuaged.

Opening her door on Sunday, I had no idea what to expect. There was Sofia, half rising out of the bed with a small white-haired lady on the other side of it. I intuitively knew it was her lifelong friend from Chicago. Sofia looked toward me, "Ay this is my good friend . . . " I almost filled in "Maria" when she said, "Peggy." Not allowing us time to respond, she said, "Look how much better I am," as she rose to sit on the side of the bed with minimal assistance. I plunked down on the closed bedside commode in front of her—speechless. As I looked up and she smiled down at me, she commented mirthfully, "The minute you left, I started to feel better." "Oh, *you* felt better," I said with a sarcastic tone remembering how totally drained I had felt. "I guess I'm a jinx." We both laughed.

She lay back down and had me check two wet spots on the bed to make sure the IV had not leaked. Then she said, "It isn't urine, or it would be yellow." I again looked at her and laughed because that was exactly what I was thinking.

Sofia thanked me profusely for spending the night with her. "You know just what to do, just how to touch me . . . " Inwardly, I smiled that she had picked up on what I had hoped to project—calm, quiet, confidence—rather than intense concentration and self-doubt.

For Sofia, the previous night had been much better. She had awakened several times but not with panic. Her friend, an evangelist, had talked to her about "Our Lord" and she found that comforting. She literally prattled on without any solicitation on my part. I was updated about the identities and lives of the family members whom I had seen the previous morning. All the while she talked, she watched me with a gentle smile and soft look. The barriers were gone. Sofia explained who from the family was coming from all over the country and what their relationship was to her. Awed, tears welling up but smiling, "I didn't want to bother them, but they are all coming." "You feel good and somewhat relieved because you and your family are together on this?" "Yes. Did you know until yesterday, my mother did not think I was going to die? Neither did Maria. But now they know."

"You were under quite a strain carrying this all around with you. But now you are relieved because you have your family's support?" "Ah yes."

I offered to give her a bed bath to help freshen up for the expected visitors and she consented. While we were engaged in the bath, she remarked that she was no longer receiving the Flagyl which had been discontinued because of her difficulty swallowing it. "Don't I need it to stop the diarrhea?" Looking her in the eye, I said, "Yesterday you felt that you were dying. Dr. Ochoa wanted to make it as easy as possible and not put you through swallowing those pills. Today is different and I guess he may want to re-assess that with you. I think we have to take these things a day at a time." "Ok," she said matter-of-factly and moved to another topic.

As I bathed her, Sofia shared a story about one of her visitors. When the woman's husband had been dying, making "a sound like people do when they are dying," the doctor had asked Sofia if they should use a tube in his throat. Sofia had deferred to the wife but said she felt that, if a person is dying and nothing can be done, it is wrong to prolong their life unnecessarily or to prolong the family's suffering. If it were a heart attack which could get better, that was different. "This is what you and I were talking about the other day." *I more than you*, I thought. "Yes. And that is why I told Dr. Ochoa: no tubes." This little story, couched as information about a visitor, was her way of saying *I heard you. I knew what you meant. I just couldn't respond then.*

When her visitors arrived en masse, I left but not before Sofia said, "Ah. God bless you, Peggy. Only Our Lord can repay you for what you have done for me." I blew her a kiss.

Sofia finally admitted to being afraid of being alone and lined up family members to be sure that she was not. She was constantly plagued with vomiting and diarrhea. I took another night shift. When the diarrhea came, her abdomen peaked like a woman in labor. In fact, she reminded me of someone in transitional labor—relatively ego-centric, little eye contact, short barked commands, no extra words, working hard. She was in transitional labor between this life and another. Typically and lovingly Sofia, she episodically rose from her state and asked, "How is your mother? How are your babies (pets)?" Sometimes, as I cleaned her or furnished the ice chips she craved, she'd mumble, "I sorry, I sorry." Gently stroking her arms was like pushing a relaxation button and she drifted off to sleep if only for a few minutes.

In the morning, when the hospital housekeeper, Juanita, entered, she was obviously saddened by Sofia's debilitated state. She felt close to Sofia who had been on that unit episodically for the better part of six months. Juanita, walked close to the bed up to the apparently out-of-it Sofia, touched her hand and said with her soft Southern accent, "Hey, honey." Sofia opened her eyes and said, "Hi Juanita. How is your little granddaughter?" Juanita smiled and said, "Getting into trouble." "Ah," said Sofia, eyes smiling and warm—then out again.

The week passed in a blur. It was impossible to imagine that she could continue, but she did—not more than an hour's sleep at a time, vomiting, diarrhea, hypotension, blood-work terribly out of whack. A family member was always with her. Sofia alternated between stupor and rising to the occasion. Her mother now accepted the inevitability of her death. Sofia worried that a crypt which she owned in Chicago would be given to her friend.

Sunday morning, at eight, as I walked toward 3NE, I saw Juanita with her cleaning equipment outside Sofia's room. Sofia had died. According to the team leader, Diane, she died peacefully in her sleep at midnight with her long-time evangelical friend by her side.

After transcribing and editing Sofia's story from the original written so many years ago, I realize that I did not include her age (sixty) or disease. And now I cannot remember her diagnosis. The disease would have been all important to me then. Intellectualizing about the disease process was my best defense mechanism. But did it really matter? Being with her moment to moment—in the moment— and letting her know that she was heard were my most valuable interventions.

Care Study: Mabel
June to October 1990

A former maternal infant nurse, I conceptualized the dying process as labor. Just like those quick labors where a policeman delivers the baby in a car on the road-side, some deaths progress with blitzkrieg rapidity. The deaths with which I was involved were usually a very personal process of evolution. No labor is the same as another's. No death is either. How the process is faced is determined by previous life experiences. There is no "right" way to labor, and no "right" way to die—regardless of some authors' proclivity to subdivide dying into particular stages or phases.

In the mid-eighties, a perceived lack of support in a conventional labor room setting gave rise to the labor doula (coach). Doulas were specialized lay people who estab-lished trust in the months prior to delivery and were present throughout the labor. The ability to stand with the patient *and, sometimes by sheer force of personality,* pull her through *in the most difficult moments characterize a good doula or a good labor nurse. Now there are death doulas. Trust is the essential element.*

Establishing trust and intervening as needed had been my modus operandi as an oncology nurse. That did not change when I encountered my first oncology patient as a home health nurse. This woman's world was as different from mine as Dorene's had been. Mabel represented the other extreme of the social spectrum.

I had just transferred to St. Anthony's Home Health Care (SAHHC) after a fourteen year stretch as Oncology Clinical Nurse Specialist. I felt stupid but excited about its alien territory of amputations, CHF, diabetes and Medicare "Greek."

A nurse-colleague returned to the office from dressing the wound of a woman with a large fungating mass, on her right chest over a previous mastectomy site. She described the patient as meticulous, perfectionistic and exacting, very anxious, and "in denial." Martha asked our supervisor if I could visit the patient because "she really needs you." The supervisor obliged.

Our patient lived in Snell Isle, a posh area of St. Petersburg. Jill, the woman's regular nurse, reported that the patient was a real dilly—scheduling daily dressing changes around social engagements. She was not very homebound—a

Medicare requirement for home health care. Jill warned that the patient did not operate in the real world and was more concerned with social obligations than with her condition.

With delight at finally being assigned to something that I knew—and with dread of dealing with an unrealistic socialite, I rang Mabel's doorbell. The door was opened by a soft-spoken woman smiling pleasantly and graciously. She wore no makeup on her pale, freckled face. Her large brown eyes smiled. She wore a printed housecoat over a hospital patient gown. Her hair was inches long, brown and coarse, combed plainly, the back pressed into the cowlick that she had not bothered to comb after sleep. Inside, her house was beautiful. It took my breath away, decorated traditionally in federalist style on beautiful hardwood floors. Avoiding comment while following her to her bedroom took all my gumption. She was nicer than I'd expected—but if she were anxious or perfectionistic, it would be unwise to appear fragmented in thought or anything less than professional.

The bedroom was large with a queen-size four poster cannonball bed. She stood on tiptoes to get into it. Her bearing as she walked to the bedroom had been regal—head erect, shoulders back. She directed me to a mahogany tea cart loaded with dressing supplies. After taking her vital signs, I performed the dressing as she directed though I had memorized Jill's directions. Dressing removed, I could see the hollow where her sternum had been removed. I watched her heart (100 bpm) beat under what was now just a layer of grafted skin. Her voice was shallow and breathless. Thanks to her sternectomy, she was breathless; had difficulty coughing or vomiting, requiring counter pressure; and difficulty rising from a recumbent position. Her arms could not be pulled since they no longer had the sternum to anchor the clavicles and rib cage. She advised me to hold my arm out in front of her like a trapeze bar and she would pull herself up that way. She recounted her recent return from MD Anderson with a "recipe" for chemotherapy that she thought would work. Before it could be administered, a vascular access device would be inserted.

Mabel obviously had an aversion to the serous fluid which drained from her doughnut-sized, red, exophytic chest lesion, cautioning me many times not to "contaminate" myself with it. A common misconception was that cancer was contagious. She also had an inflamed sub-axillary rash. I was to cleanse the wound with an iodine-based drying agent, apply cortisone cream to the rash, antibiotic ointment to the Vaseline-impregnated gauze (Adaptic®) which was then positioned on the lesion. The whole area, according to Mabel, was covered with a specific number of Kerlix® Fluff sponges, in a specific order, making a sponge "sandwich" under the ABD pad to fill in the sternal dip so that we could get a good "seal" with the ten-inch-wide flexible adhesive bandage. As I worked, her body language belied her pleasantries. She unconsciously ground her teeth. Her abdominal muscles tensed as my hand approached. Yet she lay there acquiescently vulnerable, arms bent upward and back in mock surprise to allow access.

It took an hour to do it "just so." Assured that I was proceeding slowly and wouldn't take a step without her consultation, Mabel began to talk. Her accent was soft and Southern where *want* is pronounced *wont*; *gone* is *gOhn*; and *on* is pronounced *own*. She mentioned that there was this perfectly *MAHvelous* oncology nurse at St. Anthony's who had cared for her husband when he had cancer. Thanks to the nurse's advice, she had provided her husband with good nutritional support, allowing him to remain functional until he was close to death. When was this? 1978. Funny, I had been the only "official" oncology nurse then at St. Anthony's. I wondered if I knew the nurse in question. Did she remember the nurse's name? "No. But her husband died when he was very young of cancer. Maybe her name was Nancy . . . " My heart leapt at her totally innocent and sincere praise. I said very slowly to still the inner feeling, "No, her name was not Nancy. It was Peggy. It was me." A shocked, open-mouthed expression crossed her face. Then I remembered. "Your husband was a . . . wasn't he?" "Yes. That's his picture over there," pointing to the dresser. I remembered him—but not her.

We spoke of many things that morning. I explained that I had only been in home health for one month after resigning as oncology nurse-specialist. Quietly and slowly she disclosed that, after coming home from MD Anderson, her friends had asked if there had been any miracles. She replied that there had been no big miracles but some little ones. "Today has been one of those little miracles." She asked if I would return—and I replied that I didn't know—that I didn't have a territory yet—but that I hoped so. I would make no promises that couldn't be kept.

I was assigned to visit Mabel the next day! Again, she was gracious and stiffly formal. Her body language was tense with the same unconscious teeth gnashing and reflexive abdominal rigidity. I mentioned that it might be wise to wash the intact skin area which was always under the bandage with soap and water before applying Skin Prep™ to protect it from adhesive and from moisture. She was receptive and thought so too.

Mabel viewed her lesions unflinchingly, totally repulsed by what she saw. Intellectually she was well-versed regarding her cancer. She was desperately afraid that it had an odor or would have an odor—that the "cancer fluid" which oozed from the lesion was "contaminated." She was grateful to be washed, grateful to be dry. Two plastic-backed pads stayed on her bed in case the dressing leaked overnight. That day, and each day following, I conducted a ceremony of smelling the old dressing to assure her honestly that it did not have an odor or that it smelled like normal body fluid. She was grateful that I checked. She had not noticed the other nurses doing it. They had camouflaged the maneuver, trying not to offend this very genteel lady. The legitimate point of sniffing was to detect the odor of infection.

A more complete clinical picture emerged. Unlike in the hospital, information about home patients can be sketchy. In this case, the patient was well-versed and able to fill me in. Her husband had died of a smoking-related cancer in 1978. According to her, smoking was the cause. Conversely, she was aware of nothing that she had done to cause her cancer. In fact, she had done everything right. It had started as a small, less than one-centimeter lump in her right breast in 1982. She had an immediate mastectomy. Because there were no axillary nodes involved, she was told that no further treatment was indicated. Five years later, when it recurred on her chest wall, she received a complete course of radiation therapy. She was hospitalized on an emergency basis for a pericardial effusion, a collection of fluid in the sack surrounding the heart, which was drained. The effusion could have represented a malignancy, but pathology reports were negative. The theory switched to radiation as the culprit. Her chest wall recurrence returned approximately one year ago. She had the sternectomy with a skin graft. In intensive care, a chest tube became dislodged and was re-inserted for a "collapsed lung." Recovery from the operation had been long and hard. Recurrences persisted and she had begun chemotherapy.

The previous Christmas while visiting her daughter out-of-state, Mabel experienced an acute episode of shortness of breath. Pulmonary emboli (blood clots in lungs) were the cause and she was rushed to the hospital. A DVT (blood clot) in her left leg was the source. She felt that her St. Petersburg doctors had ignored early warning signs. Mabel was treated with the blood thinner, Coumadin and compression hose both of which she still used. For a time, the chemotherapy protocol was effective. Some chest lumps disappeared. Then the primary one returned and continued to grow. Urged by friends, she sought a second opinion in early May at MD Anderson in Texas. She was disappointed with the enormity and the assembly-line character of the facility and with the absence of "hands on" examination. She returned with a letter for her oncologist from the Texas oncologist outlining alternatives.

Mabel produced the letter to share its information. She asked me to read it aloud, stopping me episodically to question medical terms. The bottom line was literally the bottom line. The oncologist predicted a forty percent chance of response to his recommended protocol. When I read that, though she had discussed it with her oncologist and had tried to read the letter before, it was as though she heard it for the first time. "Forty percent, that's not very much, is it?" My thoughts were plentiful: was he talking complete response or partial response? If there was a response, what was the expected mean duration of response? The letter seemed poorly phrased. But what should I say to her? "It *is* forty percent." I did not want to rain on her parade nor did I want to instill false hope. She was thoughtful.

When I prepared to leave, she rose from the bed and led me over to the dresser to her husband's framed picture. She picked up a faded photo, worn around the edges from use. "This was a picture of me that my husband always kept in his wallet. Many times, I asked him to replace it, but he kept it in his wallet until he died." The picture was of a vivacious, shining eyed girl of nineteen or twenty. I gazed at it thoughtfully, unsure what to say while appreciating the self-disclosure from a very private person. Finally, I said something like, it must have always made him feel good, no matter how hard the times, to reach back into his wallet and look at it. She smiled. "That's what he said."

She walked me around the bed to the wall to the right of the headboard. "That was me." A black and white portrait-sized photograph in a grand wood oval frame was of a blooming young woman with dark hair and full, dark lips. It could have been Scarlet O'Hara. The sweet, shy, innocent look of the wallet picture was replaced with guile, an awareness of her youthful womanly powers. I wanted to say, "You were beautiful," but checked myself. Was she revealing who she is, who she was or what she had lost? I thought of her mutilated chest. I thought of the fact that the picture was over forty years old—and of how much had happened in between. "That is a very beautiful young woman," I said to the woman expectantly awaiting my reaction. As Mabel walked me back to my bag and charts, she said, averting her gaze, "I really think that I need an oncology nurse-specialist, don't you?" From this proud, frightened woman I heard a plea, "Won't you please be my nurse?" My heart heard her heart and I wanted to respond—but was blunted by my own insecurity. She was Jill's patient. I didn't know where my territory would be. I wasn't sure what the managers would say. I knew that I would rather promise her very little than promise her and then not be able to deliver. Whoever worked with her needed to establish trust. I mumbled something about there being very few certified oncology clinical nurse-specialists throughout the country and most patients got along very well without them. No matter how often I was scheduled to see her, I would be available to the nurses for consultation.

Shortly thereafter, Mabel became my patient. She was on the edge of my territory. Jill was happy to abandon fitting visits between Mabel's social events. Mabel, herself, had begun to understand that her friends' support—asking her out for lunch and dinner—had become too tiring. She began to set limits. She needed rest and was already in the habit of disconnecting the phone between four and six p.m. for her "beauty rest." She grappled with guilt about possibly offending her friends by turning them down. As the summer progressed, it became less of an issue since most of her friends summered in cooler climates.

I acquired Mabel's trust by being consistent: making daily visits; arriving at the pre-arranged time of ten a.m. sharp and conforming to her rigid bandage routine. She focused less on the bandage, sharing more about herself—but always in a reserved way, a self-described private person.

Mabel had been exposed to extensive pop psychology about cancer—Bernie Siegel's book[1] lay under her TV—but she discounted most of it. She did believe that stress had contributed to the development of her cancer. The stressors were her husband's death; a long and bitter suit for her children's inheritance—which she lost; and her flooded home during Hurricane Elena in 1985—when the floors and much of the content of her beautiful and cherished home were destroyed. Repeatedly she claimed that she had "fallen through the cracks of medicine"—hinting but never accusing that, if her medical care had been different, she would never have been in this predicament. Often, she asked if I had ever seen a breast cancer like hers before but when I said that I had, she never pursued it further. *The women had all died.* She marveled that, to this point, all other tests were negative—no cancer anywhere but on the top of her chest.

Mabel had a vivid imagination—maybe wishful thinking. She imagined scenarios where the Betadine® or the Topicort® or the Bacitracin would unexpectedly put her tumors into remission. Why couldn't they be cured? Why couldn't they be cut off? Why wasn't there a magic salve to heal it? She knew the answers but asked repeatedly.

Daily, for an hour, as I methodically changed her dressing, Mabel disclosed more. She had been the youngest in a large family of children born to parents in their forties in rural North Carolina. Her closest sister was six years older. One of her sisters delivered a baby the same year Mabel was born. In many respects, she had been an only child. She described her parents as strong. Black tenant farmers worked on her father's farm where he walked among them with his German Shepherd. Ever-resourceful, her mother had nursed the wounds of a black child and ironed linens to dress them, scorching the cloth to prevent sticking. It reminded Mabel of the Adaptic® we used now. She remembered playing with black children who used spider webs from the barn to heal wounds. Would that work on hers? Her parents, upright and severe, now glowered at her from their frames at the foot of her bed.

Eighteen-year-old Mabel wore a corsage when she attended the Atlanta premier of *Gone with the Wind*.[2] It made a lasting impression. It was not accidental that those early portraits of Mabel resembled Scarlett.

After eleven years of school—high school graduation in North Carolina then— Mabel moved to Atlanta to work in a government job as a secretary living with a group of other young working women and their "black help." There she met her future husband studying at Emory after graduating from the University of Florida. When they decided to marry in 1943, his mother did not approve but "he was all grown up" and they married anyway. Their first child was born in Atlanta after her husband returned from the Navy. Their second child was born in St. Petersburg. Her husband set up his practice there and, by 1952, their permanent home was built to their specifications on Snell Isle.

Our conversations passed as social chit chat during the dressing changes. They were not very deep, just topical. Incrementally, I understood her better. The tense body language, the social smile, the politeness remained. She liked having me as her nurse and felt secure because of my "special knowledge." But when she dropped the names of multiple prominent people who were her friends, I knew that I had my "place."

Because her skin was fragile and prone to breakdown, I took meticulous care of it—beginning with the manner of removing tape, using counter pressure on the skin with one hand while pulling horizontally with the other. Cleansing and drying the skin was important before applying skin prep, and then applying no more tape than necessary to achieve the perfect "seal." I taught nutrition as supportive therapy for cancer; chemotherapy, effects and side effects; placement and use of the port; cancer basics—non-contagious, odorless, not necessarily pain-ful—Cancer 101. She was a good and receptive student. Facts more than feelings were our daily fare.

At the beginning, establishing trust was the primary goal—necessary to al-lay anxiety. It meant allowing her to control what she thought was important. Some nurses have difficulty with that—needing to be the expert whose word is followed. I have never had difficulty allowing patients to call the shots pro-vided it didn't cause harm. Mabel called the shots about how and when her wound care was performed. The doctor ordered the medication to be used on the wound—just not the method. No sense in wasting our energy struggling for control. Instead, I used my own energy by being predictable. I established a sense of sameness—same time, same order of assessment, same order of dress-ing, same nurse. She had so much unknown to fear, why create more?

Trying to win her over, Jill had engaged her in casual conversation about her friends and social engagements—recognizing their importance to Mabel. I used a different tactic. I couldn't care less who her friends were or where she or they went unless it pertained to how supported or unsupported she felt. Instead, I concentrated on her values, her experiences, her history. Rather than batting my head against the stone wall of denial or cementing it, I aimed to-ward life-review and values-clarification—both components of the grieving process—though they need not be announced as such. I was influenced by Sid Jourard who furnished a guiding premise:

> When a person has been able to disclose himself utterly to an-other person, he learns how to increase his contact with his real self, and he may then be better able to direct his destiny on the basis of this knowledge . . . .
>
> Self-disclosure requires courage. [3]

We all wear masks—maybe those of us overburdened by so-called profession-alism wear the most ornate masks of all. In my relationship with Mabel, I am grateful that caring mostly won the day—that the best things happened when I forgot to intellectualize and remembered to care. In the weeks before her ad-mission to St. Anthony's for the first of the "magic" chemo, we had both worn social masks. I learned more about her past. She learned how I would react to her wound and to her disclosures.

After the port was placed and it had healed, she was scheduled for her first chemotherapy in the hospital. The tumor grew, spreading daily. The portion which I had initially termed sub-axillary rash and which her plastic surgeon treated with the topical cortisone was obviously tumor. My own imagination was fanciful as I wondered if the cortisone cream was indeed making it spread. Mabel and I were not that different when it came to magical thinking.

On the day of admission, we finished the usual morning wound care. Her anxiety was palpable. I made a list of wound care instructions for the hospital nurses to follow. The next day at lunchtime I returned to demonstrate it for them—an act for which they were grateful. So was Mabel. She happened to be on my former unit—they knew and trusted me. She picked up on that and felt supported by the continuity of care which she was receiving. They meticulously followed the printed instructions staving off unnecessary anxiety. The chemotherapy went beautifully with only slight nausea on the last day. I had prepared her for what to expect from Adriamycin® and Vinblastine.

Throughout her hospitalization, Mabel wore and slept in a perfectly coifed chestnut colored wig. Her makeup was extreme. Yellow/beige foundation cast a jaundiced hue. Dark blue mascara and eyeliner were on lower lids only. It was my first glimpse of her war paint—a caricature of herself. Here was a woman who couldn't afford to be comfortable in the hospital lest someone see her less than perfect.

The last day of hospitalization, I dashed in for a lunchtime visit while making a lab drop for a home patient. As Mabel spoke, for lack of available space, I squatted next to her bed. She mentioned that she had a cough for which the doctor had ordered an expectorant. Her chest x-ray revealed possible fluid at her right lung base. Honestly, I listened to her with only half an ear, my mind on my next home visit. She spoke very matter-of-factly. Feeling rushed to hurry to my next visit, I did something very uncharacteristic. I grabbed her hand with both of mine assuring, "It's going to be okay . . . once you go home . . . "

The moment the words were out of my mouth, I could have bitten my tongue. I abhor false reassurance. She had a right to be worried and things would *not* necessarily be okay. But she visibly softened and relaxed, smiling up at me. Had it been something she had needed to hear or was it something which I had done—spontaneously, warmly, genuinely reaching out to her and touching her. It was the first that I had touched her for anything other than clinical reasons. There had always been that aloofness, that stiffness which silently forbade it. I suspected that walls had begun to crumble.

That evening, after her return home, I did my first Home Health "pickup" which is jargon for re-admitting the patient after she returns from the hospital. My supervisor and Jill had asked, "When is he going to make her a no code?" An inevitability to anyone familiar with the case was not so inevitable to the patient. To my knowledge, she had no living will, a component of "no code" status. Since tonight I would ask her to sign many papers, I resolved to at least introduce the topic. Besides, I was in Mabel's good graces, having paid for her trust and confidence with beyond-the-call-of-duty un-charged hospital visits on my own time. I certainly did not want to even contemplate performing CPR on her sternum-less chest!

The night began pleasantly. We talked while she donned her patient gown, open in the front for the dressing change. I asked offhandedly how, with no sternum, CPR could be done. Oh, definitely, no one should do chest compressions on her, she said. The very thought frightened her. She had taken a CPR course and knew exactly what it was. Abandoning the topic, I performed my nursing tasks and left the paper signing until last. I still felt awkward synopsizing the patient's bill of rights and responsibilities for her to sign.

She signed it and my visit note. Then I took a deep breath and broached a discussion about living wills. I felt, naïvely, that it was a piece of cake. Obviously, she did not want any part of CPR. Oh, was I wrong! From a straight-backed chair, I faced her as she sat on the side of the bed, legs dangling, peering down at me.

I never forcibly confronted people with end-of-life discussion. Gently, I thought, I returned to her statement that she did not want CPR. There was a form which people sign to protect themselves. It was called a living will. While I continued as gently as possible, her tension built—the jaw set, the respirations quickened. She did not believe in living wills; in cutting your options before you ever reached that point. Wasn't there more to CPR than just chest compressions—oxygen, medications? She did not want to eliminate those options. That was why there are doctors to use their discretion when the time came. Would I excuse her, please, she had to go to the bathroom?

I continued to sit in that straight-backed chair in the calm, emotionless manner that I had chosen as a foil for my own escalating anxiety. Had she been able to watch me from behind the closed bathroom door, that's all that she would have seen. But inside! My God, I had witnessed a *fight or flight* response before my very eyes. I had literally *scared her shitless*. Never had I caused such terror.

She returned stone-faced, avoiding my eyes but again sitting opposite me on the bed. "I've upset you . . . " She began to sob. While remaining seated, she positioned her body facing away from me, pulling her hands to her face, curling into herself.

"You must think I am going to die very soon to have brought this up." Touching her shoulder, I said "No *(???)* but I thought it was something we should talk about." She sat fingers to her mouth, swallowing her tears, trying hard to regain control. "It's okay, it's okay to cry. You've been through a lot. Just let it out." "No, crying just makes me sick. My mother told me long ago that if you cry, you get a cold chill and that makes you sick." Her body tensed, struggling for control. Making eye contact, she spoke defiantly, "I think you should know that I've thought about this before. I have made my funeral arrangements and I have talked with my minister about the services. I've had a lot of time to think about this . . . The control was giving way to tears again. My heart ached for her. I stood and asked if I could give her a hug. She nodded assent but only stiffened in response to my quick hug.

Later that night, I wondered if she had a "cold chill" after my visit. I felt unraveled and guilty. If I were to help her, I would have to re-establish our relationship somehow. My heart went out to her—so private, so lonely, so tense, so fearful, so trapped by long-ingrained, self-imposed limitations. It was only the beginning of what could become a terrible situation.

I formulated a plan and carried it out the next day. Instead of proceeding with the visit, I asked Mabel to sit down on the bed while I sat across from her. I apologized for having upset her the previous night, noting that she had looked at me as though I had betrayed her. She denied it and said that she was glad that it had come up, that it would have to come up sooner or later and that she was glad that I now knew about her funeral plans. I explained that, because we were re-admitting her last night, I had felt compelled to finish a certain amount of paperwork. I had been clumsy. I would like to explain it in a more personal way. I drew the chair closer so that we could both look at the agreement as I explained it. She followed the paper seriously as I spoke.

Under *Dignity and Respect*: I explained that she was a special and unique person whom I respected. Under *Decision Making*: I explained that my relationship with her would be open—I would tell her anything that I knew directly and honestly. She did not have to fear what I knew but was not saying. If her wound had an odor, I would say so. If I thought she was dying, I would say so. I would share any finding on physical assessment. Under *Confidentiality and Privacy*: I did not know her friends. What she said and information about her condition I would share with no one other than her doctor. Under *Quality of Care*: I explained that she was entitled to the highest quality of care that we could provide, and that cancer was my area of expertise.

Under *Patient Responsibility*: her part of this contract would be to be honest with me, not only about the symptoms but also her feelings—that I could take care of her best if I knew how she felt about what was happening; what she feared; and what worried her. I summarized by saying that the relationship that a patient has with a nurse can be a very special one—unlike any other relation-ship—but it needs work and commitment on both people's part.

Mabel looked up from time to time but mostly concentrated on the form. I asked her if we could shake on this contract. When we shook, she regarded me oddly. I asked her what she understood, fearful that it had seemed like so much gobbledygook. She turned her head, looking up at me with a broad grin and relaxed eyes. "You won't abandon me." My mouth must have dropped open. She had it in a nutshell—but where had she heard those words? Recognizing my quandary, she replied that her oncologist had told her that he wouldn't abandon her. How had that made her feel? Good. Secure. We moved on to the dressing.

Over the next few weeks, I continued our very predictable pattern of care. Mabel commented that I always left everything as I'd found it. She didn't re-alize that it was purposeful—not an obsessive-compulsive idiosyncrasy—but planned predictability geared to minimize unnecessary anxiety or distress.

I made a calendar to project when to expect which side effects from the chemo and instructed accordingly. I called her attention to the signs of tension which I had observed—the tooth grinding which resembled chewing, the physical tension. She had been unaware of the tooth grinding and smiled marveling, "No one else would have told me that." We began to talk about ways to relieve tension when she was able to admit that "I am anxious." We practiced quick and easy relaxation techniques. We practiced progressive relaxation with deep breathing and guided imagery. We hit a stumbling block when I guided her to shoulder shrug. That hurt because of her sternectomy, so we decided to do everything but that. It amazed me that she was so willing to be led. I had an-ticipated resistance.

Wondering aloud where to "take" her on our guided imagery, I discovered that the outdoor place which she loved most was outside her home under the beautiful live oaks which her husband had planted. When they first moved into the house, she had envisioned calling the house *The Oaks*—like the plantation *Tara*. At the close of each visit, instead of bounding out of bed to get dressed, she took a few minutes as I directed her to alternately contract and relax muscle groups; to take some slow deep breaths, feel her body become weightless and float outside onto the grass, look up through the oaks—watch, smell, feel various outdoor phenomena. The exercise visibly relaxed Mabel. She would lie there relaxed as I finished my notes. As the weeks passed and her hemoglobin fell, she dozed off while I completed my notes.

Was there a relationship between the guided imagery and accepting death? Of course—no matter how tangential. A behaviorist would say that I was conditioning her to relax at the sound of my voice. But neither were my immediate intentions. I just wanted her to recognize tension in her body and to be able to act herself to correct it.

I was supremely busy during each visit. From what I have written, it could be construed that I sat back in an armchair as we had lengthy conversations. Nothing could be further from the truth. There was a tremendous amount of physical care that—no matter how I did it—was too time consuming for someone like me—new to the job with four to five other visits to make. I dared not waste one second. The heaviest of conversations occurred while I was busy with assessment, the wound, the port, etc. There was very little hand holding because usually there was something else in my hand. I sweat like a fox in a forest fire—eliciting good-natured change-of-life jokes from her after I made them myself. It wasn't so much that her house was warm—it was that I was so _busy_—doing the work while processing her words.

During those weeks after chemo, we each became more transparent. She boasted that her husband had been ahead of his time and had insisted that she be liberated from the start. He expected her to keep abreast of current events. They had travelled extensively and taken archeology courses. She joked that when her body was exhumed by archeologists of the future, what would they think of the elaborate bandage?

Her husband had been hospitalized for two months before he died. One day, while she waited for the nurses to finish working with him, she sat in a little alcove, unseen. One of the nurses came out of his room crying. Another nurse tried to comfort her, remarking, "I would think as long as you've been in nursing it wouldn't get to you like this." The first nurse replied, "When it doesn't get to you, then you don't belong in nursing." When I asked Mabel how she felt about this, she replied that it had been a great comfort to know that the nurses caring for her husband cared that much about him.

Mabel called me *Peggy* but, whenever she was on the phone with her friends, I heard myself described, not by name but by category—*the visiting nurse*—just as she referred to her housekeeper, Evelyn. Though I grew to love this lady, she was not only classy but class-conscious. It was not always easy to see that her social mask hid a very warm and vulnerable heart.

To recognize her expertise in wound care—*because over the last few years she had used almost every dressing conceivable*—I teased that she had her PhD in wound care and that she could be hired out as a consultant even to MD Anderson. She took this as the compliment and gentle tease that it was. I told her that she was Nurse #1 and that I was Nurse #2. She responded to it well—seeing it as a vote of confidence, of collegiality. We were co-conspirators.

One weekend when I was off, I left detailed instructions about wound care for the weekend nurse. Mabel had been maintaining her weight. But, when I returned on Monday, I could see that the scale would reveal a loss. It did—five pounds. Her face was gaunt. Except for the nurse visits, she had been alone all weekend—and miserable. To a new nurse, seeing an advanced cancer patient for the first time, no red flags would have appeared. To me, there was a marked difference. She was weaker, increasingly short of breath. She had stomatitis (mouth sores) which was predictable. But it had prevented her from eating much of anything. She knew what to eat but didn't have the energy to prepare it. She had decided to take an old prescription for thrush (swish and swallow). I saw no signs of monilia—just severe stomatitis. Her right lower lung sounds were absent. At least she was to see her doctor on Tuesday and her daughter would arrive for a visit on Wednesday.

I reviewed types of food that were high calorie and easy on the mouth. Her housekeeper, Evelyn, would be there to help fix or buy food—an improvement on her lonely, miserable weekend. During the relaxation, she fell asleep.

Mabel made a brief MD office visit. I had left him a note about my concerns, but he picked up on none of them. The next day he was out of town. I knew the MD covering his practice and caught up to him in the hospital, outlining my concerns—particularly that she was developing a pleural effusion. He agreed that she needed to be seen in the ER.

At her home, I met Mabel's daughter in the kitchen. She was an attractive brown-eyed brunette, a few years younger than I. Mabel, unwell, had returned to bed after breakfast. During the assessment, I noted that she was dyspneic (short of breath) at rest. Her lung sounds were worse with nothing audible below mid-point. Checking for tactile fremitus, a vibration normally heard or felt when the patient repeats "ninety-nine," confirmed it.

After the assessment, I faced her, trying to center myself. The goal was to minimize fear while maximizing motivation to get to the hospital. I didn't want to leave the impression that her own physician had left us (me) holding the bag—which, indeed, he had. I shared that, in the last few days, I had begun to hear less at the base of her right lung. Today I had heard even less. I was concerned that it could be a collection of fluid at the bottom of her lung, causing shortness of breath. Her doctor was now out of town (surprised look). I had reviewed the situation with the covering oncologist who thought she should be seen in the ER for a chest x-ray.

Her reaction wasn't the hysteria I expected. She was concerned. I allowed her to listen to her own lungs with my stethoscope. She could hear the difference. She asked me to call in her daughter to participate in the decision.

They asked appropriate questions. What would be done about the fluid? They would drain it with a needle. Mabel remembered pericardiocentesis as painful—but, I pointed to where the needle would be placed, and it might not be so painful. I mentioned that her heart had been racing at one-hundred-and-twenty-five trying to keep up with the body's oxygen needs. They both agreed that the x-ray should be done. I called the doctor to confirm, feeling constrained because Mabel and daughter were listening. Mabel was concerned about being exposed to many people in the ER at a time when she was severely immuno-compromised from chemo. I placed another call from the bedside and spoke with the ER nurse specialist, Kathy Quail, asking her to look out for Mabel's special needs.

Leaving that day, I reflected that the woman whom I had expected to go to pieces looked relieved. She could handle adversity. What she could not handle was not being taken seriously. Perhaps it was my imagination that I detected in her smiling eyes—they did smile at me that day—*you cared; you investigated; you followed through. You haven't abandoned me.*

True to my suspicions, the ER discovered that she had a large right pleural effusion (later drained for 1800cc) and a hemoglobin of eight (normal:12-15). Her white blood count was also low. Mabel was discharged home because the hospital had no vacant private rooms needed for protective isolation. She was to be admitted the next day.

Away from Mabel, in the kitchen, her daughter criticized Mabel's superficiality. She and her brother had been clueless about the worsening situation because Mabel had glossed over it on the phone. She critiqued her mother being "in denial." I shared the gist of our discussion about the living will. Her daughter responded, "I would have confronted her by saying, 'That makes you angry, doesn't it?'" I simply responded that, at the end of life, I wasn't sure that confrontation is important—support would be more appropriate. Her daughter recoiled as though I had slapped her. "Is this the end of her life?" For the second time with this family, I felt like a butterfly pinned to the wall! I said. "I think we are talking months, not years . . ." Trying to be supportive and understanding, I sensed the daughter's inner conflict. She wanted to help but she did not like Mabel very much. She recalled her father's advice that, to keep the peace, it is important to remember that there are two ways: the wrong way and Mabel's way.

After Mabel was admitted, I returned to the hospital during my lunch break. It was wet that day, raining intermittently, a typical St. Petersburg summer. As usual, Mabel was decked out in full regalia—wig and makeup. She was much improved and more comfortable. Her face was fuller reflecting rehydration. Avoiding my eyes, she glanced out her window. "I have a new name for you." "What?" She looked up at me affectionately smiling and then turned away bashfully, "Mary Poppins!" She confided that, while watching the rain that morning, she had imagined me dropping into various patients' homes umbrella in hand. The umbrella part was certainly true—but I had not yet mastered the art of levitation. I smiled. "Then you don't mind that I called you that?" she asked, looking up at me. "No," I smiled. Inwardly, my thoughts were dark as I remembered the song: *Just a spoonful of sugar helps the medicine go down, medicine go down*[4] . . . I was Mary Poppins, sugar coating death.

During Mabel's hospitalization, her daughter arranged for Evelyn, Mabel's long-time housekeeper, to live with her at her home after discharge.

Meanwhile, the tumors covering Mabel's right chest were "juicier" with better hydration thanks to the IV fluids. The tumors extended to her right axilla and grew at a rapid pace. Her hair fell out in clumps. Wig remained firmly in place. This was a woman to whom appearance was everything.

Visiting on another day, I found her on the phone, pink bed jacket in place, made up, talking to her friends about "this perfectly *mahvelous* salad that they sent up." Listening, I, like her daughter, questioned her grasp of reality. She sounded as though she believed she was in an exclusive health resort—not a hospital. Had she really bought into her own fantasy or was she doing what she had done for years—glossing over the unpleasant for her loved ones' sake?

On another occasion, I dropped in on my lunch break. The staff reported that Mabel had been crying ever since her doctor's visit.

How had I known to come when she needed me? she blurted. Her lips flushed, and she began to cry, quickly apologizing, trying to staunch the flow. I took her hand, saying, "It's okay, just let it out and tell me what's happened." Her returning doctor had looked angry. Peaking under, not removing the bandage, he pronounced that the chemotherapy had not worked. The tumor was bigger. He could give her more chemo but would have to cut back on the dose to minimize drug side effects. It probably wouldn't do any good. She had told him that she wanted it anyway.

After he left, she felt as though he had physically hit her. Now she dissolved into tears repeating, "I wont (want) to live. I don't wont to die. I have done everything I could all along. I was sure that I could overcome it. I know it sounds foolish, but I thought that *I* was special. I'm too young to die. There is so much that I wont to do. I wont to see my grandchildren grow up and know what happens to them. I've had a wonderful life and I don't wont to stop now." More was said, as she clung to my hand and openly wept. A cleansing. The very private person was taking comfort in allowing herself to be known. When it was time for me to leave, Mabel, dry-eyed, marveled that I had come when I did.

The next day, Mabel was tired from having cried so much, still doubting the cleansing function of tears. I countered that it was not only good but necessary to relieve pent up feelings causing the physical tension that we had been working on for the past few weeks. Tears help us express who we really are and what we really feel. It takes a lot of energy to hide behind social masks. She gazed at me in wide-eyed, child-like innocence asking, "Do you think I wear a mask?"

We talked about her fears. I reiterated that discussing the "*what ifs*" doesn't make them happen but can help us know how to deal with them should the time come. Very honestly and openly, she shared that she was not afraid of death. She just did not want to stop living. What did she think happens to us when we die? She believed in God and his goodness. The specifics about what will happen are unfathomable to us in this life. Would she see her husband? No—at least not in that form—after all, what would happen to people with more than one spouse—how could they be perfectly happy? Would she know what was happening to her grandchildren in this life? No, she did not believe so. Her only concern was that, though she sincerely believed in God and his goodness, she could not picture Him in one specific way—like the Good Shepherd. She had asked her pastor and one of the pastoral care nuns. Both had assured her that was okay.

Mabel remained in the hospital for a few more days to receive that much-reduced chemotherapy dose. According to her, she had no choice if she wanted to live. She finally had a long talk with her doctor and had made clear that she wanted no extraordinary measures or heroics.

By this time, Mabel's hair had fallen out and she was mortified. Except with the bathroom door closed behind her, that wig had not come off once in almost two weeks in the hospital. My scalp itched for her! She admitted that it felt pretty awful. I borrowed some soft paper "shower caps" worn by the labor nurses and asked Mabel if she would try them to give her head a rest. She looked at me sheepishly. "I don't *wont* you to see me this way." "I see bald people all the time," I countered. "It's not your hair that makes you special. Come on, I'm your nurse." "Okay." She sat straight up in bed and, looking away from me out the window, slowly lifted what I had mentally dubbed "*the squirrel.*" Quickly, she stole a glance to check my reaction and bashfully covered her face with her hand. There was something about the child-like vulnerability in that action which touched me. Gently, placing two caps together, I strapped a rubber band around a section of both in the middle. I turned it inside out and replaced it on her head where it puffed beautifully. With a glance in the mirror, she pronounced that it was not only comfortable but attractive and she wore it almost exclusively for the remainder of her stay.

Here my notes stop. Mabel returned home where her housekeeper and long-time friend (unclaimed but true), Evelyn, slept in the adjoining bedroom, assuring Mabel of companionship, nutrition and hydration. Increasingly aware of her proximity to death, Mabel directed that her good silver tray be used to serve her meals in bed. She wanted to die in her own bed—that beautiful big cannonball bed.

The exophytic lesions on her right chest continued to grow under her axilla and upward. Concerned about appearances, she worried that they would continue to move up into her face. I can only describe the lesions as shiny, red and bulbous. When they outgrew their blood supply, they became necrotic, sloughed and oozed, before establishing a new blood supply and growing even larger. They were not discreet and isolated but covered a large, ten-inch by eight-inch area. Before performing wound care, I walked her into her tub to shower just to keep her as clean as possible. I silently hummed Shambala. "Wash away my troubles, wash away my pain with the rain in Shambala. Wash away my sorrow, wash away my shame with the rain in Shambala."[5]

At one point, her plastic surgeon, Dr. Gallant, met me at her home and demonstrated how to use his special concoction to cleanse her chest now twice daily to minimize the odor of rotting flesh.

Mabel's living will finally complete, a copy was sent to the funeral home which she had chosen. Her doctor called them, too, to be sure that there would be no police fanfare at the time of her home death. Her adult children arrived to stay a week before her death. Mabel basked in their presence. One evening, just as I arrived for the evening dressing change, Mabel took her last breath peacefully in the presence of her children—in her huge cannonball bed.

Endnotes

1. Bernie Siegel, *Love, Medicine and Miracles* (New York: Harper Collins Publishers, 1988).

2. Margaret Mitchell, *Gone with the Wind* (New York: MacMillan, June 30, 1936). Film: 1939 based upon the Pulitzer winning novel.

3. Sid Jourard, *The Transparent Self* (New York: D. Van Norstrand Reinhold, 1964).

4. P.L. Travers, *Mary Poppins* (London: Harper Collins, 1934). Disney Film: 1964.

5. Daniel Joseph Moore, *Shambala* sung by Three Dog Night. (Los Angeles: Dunhill, 1973).

Care Study: Mary
1991 to 1993

Her straight steel gray hair was chopped, unstylish, and institutional. A raspy, mumbled voice answered my questions inappropriately. On my last visit of the day, I was tired and had worked the downtown district long enough to anticipate the marginally cognitively-impaired elderly even at this pleasant and spacious Assisted Living Facility (ALF). At eighty, she had just been discharged from a nursing home, her room cluttered with unpacked belongings. She had lived in the same ALF when she fell, sustained a concussion and was hospitalized. Later she had been sent to a SNF for rehab. Her Foley catheter was in place. Home nursing was ordered for an open area on her right heel. I stumbled through the visit as best I could. Not always comprehending her replies, unconsciously, I began talking with her as I would with someone with a mental impairment.

Luckily, on my second visit, the home health aid who had cared for Mary prior to her nursing home stay was present. Dorothy was short, black and no-nonsense. When Dorothy heard me addressing Mary, she stood right up under my nose and whispered, "Mary is really smart—she just can't hear. Talk into her left ear. She doesn't like to be called Miss Krause. Call her Mary." I must have looked dubious because Dorothy repeated, "*Really*. She is very smart."

I made eye contact with Mary. She was stern—black/gray eyebrows knitted. She spoke in a fast mumble. But wait—only Pittsburgh people spoke at that pace. Raising my voice and speaking into her left ear, I verified that, in fact, she was from Pittsburgh. We began to compare Pittsburgh notes over a long series of visits.

In addition to providing care as ordered, I noticed small things at first. Her door was never locked. I would just knock—which she couldn't hear—and come in. No privacy. Questionable safety. But she had no choice—being chair-bound and hard of hearing. There was a string on the knob so that she could pull the door shut when she passed through it. The door to her bathroom had been removed to accommodate her electric scooter. Thus, she could be surprised in a most unceremonious position. I surprised her several times—Mary naked as a jaybird with Dorothy helping her transfer from shower to chair.

She had gadgets all around to help her accomplish activities of daily living—grabbers and hooks on sticks. She had a belt-like device with a loop that she used to raise her immobile leg over the tub side. In the bathroom, there was a commode extender and an electric tooth brush within reach of her scooter. She was dangerous with that scooter—zipping around in it speedily and professionally. I jumped a few times for fear of being plowed over.

Her room was Spartan. No photographs. Very few personal effects. A typewriter on a small table and a television were the only evidence of her activity. Her dress was Spartan, too—pants and shirts. No jewelry. No makeup. Plain cotton panties and bra. She dressed by clasping the bra in front with difficulty, then turning it around to enable her to slip her right, disabled hand through the strap—and then only—the left one. She referred to her droopy breasts as "fried eggs." I once commented that she seemed to like plain, sporty dress. She replied no, not necessarily. Pants worked better than skirts for bed-to-chair transfers. On another occasion, she mentioned that she owned a pendant on a neck chain like mine but that she had given her jewelry to her cousin since "this would not be a safe place to have things like that."

Shortly after her return to the ALF, she took advantage of the resident beautician who gave her a trim and a perm. The new look made Dorothy's contention that she was "smart" more plausible—though the truth of Dorothy's statement had already become clear.

I began to listen very closely. Perhaps it was my skillful interviewing—not likely. More likely it was a desperate soul struggling to be known. Within a few short visits, I learned that she was from Mount Lebanon, just outside of Pittsburgh. She was the daughter of a plumber and his wife—both immigrants from Europe. Hers was the first house in her area to have indoor plumbing. Her older brother was a priest but had died. Mary had never married. She had been a clerical person/translator at a chemical company in Pittsburgh. She worked with their patent attorney, translating French and German texts about polymers. During World War II, she worked for the government to translate classified documents.

I appreciated my new patient incrementally through casual conversations during wound care. Despite diligent care and the use of heel protectors, the wound, measured once weekly, was not healing. I asked for orders to do some fasting blood sugars for diabetes. There was a family history. Eventually, her peripheral vascular disease and need for a femoral-popliteal bypass graft became evident.

When twice daily wound care with different wound care products was ordered, my twice daily visits began.

Our visits were mundane—nothing unusual. On one of them, I found Mary in the lobby visiting with friends. When we returned to her room for the wound care, I discovered her left pant leg was wet with urine. The valve on her leg bag had not been completely closed. She asked me to help change the pants so that she could return to her visitors. I had no extra time. Another patient was waiting. We changed the pants as Mary sat in her chair. She lifted her body off the chair with her arms. That explained her sinewy, knotted arm muscles stretched over a boney frame.

On another visit, I placed the thermometer in her mouth, listened to her heart and was taking her blood pressure when, suddenly, I heard a muttered, raspy, "Take this damn thermometer out!" Disbelieving what I had heard, my eyes sought hers, only to find them crinkled in a humorous grin. Had I only heard, I would have cringed—but after making eye contact, all I could do was laugh— and remove the thermometer. After all, her "damn" temperature was being taken three times a day between Dorothy and me!

One morning, I swung open her door to find Mary waiting for me in her chair, reading a book. She peered up at me over glasses which had slid down over her nose. Before me was a woman whom I had taken to be practically dement- ed; a woman with so many obstacles to normalcy to confront; a woman well- groomed wearing slacks and a pink blouse, with a new perm, looking up at me over her glasses, novel in hand.

As we became better acquainted, I discovered that those knitted brows were the result of constant nerve pain down her right, spastic leg—as well as arthritic pain in her grossly deformed left knee. She recounted that, in 1954, she had entered a "famous hospital in Boston" for a cordotomy to relieve nerve pain in her right leg. Instead, on the operating table, she had felt her left leg fly up and then become motionless. Her left motor neurons had been severed. The story from the doctor had been that her spinal cord nerve fibers were reversed. She had returned to Pittsburgh with a motionless left leg and the same nerve pain in her right leg. Did I hear bitterness or anger? No. Simply acceptance.

After a month, per agency policy, I was scheduled to replace Mary's Foley cath- eter. Her legs were so contracted in an adducted position (tight together) that she warned me that I would have to do it from behind. This was my first time to insert a Foley that way—and without a high-low bed. It worked like a charm thanks to Mary's patience and Dorothy's skillful aiming of the flashlight beam.

Though we interacted daily or twice daily, Mary struck me as an independent, somewhat stiffly aloof person. I felt that she tolerated me as necessary for her wound. So, one day, when she referred me to a letter on her dresser, I was shocked. It was a form letter sent by our agency to evaluate care. Unable to write legibly with her grossly deformed right hand, she had painstakingly fed the form through her typewriter so that she could type x's in the boxes of all the superlatives. Remarkably, this was the first indication that she liked what I did. Later, she made it clear that she had liked it from the start.

Increasingly in her vocabulary, I heard the word "struggle." She struggled to make transfers, struggled to get dressed and undressed. Increasingly, as I sat with her at the end of the visit completing my notes, I realized that—unasked— she was going through life-review—specifically recounting the deaths of those who had been close to her: . . . mother . . . father . . . brother. And though I realized that it was important to *look* as though I were listening, being swamped with paperwork, too often, I was not . . .

Mary was, by far, my most memorable home health patient. Long after she returned to a nursing home setting, unable to make transfers, Mary and I continued to be friends until the day she died. In the nursing home, our Scrabble game scores set records which we vied to break. She was one of the most intelligent and courageous people I have ever met. She was trapped in a body which prompted one of the aids in the nursing home to ask, "Who is in charge of Mary?" Of course, my reply was, "Mary is in charge of Mary." Mary was not only intelligent and in charge but comfortable in her own skin; at home with what her body had become; doing what she had to do; relinquishing what could no longer be kept. Once, during a difficult time, I said to her, "You are very brave." She looked me in the eye and replied matter-of-factly, "I know."

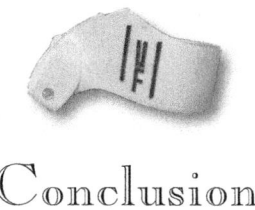

Conclusion

Any amateur psychologist will explain that people in the helping professions are really meeting their own dependency needs. Patients need us . . . but we need them more.

I benefitted from my close connection with people in my care. Their experiences during critical episodes in their lives—and how they handled them—taught me:

Life is punctuated by birth, death, and the commas in between.

Life is a journey not measured in miles but in moments.

Life is not about temporal possessions.

Our only enduring possessions rest between our ears . . .

Under the Cap.

Bibliography

Abdellah, Faye. *Patient-Centered Approaches to Nursing.* London: MacMillan, 1960.

Baggini, Julian. "In Praise of Cynicism," *St. Petersburg Times,* July 20, 2003.

Bing, Elisabeth. *Six Practical Lessons for an Easier Childbirth.* New York: Random House, 1967.

Boston Women's Health Book Collective. *Our Bodies Ourselves.* New York: Simon and Schuster, 1973.

Cuniff, John. "What is a Flum? A Manager Who Brings About Chaos," *St. Petersburg Times,* April 30,1993.

Dick-Read, Grantly. *Childbirth Without Fear.* New York: Harper, 1943.

Fitzpatrick, Elise and Nicholson Eastman. *Zabriskie's Obstetrics for Nurses,* 10th ed. Philadelphia: J.B. Lippincott, 1960, 504.

Friedan, Betty. *The Feminine Mystique.* New York: W.D. Norton and Co., 1963.

Frost, Robert. "The Road Not Taken," *Immortal Poems of the English Language.* New York: Washington Square Press, 1965.

Gilbert, W.S. and Arthur Sullivan. "Things Are Seldom What They Seem," *H.M.S. Pinafore.* [1878].

Goodrum, Randy. "You Needed Me," *Let's Keep it That Way.* Los Angeles: Capitol Records, 1978.

Henderson, Virginia. *The Nature of Nursing.* New York: National League for Nursing Press, 1966.

Holy Bible, New International Version (NIV). Grand Rapids, MI: Zondervan Bible Publishers, 2011.

Jacobs, Jacob and Sholom Scuda. "Bei Mir Bistu Shein." 1932. Andrews Sisters on Decca, 1937.

Jourard, Sid. *The Transparent Self.* New York: D. Van Norstrand Reinhold, 1964.

Karmel, Marjorie. *Thank You Doctor LaMaze.* University of Michigan: Lippincott, 1959.

Machiavelli, Niccolò. *The Prince*. [1532].

McEver, Dan. "Ode to Patient Care," *American Journal of Nursing*, (June 1979): 1083.

Mitchell, Margaret. *Gone with the Wind*. New York: MacMillan, June 30, 1936. Motion Picture: 1939.

Moore, Daniel Joseph. "Shambala," *Cyan*. Los Angeles: Dunhill, 1973.

Myers, Isabel Briggs et al. *MBTI Handbook: A Guide to the Development and Use of the Myers-Briggs Type Indicator Third Edition*. Sunnyvale, CA: Consulting Psychologists Press. 1998.

Reddy, Helen and Ray Burton. "I Am Woman," *I Am Woman*. Los Angeles: Capitol Records, 1972.

Ross, Elisabeth Kübler. *On Death and Dying*. New York: Scribner, 1969.

Rubin, Reva. "Puerperal Change," *Nursing Outlook*. (December 1961): 753-755.

Sandberg, Sheryl. *Lean In: Women, Work and the Will to Lead*. New York: Random House LLC, 2013.

Saxon, Sue and Mary Jean Etten. *Physical Change and Aging: A Guide for the Helping Professions*, 3rd ed. University of Michigan: Tiresias Press, 1994.

Sheindlin, Judge Judy. *Don't Pee on Me and Tell Me It's Raining*. New York: Harper Perennial, 1997.

Shirley, James. "Death the Leveler," *Immortal Poems of the English Language*. New York: Washington Square Press, 1965.

Siegel, Bernie. *Love, Medicine and Miracles*. New York: Harper Collins Publishers, 1988.

Simonton, O. Carl and Stephanie Matthews Simonton. *Getting Well Again*. New York: Tarcher, 1978.

Teresa, Mother. *A Gift for God*. New York: Harper Collins Publishers, 2003.

Townsend, Peter. "Baba O'Riley," *Who's Next?* Nashville: Universal Music Publishing Group, 1971.

Travers, P.L. *Mary Poppins*. London: Harper Collins, 1934. Disney film: 1964.

Wells, Helen. *Cherry Ames* Series. New York: Grosset & Dunlap, 1943-1968.

Wiedenbach, Ernestine. *Family-Centered Maternity Nursing.* New York: Putnam, 1958.

Wordsworth, William. "The Tables Turned," Lyrical Ballads. London: J. & A. Arch, 1798.

Made in the USA
Middletown, DE
26 December 2021